Pediatric Neurology:

A Case-Based Review

Tena Rosser, MD

Children's Hospital Los Angeles
University of Southern California Keck School of Medicine
Los Angeles, California

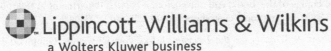
Lippincott Williams & Wilkins
a Wolters Kluwer business
Philadelphia • Baltimore • New York • London
Buenos Aires • Hong Kong • Sydney • Tokyo

KH

Acquisitions Editor: Frances DeStefano
Managing Editor: Scott Scheidt
Developmental Editor: Lisa Consoli
Project Manager: Fran Gunning
Marketing Manager: Kimberly Schonberger
Design Coordinator: Stephen Druding
Manufacturing Coordinator: Kathleen Brown
Compositor: International Typesetting and Composition
Printer: Strategic Content Imaging

Library of Congress Cataloging-in-Publication Data

Pediatric neurology : a case-based review / [edited by] Tena Rosser ;
contributing authors, Arthur Partikian . . . [et al.].
  p. ; cm.
 Includes bibliographical references and index.
 ISBN-13: 978-0-7817-7888-6
 ISBN-10: 0-7817-7888-3
 1. Pediatric neurology. 2. Pediatric neurology—Case studies. I. Rosser,
Tena. II. Partikian, Arthur.
 [DNLM: 1. Nervous System Diseases—Case Reports. 2. Nervous System
Diseases—Examination Questions. 3. Child. 4. Infant. WS 18.2 P36997
2007]
RJ486.P433 2007
618.92'8—dc22

                    2006011452

17 16
10

1/10/18

CONTRIBUTING AUTHORS

Children's Hospital Los Angeles
University of Southern California Keck School of Medicine
Los Angeles, California

Arthur Partikian, MD
Tena Rosser, MD
Kiarash Sadrieh, MD

Children's National Medical School
George Washington University School of Medicine
Washington, District of Columbia

Taeun Chang, MD
John Crawford, MD
Tammy Tsuchida, MD, PhD
Adeline Vanderver, MD

To my mentors and colleagues in the neurology department at Children's National Medical Center, Washington, DC.

To my family.

CONTENTS

PREFACE

The idea for the development of this book arose while preparing for the oral portion of the American Board of Psychiatry and Neurology board examination. I quickly came to realize that there was no current published collection of cases in pediatric neurology that might serve as a study aid. Although this book will likely appeal most to adult and pediatric neurology residents preparing for the oral board examination, it is also intended to be of interest to a broader audience of practicing adult and child neurologists, general pediatricians, and medical students.

Although it is difficult to recreate the oral board examination experience on paper, this book is written as a case-based review with discussions structured according to the format used in the neurology oral boards. Both common and rare neurologic disorders are covered in the text, but the majority of cases are based on actual patient presentations. The cases demonstrate the diverse and fascinating disease processes found in the field of child neurology. The vignettes in this book are presented randomly and not by disease category to simulate the experience of the oral boards. However, for individuals who wish to perform more focused study on a particular area of child neurology, an index by disease category is provided in the back of the book. Overall, this book is intended to help readers gain a foundation of knowledge in pediatric neurology and develop an organized approach to clinical decision making.

ABBREVIATIONS

ACTH	Adrenocorticotropic hormone
ANA	Antinuclear antibody
BAER	Brainstem auditory evoked response
BUN	Blood urea nitrogen
CBC	Complete blood count
CIDP	Chronic inflammatory demyelinating polyneuropathy
CK	Creatine kinase
cm	Centimeter
CMAP	Compound muscle action potential
CMV	Cytomegalovirus
CNS	Central nervous system
CSF	Cerebrospinal fluid
CT	Computed tomography
DNA	Deoxyribonucleic acid
DWI	Diffusion-weighted imaging
EBV	Epstein-Barr virus
ECG	Electrocardiogram
ECHO	Echocardiogram
EEG	Electroencephalogram
EMG	Electromyography
ER	Emergency room
ESR	Erythrocyte sedimentation rate
FDA	Food and Drug Administration
kg	Kilogram
HIV	Human immunodeficiency virus
HMA	Homovanillic acid
HSV	Herpes simplex virus
HTLV-1	Human T-cell lymphotropic virus type 1
ICP	Intracranial pressure
ICU	Intensive care unit
IQ	Intelligence quotient
IV	Intravenous

IVIG	Intravenous immunoglobulin
LDL	Low-density lipoprotein
MELAS	Mitochondrial encephalomyopathy with lactic acidosis and stroke-like episodes
mg	Milligram
mm	Millimeter
MRA	Magnetic resonance angiography
MRI	Magnetic resonance imaging
MRV	Magnetic resonance venography
NCS	Nerve conduction study
NCV	Nerve conduction velocity
NICU	Neonatal intensive care unit
NMDA	N-methyl-D-aspartate
NPO	Nothing per os (mouth)
PCR	Polymerase chain reaction
PT	Prothrombin time
PTT	Partial thromboplastin time
RPR	Rapid plasmin reagin
SPECT	Single-photon emission computed tomography
SSEP	Somatosensory-evoked potential
SSPE	Subacute sclerosing panencephalitis
TORCH	Toxoplasmosis, other, rubella, CMV, HIV, HSV infections
TSH	Thyroid-stimulating hormone
VDRL	Venereal Disease Research Laboratory
VER	Visual-evoked response
VLDL	Very-low-density lipoprotein
VMA	Vanillylmandelic acid

INTRODUCTION

Preparing for the oral neurology boards is a challenging task. It is important to understand from the outset that the purpose of this test is to evaluate the candidate's thinking process and to make sure that the candidate is a safe physician with good clinical judgment. Of course, this requires a basic fund of knowledge and a certain level of experience. Adequate preparation, which involves understanding what will be asked of you during the test and being familiar with a broad range of neurologic diseases in both adults and children, can significantly ease the stress of the process.

Preparation for such an important examination does not happen overnight. It will likely be insufficient to read a child neurology textbook several weeks before the test. You will need time to familiarize yourself with all aspects of this field and recall the cases in pediatric neurology that you encountered during your training. Thus, begin studying for the exam as early as possible.

Practice is another important element of preparation. During the exam, whether with a live patient or with vignettes, you are asked to review and synthesize information in an organized fashion in a limited amount of time. Although residency may prepare you for this to some degree, the oral boards demand a certain amount of succinctness that may not come naturally to everyone. Developing the clinical skills and thought processes to perform a physical exam or discuss a case in a timely fashion requires practice. Try to take a history and perform a physical examination in 30 minutes on patients whom you currently see. Also, reading through vignettes alone or with colleagues as often as possible before the exam definitely will make the task easier when you are asked to do it in front of examiners.

THE EXAMINATION

The oral neurology boards consist of three 1-hour-long parts. The first part consists of a live patient examination. You will have 30 minutes to take a history and perform a physical exam on a live patient. Candidates in child neurology examine a pediatric patient, whereas candidates in adult neurology examine an adult patient. During the remaining 30 minutes, you will be asked to present the case to the examiners. This involves summarizing important factors of the history and physical exam, localizing neurologic findings, formulating a differential diagnosis, providing the likely diagnosis, discussing a diagnostic evaluation, and giving a treatment plan. Depending on the time, examiners are also likely to ask you questions about the case or other general topics in neurology.

The vignettes form the other portions of the examination. Adult and child vignettes are structured the same way with each session lasting 1 hour. Vignettes consist of several sentences or a short paragraph describing a patient's history and pertinent physical exam findings. However, they may vary in length and the degree of detail provided. Some may be very specific, whereas others seem more open ended. Within the hour, 50 minutes are devoted to five vignettes, each lasting approximately 10 minutes. The last 10 minutes are then used to review shorter vignettes, which are often neurologic emergencies. This time might also be used to ask the candidate questions about different subjects.

Candidates are given a choice of reading the vignette aloud or in silence. Examiners may also read the case aloud for the candidate. Candidates can take notes during this process but this should not consume too much time. After the case has been read, you will be asked to discuss the case, which involves the following steps:

- Briefly summarizing the case.

- Localizing the examination findings.

- Giving the most likely diagnosis and providing a differential diagnosis.

- Discussing an appropriate diagnostic work-up.

- Discussing the management of the patient.

HELPFUL HINTS

- As with any exam, go into the experience as prepared as possible. Begin your studies early. Know what is expected of you during the test and practice exam skills as much as possible beforehand.

- Stay focused and organized. The oral boards are a timed test so always keep the time limits in mind. Try not to be distracted by a lack of response from examiners, difficult cases, or the stress of the exam.

- Identify cases as neurologic emergencies. Examiners want to know that you have a clear understanding of the urgency of diagnosis and management with emergency presentations. You need to demonstrate that you have good clinical judgment.

- Identify treatable diseases. This is also very important. Many neurologic diseases of childhood have no specific therapy. However, missing a treatable condition may result in poor neurodevelopmental outcome or significant neurologic sequelae for a child.

- Justify why you want to do certain tests. Simply providing a laundry list of possible tests that you might order in a case does not demonstrate a thorough thought process. Carefully consider the tests that you might order and give an explanation of why.

- Admit when you do not know what to do or when you do not have the knowledge to answer a question. You are not expected to know everything and it is best to be honest. Giving vapid or long-winded answers to waste time is not helpful. Examiners respect that candidates sometimes get stuck on a certain aspect of a case or may not be able to answer a question. They will help guide you through a difficult case but will not look favorably on made up or obviously incorrect statements.

FORMAT OF THIS BOOK

It is very difficult to simulate the experience of the oral boards on paper. Depending on the case, your answers, and the examiners, your experience with a live patient presentation or a vignette may take a variety of courses. Discussions may focus only on a given case or you may find yourself reviewing a completely unrelated topic. This book is intended to provide an overview of typical child neurology cases with which you should be familiar. It is not intended to be a pediatric neurology textbook. If you read a case and are not familiar with the disease process, further detailed reading in that area should be done.

This book is primarily designed to guide preparation of the clinical vignettes in child neurology. However, it is important to recognize that the vignettes presented in this book are likely longer and more detailed than those that you will encounter during the oral boards. This was done to standardize the cases in this textbook and to fully describe patient presentations for teaching purposes. On the exam, a briefer history may be given and the exam findings will not all be described in an organized fashion. In addition, the vignettes in this book are organized randomly as cases will be presented during the oral boards to help simulate the experience. However, in the back, there is a separate index by disease category for those who want to focus their studies on a particular area in child neurology. Finally, many of the cases are followed by a section containing additional questions. These questions generally cover topics that are important to know and answering them will help broaden your knowledge in these areas.

A healthy 9-year-old girl is brought to the emergency room after her parents witnessed her having an unusual event shortly after going to bed. They reported hearing gurgling noises coming from her room. When they found her, she was sitting up in bed and unable to speak. She had jerking of her right lower face with excessive drooling. She appeared awake during the spell. It stopped spontaneously after 2 minutes. She has had a cold but otherwise has been well recently.

Physical Examination General Examination: Normal. Neurologic Examination: Mental Status: Alert and cooperative. Language: Fluent without dysarthria. Cranial Nerves: II through XII intact. Motor: She has normal bulk and tone with 5/5 strength throughout. Coordination: There is no dysmetria on finger-to-nose testing. Sensory: No deficits are noted. Gait: She has a normal heel, toe, flat, and tandem gait. Reflexes: 2+ throughout with bilateral plantar flexor responses.

Guide to Case Discussion

■ Briefly summarize this case.

■ Localize the examination findings.

■ Give the most likely diagnosis and provide a differential diagnosis.

■ Discuss an appropriate diagnostic work-up.

■ Discuss the management of this patient.

Diagnosis Benign childhood epilepsy with centrotemporal spikes.

Discussion Benign childhood epilepsy with centrotemporal spikes (BECTS) or benign rolandic epilepsy is the most common form of idiopathic epilepsy in childhood. The peak ages of onset are between 5 and 10 years. However, onset may occur in children as young as 3 years or as old as 13 years. Affected children are typically developmentally and intellectually normal. There is a strong genetic predisposition to epilepsy in BECTS. A gene on chromosome 15q14 has been implicated in some families.

The seizures in BECTS are brief and infrequent. Approximately 10% of children will experience only one seizure. In the majority of children (70%), seizures will occur only two to six times. Twenty percent of patients will experience more frequent seizures. In approximately 70% of children, seizures occur only at night. The seizures in BECTS have a characteristic semiology, involving hemifacial clonic movements, speech arrest, dysarthria, and excessive drooling. Preceding paresthesias around the mouth, gums, cheek, or lips may occur. During the seizure, there may be involvement of the ipsilateral arm or leg, as well as secondary generalization. The seizures usually last 1 to 2 minutes.

The EEG background in BECTS is normal in the awake and sleep states. Epileptiform paroxysms are described as focal, diphasic spike-and-slow-wave activity of medium to high voltage located over the rolandic or centrotemporal regions. Epileptiform discharges may occur either unilaterally or independently and bilaterally. A horizontal dipole with maximum spike negativity over the central and temporal regions with positivity in the frontal regions is also a classic EEG finding. Characteristically in this disorder, spike-and-wave activity increases in frequency and amplitude during drowsiness and nonrapid eye movement (REM) sleep. Centrotemporal spikes may occur only during sleep in approximately 30% of children.

Spontaneous resolution of seizures by adulthood (18 years of age) occurs in almost all patients with BECTS and, thus, it is given the designation of a "benign" epilepsy. Some academic and behavioral problems have been reported in children with BECTS, but the overall prognosis for intellectual and neurologic outcome is excellent.

Summary The patient is a healthy 9-year-old girl who presents after a simple partial seizure involving right facial jerking, drooling, and speech arrest. Her neurologic exam is normal.

Localization Right facial twitching as well as speech arrest localize to the left centrotemporal, rolandic region.

Differential Diagnosis The patient in this case presents with the classic features of a focal seizure in the setting of BECTS, but the diagnosis of BECTS can be made only when both the clinical history and the EEG findings are consistent with this syndrome. Other localization-related epilepsies caused by underlying structural lesions (trauma, cerebrovascular disease, tumor, neuronal migration abnormalities, mesial temporal sclerosis) should also be considered.

Evaluation For a patient who presents to the emergency room with a new-onset focal seizure, a head CT scan, as well as basic laboratory work (basic chemistries, CBC, toxicology screen), may be warranted. A referral (inpatient or outpatient) for an awake and sleep EEG is indicated to evaluate for focal epileptiform activity. The diagnosis of BECTS may be assigned only when the clinical history as well as the EEG are consistent.

The role of neuroimaging in a patient with BECTS is controversial. If the clinical history is consistent and classic bilateral, independent centrotemporal spike-and-wave activity is found on the EEG, a brain MRI is not always performed. However, if there are atypical clinical features or the EEG shows unilateral or atypical epileptiform activity, a brain MRI is typically recommended to rule out structural abnormalities.

Management Treatment with anticonvulsants is often unnecessary in BECTS as seizures are typically infrequent and occur primarily in sleep. However, when seizures are more frequent or occur during wakefulness, they may be disruptive to a child's quality of life. A variety of anticonvulsants have been used in the treatment of BECTS and most are efficacious. However, carbamazepine, oxcarbazepine, and gabapentin have tolerable side effects and are most commonly used in clinical practice.

Additional Questions

1. How would your management be different if this patient had been ill for several days with a high fever?
2. Can children with BECTS have other EEG abnormalities?

References

Berbardina BD, Sgro V, Fejerman N. Epilepsy with centro-temporal spikes and related syndromes. In: Roger J, Bureau M, Dravet C, et al., eds. *Epileptic Syndromes in Infancy, Childhood and Adolescence.* 3rd ed. Eastleigh, UK: John Libbey; 2002:181–202.

Gelisse P, Corda D, Raybaud C, et al. Abnormal neuroimaging in patients with benign epilepsy with centrotemporal spikes. *Epilepsia.* 2003;44(3):372–378.

Willmore LJ. Treatment of benign epilepsy syndromes throughout life. *Epilepsia.* 2001; 42(suppl 8):6–9.

You are contacted by the emergency room to see **a previously healthy 15-year-old girl** who presents with complaints of worsening headache for 3 weeks and blurred vision for 2 days. The headache began several weeks ago and has gotten more severe over the last several days. She now describes it as a constant, pounding sensation all over her head. Two days ago she also developed blurred vision. She does not have a prior history of headaches or migraines. She denies photophobia, sonophobia, nausea, and vomiting. She has not had any recent fever, cough, or congestion.

Physical Examination Vital Signs: Afebrile. General Examination: The patient appears to be in moderate discomfort. There is no nuchal rigidity or back pain to palpation. Funduscopic examination reveals obscuration and elevation of optic disc margins, absence of venous pulsations and tortuous vessels bilaterally. Neurologic Examination: Mental Status: Alert. Language: She has normal naming, repetition, and comprehension. Cranial Nerves: Her pupils are equal, round, and reactive to light. Her extraocular muscles are intact except for difficulty completely abducting her left eye. Diplopia is reported on left lateral gaze. Visual field testing demonstrates enlarged blind spots bilaterally but is otherwise normal. Facial sensation and expression are intact symmetrically. Her gag is present. The tongue and uvula are midline. Motor: She has normal bulk and tone with 5/5 strength throughout. Coordination: There is no dysmetria. Sensory: No deficits are noted. Gait: She has a normal heel, toe, flat, and tandem gait. Reflexes: 1+ throughout with bilateral plantar flexor responses.

Guide to Case Discussion

- Briefly summarize this case.

- Localize the examination findings.

- Give the most likely diagnosis and provide a differential diagnosis.

- Discuss an appropriate diagnostic work-up.

- Discuss the management of this patient.

Diagnosis Idiopathic intracranial hypertension (pseudotumor cerebri).

Discussion Idiopathic intracranial hypertension (IIH) is a headache syndrome characterized by elevated intracranial pressure (ICP) in the absence of ventricular dilatation, intracranial mass lesion, or CSF abnormalities. The diagnosis requires an ICP greater than 250 mm of water as measured on lumbar puncture in addition to normal neuroimaging and CSF studies.

IIH is seen in 0.9 per 100,000 persons of the total population. It is most common in obese females between 15 and 44 years of age. In childhood, boys and girls are affected equally. After puberty, IIH is found nine times more frequently in women than in men. IIH is a diagnosis of exclusion and many secondary causes have been identified (Table 2.1), including CNS infections, cerebral sinus venous thrombosis, malnutrition, endocrine abnormalities, systemic autoimmune disorders, and medications such as vitamin A, antibiotics (tetracyclines, Bactrim, Macrobid), lithium, growth hormone, levothyroxine, and corticosteroids.

Headache is present in 90% of affected patients and is often the presenting symptom. Descriptions of the headache vary and it may be throbbing or dull. It may worsen with eye movement. Associated nausea, vomiting, and photophobia may occur, making the condition difficult to clinically distinguish from a migraine. Neck and back pain are also commonly reported. Pulsatile tinnitus is an often overlooked symptom, seen in 60% of patients. Visual complaints such as transient visual

---

TABLE 2.1

Secondary Causes of Intracranial Hypertension in Childhood

Central nervous system infection
Cerebral sinus venous thrombosis
Malnutrition
Head trauma
Endocrine abnormalities
  Hypoparathyroidism
  Hypothyroidism
  Obesity
  Addison disease
Medications
  Corticosteroids
  Lithium
  Vitamin A
  Tetracyclines
  Cis-retinoic acid (Accutane)
  Bactrim
  Levothyroxine
  Growth hormone
Systemic autoimmune disease
  Systemic lupus erythematosus
  Sarcoidosis
  Behçet disease

obscurations, blurry vision, vision loss, and diplopia are frequently reported. Transient visual obscurations appear as brief episodes of monocular or binocular vision loss and are caused by optic disc edema, leading to transient ischemia of the optic nerve head. Diplopia is typically caused by unilateral or bilateral abducens nerve palsy.

On physical exam, varying degrees of papilledema are typically seen at presentation. However, it is important to be aware that there are case reports of IIH without papilledema. A loss of venous pulsations may also subtly indicate elevated ICP. As papilledema progresses, visual acuity may deteriorate. Enlargement of physiologic blind spots is very common. Inferonasal defects, generalized visual field restriction, and scotomas (central, paracentral, arcuate, and altitudinal) are also frequently seen. If increased ICP is allowed to progress, blindness may ensue.

The pathophysiology of IIH is poorly understood. Most likely IIH represents a disorder of CSF homeostasis and is related to either increased CSF production or decreased CSF absorption. The most widely accepted theory hypothesizes that there is decreased CSF absorption at the level of the arachnoid granulations.

Summary The patient is a previously healthy 15-year-old girl who presents with a 3-week history of worsening headaches and a 2-day history of blurred vision. On neurologic exam, she is found to have bilateral papilledema, a left abducens nerve palsy, and enlarged blind spots on visual field testing.

Localization The patient's headache is likely caused by the displacement of the intracranial pain sensitive structures (cerebral arteries, dural arteries, large veins, venous sinuses) by elevated ICP. Pain sensation in the supratentorial intracranial blood vessels is mediated through the trigeminal nerve.

The presence of papilledema indicates increased ICP. The isolated left abducens nerve palsy is a nonspecific sign often seen with elevated ICP. Increased ICP leads to downward displacement of the brainstem, which stretches the abducens nerve as it passes out of the brainstem and through the subarachnoid space. This, in turn, produces weakness of the ipsilateral lateral rectus muscle, causing diplopia on left lateral gaze. Enlarged blind spots localize to the retinal cells adjacent to the optic disc and can occur with any cause of optic disc swelling.

Differential Diagnosis The patient in this case presents with the primary complaints of worsening headache with blurry vision and is found to have evidence of elevated ICP on exam. There are many potential causes of her symptoms but some diagnoses can be easily ruled out. Her presentation is not consistent with a headache syndrome such as a migraine, tension headache, or cluster headache. There are no complaints of fever, photophobia, or nuchal rigidity that would suggest an infectious process such as meningitis or encephalitis. Trauma could lead to headache and elevated ICP with a subdural hematoma but the adolescent in this case has no history of head injury. Hydrocephalus from a brain tumor could cause this clinical picture but might be expected to cause more neurologic deficits. A slowly progressive subarachnoid bleed or sinus venous thrombosis should be considered. However, the initial differentiation of diagnostic possibilities requires neuroimaging.

Evaluation The patient's evaluation should begin with a head CT with and without contrast performed in the emergency room. This helps rule out hydrocephalus, hemorrhage, masses, stroke, sinus venous thrombosis, and infection. Follow-up neuroimaging with a brain MRI (with and without gadolinium) and magnetic resonance venogram (MRV) is then required. Although the head CT is an adequate screening tool, an MRI is needed to better evaluate for underlying structural abnormalities that may be responsible for the patient's symptoms.

Next, a lumbar puncture should be performed if the head CT is unremarkable. The lumbar puncture should be done with careful measurement of the opening pressure with the patient in a lateral decubitus position with the legs extended. A pressure greater than 250 mm of water is diagnostic of IIH. Routine CSF studies, including cell count, glucose, protein, and bacterial culture should be sent to exclude an infectious process.

Serum studies including a basic chemistry panel, liver function tests, thyroid function tests, erythrocyte sedimentation rate, ANA, parathyroid hormone level, and CBC should be performed to screen for common conditions associated with IIH. A thorough medication history, in particular acne medication in adolescents, should be reviewed as a possible secondary cause of IIH.

Once the presence of IIH has been identified, an ophthalmologic evaluation with visual acuity, funduscopic examination, and visual field testing (Humphrey or Goldmann field testing) is required to characterize and detect visual loss. Serial examinations and perimetry testing is used to follow the course of IIH and its response to treatment.

Management   With the presentation of a subacute headache with papilledema and an isolated abducens nerve palsy, immediate work-up for causes of elevated ICP should be performed. In this case, the patient should have her initial evaluation through the emergency room. As discussed above, neuroimaging and a lumbar puncture are first required. Upon confirmation of an elevated opening pressure in IIH, an appropriate amount of spinal fluid should be removed to lower the closing pressure to less than 200 mm of water.

The presence of malignant IIH as identified by overt visual field loss, significant diplopia, and elevated ICP may warrant hospitalization for close and aggressive inpatient ophthalmologic evaluation and serial therapeutic lumbar punctures. For the patient who presents with mild symptoms or an incidentally noted papilledema on ophthalmologic examination, the above work-up can be performed on an outpatient basis.

Potentially causative medications should be stopped. Weight loss and exercise should be recommended in the case of obesity. Underlying medical conditions such as hypothyroidism should be treated appropriately. Relief of symptoms as well as restoration of the baseline visual exam and function are the goals of medical and surgical treatment. The presence of papilledema and visual abnormalities (diplopia, enlarged blind spot, visual field defects, visual acuity loss) warrant medical treatment with carbonic anhydrase inhibitors (acetazolamide) and/or diuretic therapy (furosemide).

The use of acetazolamide has been studied most thoroughly and is thought to decrease the production of CSF in the choroid plexus. A dose of at least 20 mg/kg/day divided twice a day is recommended in children. Adults may require 1 to 4 g of acetazolamide per day. Also, using the long-acting formulation anecdotally has been beneficial. Common side effects include paresthesias and altered taste. Acidosis and dehydration can also occur with its use. Furosemide and other diuretics have been tried with some success.

The use of topiramate has not been comparatively examined as a monotherapy agent in IIH in adults or children. However, the side effect of appetite suppression can make topiramate an effective adjunct agent in those individuals with obesity. Serial therapeutic lumbar punctures may be performed for flare-ups. Corticosteroids are typically used only for emergent management of impending visual loss. However, rebound rise in ICP is common with its withdrawal.

Surgery is reserved for patients with rapidly deteriorating vision due to papilledema. Surgical options include optic nerve sheath decompression and CSF shunting. No direct comparative studies have been performed. Local resources (and/or preferences) usually dictate which procedure is chosen. Both have advantages and disadvantages. Optic nerve sheath fenestration may relieve local CSF pressure on the optic nerve and improve visual function. Unilateral decompression has been reported to improve visual function in both eyes. This procedure has not been shown to be as effective with chronic papilledema. CSF shunting by placement of a lumboperitoneal or a ventriculoperitoneal shunt can also be done. However, shunt failures and infections require revisions resulting in a high failure rate, particularly in obese individuals.

Additional Questions

1. Describe the ophthalmologic findings consistent with mild, moderate and severe papilledema.

2. Describe how to perform a lumbar puncture. What size and type of needle should one use in each age group? What direction should the bevel be?

References

Banta JT, Farris BK. Pseudotumor cerebri and optic nerve sheath decompression. *Ophthalmology.* 2000;107(10):1907–1912.

Bynke G, Zemack G, Bynke H, et al. Ventriculoperitoneal shunting for idiopathic intracranial hypertension. *Neurology.* 2004;63(7):1314–1316.

Fenichel GM. *Clinical Pediatric Neurology: A Signs and Symptoms Approach.* 4th ed. Philadelphia, Pa: WB Saunders; 2001:77–89.

Friedman DI. Pseudotumor cerebri. *Neurol Clin* 2004;22:99–131.

Friedman DI, Jacobson DM. Diagnostic criteria for idiopathic intracranial hypertension. *Neurology* 2002;59(10):1492–1495.

Kline LB, Bajandas FJ. *Neuro-ophthalmology.* 5th ed. Thorofare, NJ: Slack; 2001:1–44, 93–102.

A healthy 2-year-old boy is brought to the emergency room after waking up in the morning with a wobbly gait. He had been fine the night before but is now having difficulty sitting up. He is also unable to walk independently. There is no history of trauma. He is not in any apparent pain. Approximately 2 weeks ago he had a low-grade fever with cold symptoms but has been well since. He has a good appetite and is not irritable. He was born at full term by vaginal delivery without complications. His development has been normal. There is no family history of neurologic disease.

Physical Examination Vital Signs: Afebrile. General Examination: There are no dysmorphic facial features. His neck is supple. His fundi could not be visualized. Neurologic Examination: Mental Status: Alert and playful. Language: He uses short phrases with age-appropriate pronunciation. Cranial Nerves: His pupils are equal, round, and reactive to light. He tracks objects in all directions. Nystagmus is noted on lateral gaze bilaterally. His face is symmetric. The tongue is midline. Motor: He has normal bulk and tone. He moves all extremities against gravity. Coordination: Significant truncal ataxia is noted when he is in a sitting position. Dysmetria is appreciated bilaterally when he tries to pick up Cheerios from the examiner's hand. Gait: He supports himself on his legs but is unable to walk unassisted due to ataxia. Reflexes: 2+ throughout with bilateral plantar flexor responses.

Guide to Case Discussion

▨ Briefly summarize this case.

▨ Localize the examination findings.

▨ Give the most likely diagnosis and provide a differential diagnosis.

▨ Discuss an appropriate diagnostic work-up.

▨ Discuss the management of this patient.

Diagnosis Acute cerebellar ataxia.

Discussion Acute cerebellar ataxia is a relatively common, benign clinical syndrome in children, defined as the rapid onset of cerebellar dysfunction. It typically occurs in otherwise healthy children during the second year of life but may be seen in the 1- to 6-year-old age group. Acute cerebellar ataxia is likely a postinfectious, immune-mediated process, presenting several weeks after a flu-like illness. It most often occurs after a varicella infection. However, symptoms are reportedly caused by numerous infectious diseases such as EBV, *Mycoplasma pneumoniae*, mumps, enterovirus, and coxsackievirus. It may also happen after immunizations. It is suspected that the mechanism of pathogenesis involves autoantibodies against cerebellar tissues, resulting in inflammation or focal cerebellar vasculitis.

Clinically, affected children develop acute cerebellar symptoms such as gait ataxia, dysmetria, nystagmus, hypotonia, tremor, dysarthria, and scanning speech. Focal features on the neurologic examination suggest an alternate diagnosis. Additional noncerebellar symptoms of headache and photophobia also have been reported but raise the suspicion of a meningoencephalitis.

The CSF is usually normal but a mild pleocytosis with lymphocytic predominance can be seen. CSF protein is normal early in the disease course but may later be mildly elevated. Typically, neuroimaging is normal but inflammatory changes may occur in the cerebellum. For example, cerebellar edema and increased MRI signal intensity have been reported. There may be some overlap with demyelinating conditions such as acute disseminated encephalomyelitis (ADEM).

Acute cerebellar ataxia is typically a self-limiting disease. The majority of children recover completely within 2 months and only a minority of children experience persistent ataxia with other cerebellar deficits. Older children and patients with EBV infection tend to have a poorer prognosis.

Summary The patient is a 2-year-old, previously healthy, developmentally normal boy who presents with acute cerebellar ataxia 2 weeks after a viral illness. His neurologic exam is remarkable for nystagmus and bilateral dysmetria, as well as significant truncal and gait ataxia.

Localization The neurologic findings on this patient's exam localize to the cerebellum diffusely as he has appendicular, as well as truncal/gait, ataxia. This likely represents a pancerebellar syndrome. There are no focal features.

Differential Diagnosis The causes of acute ataxia in childhood are many and may depend on the age of the child (Table 3.1). Toxic ingestion is the most common cause of acute ataxia in toddlers. It should be immediately determined whether any prescription or over-the-counter medications are present in the house. Central nervous system infections such as bacterial meningitis, encephalitis, and cerebellitis also commonly present with acute cerebellar abnormalities. Other postinfectious processes, such as ADEM, deserve consideration. However, these possibilities seem unlikely as the patient appears so well.

Opsoclonus-myoclonus syndrome is a paraneoplastic syndrome associated with neuroblastoma and is an important cause of acute ataxia in young children.

TABLE 3.1

Causes of Acute Ataxia in Childhood

Toxic ingestion
Acute cerebellar ataxia
Bacterial meningitis
Encephalitis
Acute disseminated encephalomyelitis
Opsoclonus-myoclonus syndrome
Acute inflammatory demyelinating polyneuropathy
Seizure/postictal state
Migraine
Cerebellar stroke/thrombosis/hemorrhage
Trauma
Acute hydrocephalus
Intermittent ataxias
    Episodic ataxia type 1 and type 2
    Maple syrup urine disease
    Hartnup disease
    Mitochondrial diseases
    Urea cycle defects

Extreme irritability in addition to opsoclonus, myoclonus, and ataxia may be seen. However, associated opsoclonus is not always present in the early stages of the disease, so a clinician must have a high index of suspicion for this disease. Young children with acute inflammatory demyelinating polyneuropathy (Guillain-Barré syndrome) may be difficult to examine, and present with a seemingly ataxic gait that is caused by muscle weakness. The presence of deep tendon reflexes and clinical history in this case help rule this condition out.

Seizures and/or the associated postictal state may also cause an acute ataxia. Less commonly, these symptoms may be associated with migraines. Stroke, thrombosis, and hemorrhage involving the cerebellum are rare in children. They also cause encephalopathy and other neurologic abnormalities, making these unlikely etiologies for this child's symptoms. Trauma causing cerebellar edema or a subdural hematoma should also be considered.

Intermittent ataxias caused by inborn errors of metabolism are another important consideration in the differential of the acute onset of ataxia. Episodic ataxia type 1 and 2 (EA1, EA2) are channelopathies with an autosomal dominant inheritance pattern. EA1 is characterized by the acute onset of brief episodes of ataxia precipitated by stress, fatigue, exercise, or illness. Myokymia is frequently noted in periorbital and small hand muscles. EA1 is a result of a mutation on chromosome 12 and is caused by a potassium channel abnormality. EA2 is caused by an abnormality in a calcium channel and is related to the defect found in familial hemiplegic migraine. A mutation on chromosome 19 is responsible. In contrast to EA1, attacks of ataxia and other cerebellar symptoms last minutes to days. Both disorders are responsive to acetazolamide. Other inborn errors of metabolism, such as mitochondrial disease, Hartnup disease, maple syrup urine disease, and urea cycle defects, can also be associated with episodes of acute ataxia and may be precipitated by an acute illness.

Acute hydrocephalus may also cause cerebellar signs and may be associated with a variety of posterior fossa tumors. Structural abnormalities, such as posterior fossa tumors, however, rarely present acutely. This also holds true for other developmental anomalies of the posterior fossa (Dandy-Walker malformation, Arnold-Chiari malformation, cerebellar agenesis, Joubert syndrome). In addition, chronic, hereditary ataxias such as Friedreich ataxia, ataxia-telangiectasia, and spinocerebellar ataxia can be considered, but again do not produce acute symptoms.

Evaluation   The diagnosis of acute cerebellar ataxia is one of exclusion. First, it must be determined whether the patient has had a toxic ingestion. The family should be asked if the child may have taken any medications that are in the house. A urine toxicology screen is indicated in all cases. If there are concerns for a specific medication, poison control may be contacted and serum levels are sometimes available, depending on the medication ingested. Basic serum chemistries, liver function tests, and a CBC are also indicated on an initial screening evaluation. Abnormalities may help lead to a diagnosis. For example, metabolic acidosis may suggest an ingestion, whereas elevated liver function tests may support the diagnosis of an acute or resolving EBV infection.

Neuroimaging is indicated to rule out structural abnormalities. Although a head CT is more easily obtained in an emergency room setting, there is limited ability to identify white matter abnormalities such as ADEM, and the posterior fossa may not be well visualized. Thus, a brain MRI with and without gadolinium is most helpful to rule out specific structural, demyelinating, and infectious pathology. After documentation of normal neuroimaging, a lumbar puncture should be obtained. Assessment of CSF cell count, glucose, protein, and bacterial culture is mandatory. Extra CSF may be saved for evaluation of specific infections if necessary. For example, PCR testing for EBV, varicella, *Mycoplasma pneumoniae*, or other viruses can be performed. Evaluation of acute and chronic serum immunoglobulin titers for specific viruses may also be helpful in confirming the presence of a suspected virus.

If the patient presents with atypical features, further work-up may be indicated. An EEG can be performed if seizures are suspected. A metabolic work-up or specific genetic testing may be indicated if there are concerns for an inborn error of metabolism.

Management   There are no specific interventions for acute cerebellar ataxia. Once other conditions have been ruled out, management is primarily symptomatic. Affected children may often benefit from physical and occupational therapy during the recovery phase of their illness. For refractory cases, corticosteroids as well as intravenous immunoglobulin have been tried but reports of efficacy are mainly anecdotal and randomized, controlled trials have not been performed.

Additional Questions

1. What is myokymia and what causes it?
2. What is Joubert syndrome?
3. What is Hartnup disease?

References

Davis DP, Marino A. Acute cerebellar ataxia in a toddler: case report and literature review. *J Emerg Med.* 2003;24(3):281–284.

Keller C, Shapira SK, Clark GD. A urea cycle defect presenting as acute cerebellar ataxia in a 3-year-old girl. *J Child Neurol.* 1998;13(2):93–95.

Maggi G, Varone A, Aliberti F. Acute cerebellar ataxia in children. *Childs Nerv Syst.* 1997;13:542–545.

Nussinovitch M, Prais D, Volovitz B, et al. Post-infectious acute cerebellar ataxia in children. *Clin Pediatr.* 2003;42:581–584.

Swaiman KF. Muscular tone and gait disturbance. In: Swaiman KS, Ashwal S, eds. *Pediatric Neurology: Principles and Practice.* 3rd ed. St. Louis, Mo: Mosby; 1999:54–62.

Swaiman KF, Zoghbi H. Cerebellar dysfunction and ataxia in childhood. In: Swaiman KS, Ashwal S, eds. *Pediatric Neurology: Principles and Practice.* 3rd ed. St. Louis, Mo: Mosby; 1999:787–800.

You are called to the emergency room to see **a previously healthy 8-year-old girl** for complaints of a new-onset seizure. She was on the playground with her friends when she experienced an episode of eye deviation, staring, right-sided jerking, and unresponsiveness for 2 minutes. She has been very sleepy for the last 2 hours since the event occurred and the intern in the emergency room reports that she also has a right-sided Todd paralysis that has not yet resolved. Adults who witnessed the event deny any trauma or falls, although she was seen playing on the monkey bars shortly before the seizure began. She is an otherwise healthy child. There is no family history of seizures.

Physical Examination General Examination: Normal. Neurologic Examination: Mental Status: Sleepy but arousable. Language: She has difficulty following commands and attempts to say a few words that are slurred. Cranial Nerves: Both pupils react to light but the left pupil is smaller than the right, particularly when the lights are dimmed. There is a mild left ptosis. Her extraocular muscles appear intact. There is flattening of the right nasolabial fold with facial movements. A gag is present. The tongue is midline without fasciculations. Motor: Normal bulk. The right arm and leg are hypotonic. Formal motor testing is difficult but she is able to move the left arm and leg purposefully off the bed. There is some withdrawal of the right arm and leg to deep pain stimuli but she does not have antigravity strength. Coordination: No dysmetria or tremor is noted. Reflexes: 2+ on the left and 1+ on the right. There is a left plantar flexor and a right plantar extensor response.

Guide to Case Discussion

▨ Briefly summarize this case.

▨ Localize the examination findings.

▨ Give the most likely diagnosis and provide a differential diagnosis.

▨ Discuss an appropriate diagnostic work-up.

▨ Discuss the management of this patient.

Diagnosis   Left carotid artery dissection causing a left Horner syndrome and left-middle cerebral artery infarction.

Discussion   Spontaneous and traumatic carotid artery dissection is an uncommon cause of stroke in the pediatric population. Dissections may occur in the anterior as well as the posterior circulation. They may affect intracranial or extracranial vasculature. A dissection occurs when blood enters the arterial wall and may be caused by direct trauma, a tear in the intima, or a disruption of the internal elastic lamina. A subintimal hematoma may develop, causing cerebral ischemia either by hypoperfusion or by thromboembolism from the damaged arterial wall. A double lumen may also occur if the dissection rejoins the main arterial lumen.

Spontaneous dissections suggest an underlying vascular abnormality, but most often there is no obvious cause. Multiple contributing risk factors have been identified, including participation in sports, fibromuscular dysplasia, chiropractic manipulation, connective tissue disorders like Marfan syndrome, head or neck trauma, infection, migraine, Valsalva maneuvers, and vascular anomalies.

Headache, neck pain, and stroke are the most common presenting symptoms of extracranial carotid artery dissection. Some patients may experience transient ischemic attacks prior to having a stroke. Horner syndrome can frequently be seen with extracranial carotid artery dissections.

Intracranial carotid artery dissections are much less common but carry a significantly higher morbidity and mortality rate. They tend to affect the anterior circulation in children, with the supraclinoid internal carotid and middle cerebral arteries most often involved. Affected children typically present with headaches, seizures, stroke and subarachnoid hemorrhage. Brainstem and cerebellar dysfunction occur commonly with intracranial as well as extracranial vertebral and basilar artery dissection. Seizures accompany stroke in approximately 50% of children with an arterial ischemic stroke.

Summary   The patient is a healthy 8-year-old girl who developed a new-onset right focal seizure and right hemiparesis while on the playground. Her examination is remarkable for a left Horner syndrome, aphasia (expressive and receptive), and dense right hemiparesis involving her face, arm, and leg, with depressed reflexes and a right plantar extensor response.

Localization   The patient demonstrates left-sided miosis and ptosis, which is indicative of a Horner syndrome. The patient's anisocoria is more prominent in the dark, which occurs with a Horner syndrome, as the normal pupil dilates to accommodate for the darkness. Horner syndrome is caused by a disruption in the three-neuron sympathetic pathway of pupillary innervation. First-order neurons lie in the posterolateral hypothalamus and synapse with second-order neurons in the intermediolateral cell column in the lower cervical and upper thoracic spinal cord. These neurons then pass to the superior cervical ganglion where they synapse with the third-order neurons, which innervate the Müller muscles (which cause ptosis when weak) and the pupillary dilators of the eye. Anhydrosis is a variable feature of Horner syndrome and typically occurs if the lesion involves the sympathetic nerves proximal to the bifurcation of the common carotid artery. This occurs because these fibers travel along the external carotid artery.

This patient does not have any additional brainstem abnormalities to suggest a central cause for her Horner syndrome. Cortical signs (aphasia, encephalopathy, seizure), as well as the time course and possible mechanism of action, argue against the lesion being at the level of the spinal cord. Thus, most likely the child in this vignette has experienced a lesion of the cervical sympathetic chain in the neck affecting the third-order neuron.

The patient also has an expressive and receptive aphasia, dense right hemiparesis, depressed right-sided reflexes, and right plantar extensor response. These findings localize to the left cerebral hemisphere in the distribution of the left-middle cerebral artery. Her right focal seizure also localizes to the left cerebral cortex. Thus, the patient has suffered a dissection of the left carotid artery, possibly caused by neck movement or minor trauma, which has resulted in a left hemispheric stroke and focal seizure.

Differential Diagnosis There are multiple, diverse etiologies for stroke in childhood. The differential diagnosis in this case is relatively straightforward as this patient presents with a Horner syndrome in addition to a stroke. However, in general, broad categories of causes of stroke in childhood include:

- Trauma (head or neck trauma, arterial dissection, nonaccidental trauma);

- Congenital heart disease (atrial septal defect, ventricular septal defect);

- Acquired heart disease (arrhythmias, cardiomyopathy, myocarditis);

- Vasculitis (systemic lupus erythematosus, primary cerebral angiitis);

- Vasculopathy (moyamoya disease, Ehlers-Danlos syndrome, Marfan syndrome);

- Hematologic disorders/coagulopathy (antithrombin III deficiency, oral contraceptive pills, protein C or S deficiency, sickle cell disease);

- Congenital cerebrovascular abnormalities (arteriovenous malformation);

- Inborn errors of metabolism (homocystinuria, mitochondrial disease);

- Other (migraine, radiation vasculitis).

Evaluation This patient first requires an emergent head CT to evaluate the extent of her stroke. An ECG is also indicated in the emergency room to help rule out a cardioembolic event secondary to an arrhythmia as the mechanism of action may not initially be clear. Baseline labs should be drawn, including a CBC, basic chemistry panel, and PT/PTT.

Further management should include a brain MRI with diffusion-weighted imaging, again to assess the extent of her stroke. In extracranial carotid artery dissection, MRI may also demonstrate absence of flow void, altered luminal signal intensity, or an asymmetric vascular lumen, which supports the diagnosis of a dissection. Magnetic resonance angiogram of the brain and the neck should be performed to evaluate vasculature and to determine the site of the dissection. CT angiography is another useful noninvasive test to evaluate the brain and neck blood vessels, but catheter angiography is also often required if there is a high level of suspicion and the area of dissection is not identified by other means. The typical angiographic findings include a tapered arterial lumen followed by a small string sign.

An extraluminal pouch, pseudoaneurysm, intimal flap, or distal branch occlusion may also be seen.

This patient also requires an EEG to evaluate her seizure. She should also undergo an ophthalmologic examination given the presence of the Horner syndrome.

Management   As noted above, the patient should first be medically stabilized, which involves placing her on a cardiorespiratory monitor and pulse oximeter. An IV line should be placed and appropriate labs should be drawn. Maintenance IV fluids should be started with non–dextrose-containing isotonic solution, with a goal of normovolemia. Blood pressures should be maintained above the 50% for age-related norms. She should be monitored closely for decompensation; if her respiratory status becomes depressed, she should be intubated. Precautions for aspiration should be taken until she is stable. This may involve placement of a nasogastric tube for feeding initially. She should be monitored closely for hypo- or hyperglycemia as blood sugar abnormalities are associated with a worse outcome in adults. Transfer to the intensive care unit for close observation is appropriate.

Management of carotid artery dissection is typically the same in children as in adults. However, randomized, controlled trials have not been performed, so the ideal treatment is still controversial. Patients may require medical, vascular, and/or surgical therapeutic interventions.

Typically, patients with extracranial and intracranial carotid artery dissections are anticoagulated because of concerns about the risk of artery-to-artery thromboembolism and subsequent stroke. However, in a patient with a sizable stroke, the risk of bleeding with anticoagulant therapy must be balanced against the potential benefits. Heparin is used initially with transition to warfarin for 3 to 6 months. If recannulization does not occur after 6 months, warfarin may be continued for an additional 3 months, with reassessment at that time. Low-molecular-weight heparin and antiplatelet therapy are also prescribed in certain circumstances. The experience with endovascular treatment in children is limited, but angioplasty, stent placement, vascular occlusion, and pseudoaneurysm coiling are possible options that are frequently used in adults. Surgical intervention is rarely required and is only used to manage life-threatening lesions in accessible vasculature. At this time, decisions regarding appropriate treatment are usually made on a case-by-case basis.

Given that the patient has experienced a seizure secondary to her stroke, she should be loaded with phenytoin and placed on a maintenance dose in the acute setting. The need for chronic anticonvulsants can be assessed during the recovery period, and if deemed necessary, a switch to a more appropriate anticonvulsant, such as carbamazepine, can be made.

Finally, the child in this case is likely to experience long-term neurologic sequelae from her stroke. She should receive physical, occupational, and speech therapy early in the course of her hospitalization. She should also be assessed to determine if she is a candidate for inpatient rehabilitation once she is medically stable for discharge. Ongoing therapies, as well as accommodations with the school system, are frequently required for children who have experienced a significant stroke.

Additional Questions

1. How can pharmacologic testing be used to localize the causative lesion in Horner syndrome?
2. Describe the work-up for a child with an idiopathic stroke.

References

Camacho A, Villarejo A, de Aragón AM, et al. Spontaneous carotid and vertebral artery dissection in children. *Pediatr Neurol.* 2001;25:250–253.

Hutchison JS, Ichord R, Guerguerian AM, et al. Cerebrovascular disorders. *Semin Pediatr Neurol.* 2004;11(2):139–146.

Patten J. *Neurological Differential Diagnosis*, 2nd ed. London, UK: Springer-Verlag; 1996:6–15.

Roach ES. Etiology of stroke in children. *Semin Pediatr Neurol.* 2004;11(4):244–260.

Silverboard G, Tart R. Cerebrovascular arterial dissection in children and young adults. *Semin Pediatr Neurol.* 2000;7(4):289–300.

A **9-month-old boy** is referred to your office for evaluation of developmental delay. He was born at 37 weeks to a 26-year-old G_2P_1 mother by normal spontaneous vaginal delivery. The pregnancy was uncomplicated and fetal movements in utero seemed normal. The patient remained in the nursery for several weeks after birth because he required oxygen and feeding support. Because he had a poor suck and swallow, he required a nasogastric tube for the first 2 months of life. Now he is just starting to sit up, but has not attempted to crawl. He babbles appropriately. He can eat some pureed foods and drink from a bottle, but is not gaining weight well. He often has a cough and was hospitalized once at 6 months for pneumonia.

Physical Examination General Examination: He has an elongated face but no dysmorphic features. There is no hepatosplenomegaly. Neurologic Examination: Mental Status: Alert. Cranial Nerves: The pupils are equal, round, and reactive to light. He tracks objects in all directions. His facial movements are weak but symmetric. A gag is present but there is excessive drooling. The tongue is midline without fasciculations. Motor: There is normal bulk with moderate diffuse hypotonia. He is able to move all four extremities against gravity but has some mild difficulty holding his head up against gravity. He sits only with support. Coordination: He picks up small objects with a raking motion and does not use a pincer grasp. There is no dysmetria. Reflexes: Trace throughout with bilateral plantar flexor responses.

Guide to Case Discussion

- Briefly summarize this case.
- Localize the examination findings.
- Give the most likely diagnosis and provide a differential diagnosis.
- Discuss an appropriate diagnostic work-up.
- Discuss the management of this patient.

Diagnosis Nemaline myopathy.

Discussion The congenital myopathies are a relatively rare, heterogeneous group of disorders that affect the skeletal muscle. Many are hereditary. Clinically they are almost indistinguishable and most commonly present as "floppy infant syndrome" or congenital hypotonia. Other clinical presentations include muscle weakness, delayed motor developmental milestones, feeding difficulties when there is facial involvement, and arthrogryposis. Many affected children may have a relatively benign course with static weakness and hypotonia. Severe infantile presentations may be associated with rapidly progressive weakness and death from respiratory insufficiency.

Histologically, most congenital myopathies demonstrate type 1 myofiber predominance and atrophy but superimposed characteristic morphologic features help differentiate them. Serum CK levels may be normal or mildly elevated, and deep tendon reflexes are usually depressed or absent. Although multiple congenital myopathies have been described, nemaline myopathy, central core disease, and centronuclear myopathy are encountered most frequently and appear to be distinct clinical entities.

More specifically, nemaline myopathy (nema = thread) is classified clinically by age at presentation and severity of disease. Severe, intermediate, and typical congenital forms are recognized. There is much overlap between these groups, however. In the most severe cases, neonates present with profound weakness, little spontaneous movement, respiratory compromise, and abnormal feeding. These children often die of respiratory failure in the first few weeks or months of life. In typical congenital cases, the weakness and hypotonia are less profound. Although motor milestones may be delayed, these patients can often gain ambulatory abilities. With childhood onset, affected children present with delayed motor milestones, proximal weakness, and hypotonia. A long, narrow face, high-arched palate, kyphoscoliosis, and club feet may be noted. Facial, palatal, and pharyngeal muscles can be involved. However, eye musculature is typically spared and often helps differentiate nemaline myopathy from other congenital myopathies. Cardiomyopathy has been reported, but is not a typical feature of nemaline myopathy. Intelligence is usually normal. Rarely, adults present with this myopathy with a wide spectrum of clinical severity.

The muscle biopsy in nemaline myopathy typically demonstrates type 1 fiber predominance or a normal distribution of fiber types with type 1 atrophy. However, the diagnosis rests on the presence of subsarcolemmal, intermyofibrillar, or intranuclear rodlike structures. There is no correlation between the number of rods and the clinical severity of the patient. Nemaline rods are not completely specific for nemaline myopathy as they can be seen in other neuromuscular disorders or at tendinous insertions.

Several genetic abnormalities are associated with nemaline myopathy and both autosomal dominant and autosomal recessive inheritance patterns have been seen. Defects in genes coding for slow alpha-tropomyosin, beta-tropomyosin, nebulin, troponin T1, and skeletal muscle alpha-actin have been involved, primarily on chromosomes 1 and 2. These genes code for components of muscle thin filaments.

Summary The patient is a 9-month-old boy with a history of respiratory and feeding problems at birth who presents with fine and gross motor delays, as well as persistent respiratory and feeding difficulties. His exam is remarkable for a long face, facial diplegia, neck flexor weakness, oropharyngeal weakness with excessive drooling, hypotonia, and hyporeflexia.

Localization The patient's symptoms localize to the peripheral nervous system and disorders of the anterior horn cell, peripheral nerve, neuromuscular junction, and muscle should be considered. There is no history of cognitive delay or other features, such as seizures, that point to a central cause. Given the presentation, it is also unlikely that a spinal cord abnormality could explain the constellation of symptoms.

There are no tongue fasciculations to suggest anterior horn cell involvement as in spinal muscular atrophy. Polyneuropathies are extremely rare as a neonatal presentation. They cause distal more than proximal weakness and generally do not affect facial musculature. Congenital neuromuscular junction diseases such as myasthenia gravis typically cause ptosis in addition to muscle weakness. Thus, it seems that a disorder of the muscle is most likely in this case.

Differential Diagnosis The differential diagnosis of a floppy or hypotonic infant is broad (Table 5.1). Hypotonia may be caused by central, as well as peripheral nervous system disorders. It must first be determined whether the hypotonic patient is clinically weak. Central causes may result in hypotonia but do not typically cause true muscular weakness unless there has been a central nervous system injury, such as a neonatal stroke or spinal cord transection from a difficult delivery. In contrast, diseases of the anterior horn cell, peripheral nerve, neuromuscular junction, and muscle most often manifest with weakness. Taking an initial thorough birth, medical, and developmental history, as well as performing a physical examination are mandatory. Taking a family history is also essential as many of these disorders are hereditary. Testing such as neuroimaging of the brain and/or spine, measurement of serum CK levels, CSF evaluation, EMG, NCS, Tensilon testing, or muscle biopsy may be required, however, to arrive at a definitive diagnosis.

Central causes of hypotonia are often associated with dysmorphic features suggestive of a genetic disorder. The possibility of Prader-Willi syndrome should be given special consideration in hypotonic infants as it can present with hypotonia and feeding abnormalities. It can easily be ruled out with genetic testing for a mutation on chromosome 15q11-13. Additional symptoms, such as lethargy, seizures, or hemiparesis, may point to a central etiology. Also, a history of traumatic birth may suggest cerebral and spinal cord abnormalities such as hypoxic-ischemic change.

Anterior horn cell disease is an important consideration in a hypotonic infant. Babies with spinal muscular atrophy type 1 (Werdnig-Hoffmann disease) can present at birth with profound weakness and areflexia in addition to feeding and respiratory difficulties. These patients are alert and interactive. They have no sensory or sphincter deficits. However, the presence of tongue fasciculations (indicative of denervation) is usually present and can be very helpful in making the diagnosis. Infantile poliomyelitis is a rare occurrence in an industrialized nation where children are routinely vaccinated but remains in the differential diagnosis.

Axonal and demyelinating peripheral neuropathies rarely manifest during the neonatal period or in infancy. However, congenital forms of hereditary motor and sensory neuropathies (congenital hypomyelination neuropathy, Dejerine-Sottas syndrome), familial dysautonomias, giant axonal neuropathy and neuropathies associated with metabolic diseases (mitochondrial disease, leukodystrophies, lysosomal storage diseases, peroxisomal disorders) are all in the differential diagnosis of a hypotonic infant. Acute inflammatory demyelinating polyneuropathy (Guillain-Barré syndrome) has also been reported in this age group.

TABLE 5.1

Causes of Neonatal Hypotonia

Central Nervous System
  Benign congenital hypotonia
  Genetic syndromes (Prader-Willi syndrome, trisomies, many others)
  Hypoxic-ischemic encephalopathy
  Cerebral malformations
  Cortical migration abnormalities (lissencephaly, schizencephaly)
  Inborn errors of metabolism

Spinal Cord
  Trauma
  Spinal cord ischemia

Anterior Horn Cell
  Spinal muscular atrophy
  Neonatal poliomyelitis

Neuromuscular Junction
  Infantile botulism
  Transient neonatal myasthenia gravis
  Congenital myasthenia gravis

Peripheral Nerve
  Hereditary motor and sensory neuropathies
  Acute inflammatory demyelinating polyneuropathy
  Familial dysautonomia syndromes
  Giant axonal neuropathy
  Inborn errors of metabolism

Muscle
  Congenital myopathy
    Central core disease
    Nemaline myopathy
    Centronuclear myopathy
    Congenital fiber-type disproportion
  Congenital muscular dystrophy
    Without cerebral involvement
        Merosin-positive CMD
        Merosin-negative CMD
    With cerebral involvement
        Walker-Warburg CMD
        Fukuyama CMD
        Muscle-eye-brain disease
  Congenital myotonic dystrophy
  Metabolic myopathy
    Mitochondrial myopathy
    Glycogen storage diseases

CMD = Congenital muscular dystrophy

Peripheral neuropathies manifest with clinical features similar to those of other motor unit disorders, but facial weakness is unusual. Distal weakness may be more prominent than proximal weakness, which is in contrast to other motor unit disorders. An abnormal sensory examination may also be seen in peripheral neuropathies. CSF protein is often elevated. An NCS will be abnormal, possibly demonstrating slowing of motor nerve conduction, low compound muscle action potential amplitudes, or low/absent sensory nerve action potentials. A muscle biopsy may show evidence of denervation. A nerve biopsy may also be abnormal.

Neuromuscular junction diseases, such as transient myasthenia gravis and congenital myasthenia gravis, may cause congenital hypotonia. Transient myasthenia gravis occurs in infants born to mothers affected by myasthenia gravis and resolves by 6 weeks of age. Congenital myasthenia gravis syndromes are associated with presynaptic, synaptic, and postsynaptic acetylcholine transmission defects. Although neuromuscular junction diseases can also cause hypotonia, generalized weakness, feeding problems, and respiratory compromise, ptosis is usually noted on examination.

A heterogeneous group of muscle disorders must also be considered in the differential diagnosis of a patient with congenital hypotonia. These diseases include congenital myopathies, congenital muscular dystrophies, and congenital myotonic dystrophy, as well as metabolic myopathies.

Congenital myopathies are discussed above but in addition to central core disease, nemaline myopathy, and centronuclear myopathy, other less-common myopathies occur and have similar presentations. Examples include congenital fiber-type disproportion, multicore disease, reducing body myopathy, and fingerprint body myopathy.

Important clinical differences exist between central core disease, nemaline myopathy, and centronuclear myopathy that deserve mention. Central core disease is not associated with facial weakness, oculomotor palsies, or cardiomyopathy, but does carry a susceptibility to malignant hyperthermia. Nemaline myopathy frequently causes facial weakness, but oculomotor abnormalities and cardiomyopathy occur only rarely. Finally, centronuclear myopathy often causes facial and oculomotor weakness, but no cardiomyopathy.

Congenital muscular dystrophies clinically overlap with congenital myopathies. There are also a heterogeneous group of diseases that present with hypotonia, weakness, and arthrogryposis. They are differentiated from myopathies by a more elevated CK level and dystrophic myopathic changes on muscle biopsy. They are classified according to the presence or absence of cerebral involvement. Congenital muscular dystrophies without cerebral involvement are further subdivided into those patients with or without merosin (laminin α_2). Merosin is a major structural component of the myofiber basal lamina, serving to connect the muscle cytoskeleton to the extracellular matrix. The merosin-positive form is much more common and generally has a better prognosis. Merosin-negative congenital muscular dystrophy is an autosomal recessive disorder with a genetic defect on chromosome 6, and carries a much worse prognosis. White matter changes may also be seen on neuroimaging in these patients. Congenital muscular dystrophies with cerebral involvement include Walker-Warburg muscular dystrophy, Fukuyama muscular dystrophy, and muscle-eye-brain disease. These infants are usually severely affected with cerebral dysgenesis (lissencephaly, polymicrogyria, pachygyria), migrational abnormalities, intractable seizures, and a variety of ocular abnormalities in addition to weakness.

Congenital myotonic dystrophy has an autosomal dominant inheritance pattern and is caused by an unstable trinucleotide repeat sequence on chromosome 19q13. It is typically seen in infants born to mothers with myotonic dystrophy. In utero, poor fetal movement and polyhydramnios may be reported. Clinical features may include proximal weakness, hyporeflexia, respiratory compromise, poor suck, feeding difficulties, facial diplegia, arthrogryposis, and bilateral club feet. The diagnosis is most easily made by identifying myotonia in the mother, but genetic testing is also now clinically available for this condition.

Finally, metabolic myopathies may present with similar symptoms. Most commonly, mitochondrial myopathies and glycogen storage diseases should be considered. For example, Pompe disease is an autosomal recessive disorder that is caused by a mutation on chromosome 17. Pompe disease results from a deficiency of acid maltase, a lysosomal enzyme that converts maltose and other glycogen branches to glucose. The infantile form may present in the first months of life with profound weakness and fatal cardiomyopathy.

Evaluation A serum CK level may initially be sent to screen for muscle diseases. In congenital myopathies, the CK level is usually normal or only mildly elevated. A markedly elevated CK is more indicative of a congenital muscular dystrophy. EMG is also usually normal but may show mild and nonspecific myopathic features. NCSs are normal and help rule out peripheral neuropathies. Obtaining reliable EMGs and NCSs in infants and young children can be very difficult. But when performed by an experienced clinician, they can help refine the differential diagnosis in a hypotonic patient. In these cases, however, the diagnosis is usually clarified most easily with a muscle biopsy. In the future, as these diseases are better characterized, establishing a diagnosis through genetic testing may be possible.

Management There are no specific treatments for congenital myopathies at this time. Patients require varying degrees of supportive care, depending on the severity of their disease. Close monitoring by a multidisciplinary team helps prevent complications.

After the diagnosis is made, the patient in this vignette should be referred to a geneticist to review the diagnosis and to provide genetic counseling. Testing for specific genetic abnormalities associated with nemaline myopathy may be available. Prenatal testing is available in many instances were the parents to consider having additional children. The patient should also be referred to a pulmonologist to help manage the anticipated chronic respiratory problems. The input of a nutritionist and a gastroenterologist would also be helpful to promote weight gain and monitor his overall nutritional status. The patient is at risk for the development of scoliosis and contractures, so an orthopaedic surgeon may also eventually need to be involved in the patient's care. Finally, he should receive a thorough developmental evaluation with ongoing physical, occupational, and speech therapy.

Additional Questions

1. What genetic defect is associated with malignant hyperthermia?
2. What are the clinical features of Prader-Willi syndrome?
3. What is arthrogryposis?

References

Fenichel GM. *Clinical Pediatric Neurology: A Signs and Symptoms Approach*. 4th ed. Philadelphia, Pa: WB Saunders; 2001:149–169.

North K, Goebel HH. Congenital myopathies. In: Jones HR, De Vivo DC, Darras BT, eds. *Neuromuscular Disorders of Infancy, Childhood, and Adolescence: A Clinician's Approach*. Philadelphia, Pa: Butterworth-Heinemann; 2003:601–632.

Riggs JE, Bodensteiner JB, Schochet SS. Congenital myopathies/dystrophies. *Neurol Clin*. 2003;21:779–794.

Ryan MM, Schnell C, Strickland CD, et al. Nemaline myopathy: a clinical study of 143 cases. *Ann Neurol*. 2001;50:312–320.

Taratuto AL. Congenital myopathies and related disorders. *Curr Opin Neurol*. 2002;15: 553–561.

Tubridy N, Fontaine B, Eymard B. Congenital myopathies and congenital muscular dystrophies. *Curr Opin Neurol*. 2001;14:575–582.

Volpe JJ. Neonatal hypotonia. In: Jones HR, De Vivo DC, Darras BT, eds. *Neuromuscular Disorders of Infancy, Childhood, and Adolescence: A Clinician's Approach*. Philadelphia, Pa: Butterworth-Heinemann; 2003:113–122.

You are consulted by the NICU to see **a 3,500-g newborn male infant** born at 39 weeks gestation via spontaneous vaginal delivery with vacuum assistance to a mother with insulin-dependent diabetes mellitus. The infant was large-for-gestational-age. The delivery was complicated by nuchal cord and shoulder dystocia, which fractured the left humerus. His Apgar scores were 0, 2, and 6 at 1, 5, and 10 minutes of life, respectively. The patient was resuscitated, intubated, and brought back to the NICU. Shortly afterwards, decreased movement of the right upper extremity was noted.

Physical Examination General Examination: The infant is intubated and on a mild amount of sedation. Neurologic Examination: Mental Status: He is sedated but responsive to stimuli. Cranial Nerves: The pupils are equally round and reactive to light. The extraocular muscles are intact as assessed by oculocephalic maneuver. Facial expression is intact. His gag is present. The tongue is midline. Motor: The left upper arm and forearm have been boarded as a single cast by orthopaedics. The distal aspects of his fingers are exposed and move well in response to stimuli. The nurses report that the patient may occasionally raise his left arm against gravity when agitated. The right arm is noted to have decreased tone and to be internally rotated with elbow extension and forearm pronation. Muscle tone, bulk, and strength are intact and symmetric in the lower extremities. Sensory: Although there is limited ability to examine the left upper extremity because of the board, sensation to pinprick is noted in the fingers and shoulder. There is a lack of response to painful stimuli in the right upper extremity from the shoulder to the midforearm. Reflexes: 2+ in the lower extremities but difficult to appreciate in the right upper extremity. Bilateral plantar flexor responses are present.

Guide to Case Discussion

▓ Briefly summarize this case.

▓ Localize the examination findings.

▓ Give the most likely diagnosis and provide a differential diagnosis.

▓ Discuss an appropriate diagnostic work-up.

▓ Discuss the management of this patient.

Diagnosis   Brachial plexus palsy (Erb palsy).

Discussion   Brachial plexus palsy is caused by an injury to the brachial plexus as a result of traction, compression, tear, or avulsion of the nerve roots arising from C5 through T1. Brachial plexus palsy is seen in 0.5 to 1.9 per 100 livebirths. It occurs more commonly in term infants and in the right upper extremity. It is associated with large-for-gestational-age infants, diabetes (both gestational and pregestational), older maternal age, traumatic deliveries, shoulder dystocia (26%), and clavicular fracture (11%). Although lateral deviation of the head during delivery is presumed to cause traction of the nerves, cases have been reported of in utero brachial plexus palsy. Brachial plexus palsy also can occur following cesarean sections or routine nontraumatic deliveries.

There are several presentations of brachial plexus palsy (Table 6.1). A Duchenne-Erb palsy (Erb palsy) results from damage to the superior trunk or fifth and sixth cervical ventral rami. It is the most common brachial plexus palsy. Arm positioning with internal shoulder rotation, adduction, elbow extension, forearm pronation, and finger flexion (waiter's tip sign) is pathognomonic. Klumpke palsy is rare. It results from injury to the inferior trunk or eighth cervical and first thoracic ventral rami. The classic upper extremity posture involves elbow flexion (triceps weakness), forearm supination (pronator quadratus weakness), wrist extension (wrist flexor weakness), and a claw deformity of the hand (weakness of lumbricals and intrinsic hand muscles). Some patients are described as having a floppy hand. Sympathetic fibers may also be involved, causing a Horner syndrome.

A complete brachial plexus palsy can occur with involvement of the ventral rami that form the brachial plexus. Sympathetic fibers also may be involved in these cases. A flaccid limb is noted on exam. In addition, bilateral brachial plexus palsies have been described.

TABLE 6.1

Erb and Klumpke Brachial Plexus Palsy

	Erb Palsy	**Klumpke Palsy**
Involved trunk	Superior trunk	Inferior trunk
Involved nerve roots	C5-6	C8-T1
Weakness (muscles)	Shoulder abduction (deltoid, supraspinatus)	Elbow extension (triceps)
	Shoulder external rotation (infraspinatus)	Forearm pronation (pronator quadratus)
	Elbow flexion (biceps, brachioradialis)	Wrist flexion (wrist flexor group)
	Forearm supination (biceps, supinator)	Finger extension (lumbricals, hand intrinsics)

C = Cervical
T = Thoracic

Outcome in brachial plexus palsies is determined by the distribution of nerve involvement and the degree of injury. The majority of newborns will recover in 3 to 6 months. The recovery process during the first few weeks is usually the best indicator of the ultimate outcome. Those infants who show no or minimal signs of recovery during the initial 3- to 6-month period may require additional work-up and surgery to reanneal or graft the injured nerves. Those infants with associated phrenic nerve injury are more likely to require surgery. Earlier repair (by 6 months of age) may improve functional outcome.

Summary   The patient is a large-for-gestational-age full-term male infant born to a diabetic mother via vacuum-assisted vaginal delivery with shoulder dystocia resulting in left humeral fracture and right upper extremity brachial plexus palsy.

Localization   The distribution of sensory deficits and motor weakness in the right arm in the absence of long tract signs suggests a disorder of the peripheral nervous system. An Erb palsy as seen in this case localizes to either the superior trunk or the fifth and six cervical nerve roots. Classically, there is weakness of shoulder abduction (supraspinatus, deltoid), shoulder external rotation (infraspinatus), elbow flexion (biceps, brachioradialis), and forearm supination (biceps, supinator).

Differential Diagnosis   In large-for-gestational-age infants born with a traumatic birth history, the diagnosis of an obstetrical brachial plexus palsy may be relatively straightforward. The specific motor and sensory deficits noted on physical exam may suggest involvement of certain nerve roots as discussed above. An affected neonate should also be evaluated for the possibility of additional injury to associated structures such as the cervical spine, upper extremity, or phrenic nerve. Other causes of brachial plexus injury include intrauterine compression, humeral osteomyelitis, compressive neonatal hemangioma, exostosis of the first rib, neck compression, and neoplasms of the brachial plexus (neuromas, rhabdoid tumors).

The differential diagnosis of a brachial plexus palsy also includes pseudoparesis as a result of limb pain or deformity and anterior horn cell disorders (congenital cervical spinal cord atrophy, congenital varicella). Finally, brachial plexus palsies need to be differentiated from central nervous system causes of weakness such as stroke. Cortical stroke, however, would be likely associated with unilateral face, arm, and leg involvement in addition to long tract signs such as plantar extensor responses. The patient in this case does not have any signs of an upper motor neuron lesion.

Evaluation   Acute evaluation begins with a thorough neurologic examination to assess the distribution of weakness and the level of involvement. In mild cases, no diagnostic work-up may be required. For more extensive injuries, however, postganglionic brachial plexus lesions must be differentiated from avulsion of nerve roots from the spinal cord. In these cases, MRI of the brachial plexus and cervical/ upper thoracic spine may be necessary. A pseudomeningocele in the subarachnoid space is characteristic of an avulsion. EMG and NCS can also be used to evaluate the distribution and degree of injury. They may also help with prognosis. MRI of the brain is also indicated if there is a concern of a central lesion causing upper extremity weakness.

Management   Management of obstetrical brachial plexus palsy begins with a careful neurologic and general physical exam to evaluate for additional injuries. Seven days of rest are then recommended, usually with the elbow in a flexed position. Parents are asked to pin the sleeve to the opposite side of the shirt for stabilization. Passive range of motion and electrical muscle stimulation may be started 1 week later. Consultation with occupational and physical therapy can be helpful in the recovery period. In select cases, surgical intervention with nerve grafts or brachial plexus reconstruction may be required.

Additional Questions

1. What are the components of the brachial plexus?
2. What EMG and NCS findings would you expect to find with brachial plexus palsy?
3. What do Apgar scores measure?
4. What is Horner syndrome? What are the potential causes?

References

Alfonso I, Alfonso DT, Papazian O. Focal upper extremity neuropathy in neonates. *Semin Pediatr Neurol.* 2000;7(1):4–14.

Bar J, Dvir A, Hod M, et al. Brachial plexus injury and obstetrical risk factors. *Int J Gynaecol Obstet.* 2001;73(1):21–25.

Benjamin K. Part 1. Injuries to the brachial plexus: mechanisms of injury and identification of risk factors. *Adv Neonatal Care.* 2005;5(4):181–189.

Benjamin K. Part 2. Distinguishing physical characteristics and management of brachial plexus injuries. *Adv Neonatal Care.* 2005;5(4):240–251.

Noetzel MJ, Part TS, Robinson S, et al. Prospective study of recovery following neonatal brachial plexus injury. *J Child Neurol.* 2001;16:488–492.

Yilmaz K, Caliskan M, Oge E, et al. Clinical assessment, MRI, and EMG in congenital brachial plexus palsy. *Pediatr Neurol.* 1999;21(4):705–710.

A 3-year-old boy was referred to your office for evaluation of developmental delay. He was born at full-term to a 28-year-old G_2P_1 woman. The pregnancy was uncomplicated, although a cesarean section was performed because the patient weighed 9 pounds at birth. His mother became concerned about his development around 10 months of age when he was not crawling or pulling up to stand. At 3 years of age, he now walks, runs, and throws a ball but is clumsy. He has a vocabulary of approximately 25 words and does not form sentences. His mother also thinks he may have some difficulty understanding things she tells him. He does not point to body parts or identify colors. His 7-year-old sister is in special education classes but otherwise the family history is unremarkable.

Physical Examination General Examination: The head circumference is over 98%. Healthy appearing 3-year-old boy with prominent ears and long face. He is very active and has trouble cooperating with the examiner. Neurologic Examination: Mental Status: Alert. Language: He says "no," mama," and "truck," but does not form sentences. Cranial Nerves: His pupils are equal, round, and reactive to light. He tracks objects in all directions. His face is symmetric. His tongue is midline without fasciculations. Motor: There is normal bulk. He has moderate diffuse hypotonia with symmetric limb movement against gravity. Coordination: There is no dysmetria, but he picks up coins with a raking movement. Gait: His gait is slightly clumsy but not ataxic. Reflexes: 1+ throughout with bilateral plantar flexor responses.

Guide to Case Discussion

- Briefly summarize this case.

- Localize the examination findings.

- Give the most likely diagnosis and provide a differential diagnosis.

- Discuss an appropriate diagnostic work-up.

- Discuss the management of this patient.

Diagnosis   Fragile X syndrome.

Discussion   Fragile X syndrome is the most common genetic abnormality associated with mental retardation. It has a prevalence of approximately 1 in 4,000 males. Fragile X syndrome is caused by an expansion of a CGG triplet repeat sequence in the *FMR1* gene on Xq27.3. Normal individuals have 5 to 50 CGG repeats, but in some families the CGG repeat becomes unstable and expands when passed to offspring. Premutation carriers exist and typically have 61 to 200 repeats. At a threshold of 200 repeats, the *FMR1* gene is silenced, resulting in an absence of the fragile X mental retardation protein (FMRP) and subsequent associated clinical abnormalities.

Fragile X syndrome may occur in both males and females, but the clinical phenotype is most easily recognized in males with the full mutation. Affected males typically have a triad of large ears, a long, narrow face, and macroorchidism. Macroorchidism is more apparent in pubertal and postpubertal males. High birth weight and large anterior fontanelle may be seen in infancy. Macrocephaly, hyperextensible joints, hypotonia, and soft skin are also common. Cognitive abilities vary from borderline normal to severe mental retardation with IQs typically ranging from 20 to 70. Receptive and expressive language development appears to be frequently involved. Behavioral abnormalities are also commonly noted. Attention problems, hyperactivity, social anxiety, gaze aversion, and stereotypies (hand flapping or hand biting) may be seen. In addition, within the spectrum of behavioral abnormalities, as many as 30% of affected males meet the diagnostic criteria for autism.

Females with the full mutation are typically more mildly cognitively affected than full-mutation males, as phenotypic expression is influenced by inactivation of the X chromosome. Affected females then may have normal intelligence or have a wide spectrum of developmental problems, learning disabilities, or mental retardation. Behavioral abnormalities may be more subtle but can include shyness, social avoidance, and anxiety. Autism may also occur.

Premutation carriers often do not experience cognitive deficits or behavioral abnormalities. However, they may develop fragile X–associated tremor/ataxia syndrome (FXTAS) and/or premature ovarian failure. FXTAS typically occurs in males between the ages of 50 and 70 years and is characterized by progressive intention tremor, ataxia, and parkinsonian symptoms such as masked facies, resting tremor, and mild rigidity. This syndrome has also been reported in premutation females, but symptoms are less severe. Premature ovarian failure prior to 40 years of age may affect as many as 21% to 33% of women with the premutation.

Summary   The patient is a 3-year-old boy with a history of high birth weight who presents with global developmental delay and dysmorphic features including macrocephaly, prominent ears, and a long, thin face. His neurologic exam demonstrates an increased activity level and mild hypotonia as well as gross motor, fine motor, cognitive and receptive/expressive language delays but has no focal features. The family history is remarkable for a sister with a learning disability.

Localization   This patient's global developmental delay suggests diffuse cerebral involvement. This patient does not have focal features on his examination. Hypotonia is often a nonspecific finding but may be seen with central or peripheral disorders. It is most likely central in this case as there are no specific neurologic findings suggestive of anterior horn cell disease, neuromuscular junction disorders, peripheral neuropathy or muscle disease.

Differential Diagnosis   The child in this case presents as a typical case of fragile X syndrome. His high birth weight, global developmental delay, behavioral abnormalities, and physical features all point to the diagnosis. In addition, his sister also demonstrates a cognitive disability, making it likely that his mother is a premutation carrier. Of note, autistic features were not described in this child. The physical characteristics and clinical features of fragile X syndrome may be subtle in infancy and early childhood. The diagnosis should be considered in any child presenting with developmental delays, especially in speech and language skills. A maternal family history of mental retardation, learning disabilities, or developmental disabilities may be an additional clue to the diagnosis.

The differential diagnosis of a child with global developmental delay is extensive and can be overwhelming to consider. However, it can be narrowed considerably when considering a few factors. He has slightly dysmorphic facial features that suggest an underlying genetic syndrome. He appears to have a static encephalopathy. He is slowly making progress with his milestones and there is no history of regression. He does not have organomegaly, other organ involvement, or seizures. His neurologic exam shows nonspecific features of hypotonia and motor delays, but there is no weakness to suggest muscle involvement. Reflexes are present, making peripheral nerve involvement unlikely. There are no cerebellar or long tract signs. These factors all make neurodegenerative disorders much less likely.

Although macrocephaly is present and can be caused by numerous acquired (communicating or noncommunicating hydrocephalus) and inherited conditions (leukodystrophies, neurocutaneous disorders, metabolic storage diseases), these etiologies seem unlikely given his clinical presentation. Acquired disorders, such as lead toxicity and hypothyroidism, are also in the differential diagnosis, but there are no known exposures to lead in this case and congenital hypothyroidism is generally detected on newborn screening. This patient's presentation, then, is most consistent with an X-linked mental retardation syndrome.

X-linked mental retardation is a heterogenous group of disorders that are primarily divided into syndromic and nonsyndromic categories based on clinical features. More than 100 syndromic X-linked mental retardation conditions have been described. X-linked factors may account for approximately 10% to 12% of males with mental retardation. Fragile X syndrome is the cause of 20% to 25% of cases of X-linked mental retardation. Other genes commonly associated with X-linked mental retardation include *MECP2* (Rett syndrome), *ARX* (multiple clinical syndromes including isolated mental retardation), and *SLC6A8* (creatine transporter gene). Memorization of a long list of these syndromes is unnecessary; it is important to understand the concept and that a wide range of X-linked mental retardation associated conditions exist.

Evaluation   Global developmental delay affects 1% to 3% of children and there are published practice parameters to guide the diagnostic evaluation in these cases. However, diagnostic testing may be done in a stepwise fashion and should be tailored to the individual patient (Table 7.1).

TABLE 7.1

Diagnostic Evaluation of a Child with Global Developmental Delay

The following tests may be considered in the diagnostic evaluation of a child with global developmental delay.

Testing for inborn errors of metabolism
  Cytogenetic studies
    Karyotype
    Fragile X syndrome (*FMR1* gene)
    Rett syndrome (*MECP2* gene)
    Subtelomeric chromosomal rearrangements
  Lead level
  Thyroid function tests
  Neuroimaging with CT or MRI
  EEG
  Vision screening
  Audiometric assessment

Routine screening for inborn errors of metabolism has a very low yield of approximately 1% and is not generally recommended provided that appropriate newborn screening was performed. It is important to realize, however, that newborn screening is not standardized across the country and may vary from state to state. Metabolic testing should be performed when the history and/or physical exam are suggestive of a specific etiology. Screening labs may include capillary blood gas, serum lactate/pyruvate, serum ammonia, plasma amino acids, urine organic acids, and thyroid function tests.

The yield of routine cytogenetic studies is higher in children with global developmental delay, even in the absence of dysmorphic features. A karyotype may be useful when dysmorphic features are present, as with Down syndrome. Testing for fragile X syndrome, especially in the setting of a family history of cognitive or developmental delay, should be performed. Both males and females may be tested, although males are typically more frequently and more severely affected. The diagnosis of Rett syndrome should be considered in any female with unexplained moderate to severe mental retardation. Specific testing for a mutation in the *MECP2* gene can be sent. It is unclear whether females with mild mental retardation or males with moderate to severe delays should undergo testing for Rett syndrome. Finally, new molecular genetic techniques to assess subtelomeric chromosomal rearrangements may also be considered in children with unexplained moderate to severe global developmental delay.

Screening for lead toxicity should be targeted toward children with identifiable risk factors for environmental exposure. Screening for hypothyroidism is not routinely recommended if appropriate newborn screening was performed in the past.

Neuroimaging can be very useful in the diagnosis of children with global developmental delay. Head CT has a yield of finding an underlying cause for developmental delay in approximately 30%, whereas MRI may determine an underlying etiology in as many as 46.8% to 65.5% of children. Abnormalities are most likely when the neurologic examination is abnormal, as with microcephaly or cerebral palsy. Thus, neuroimaging is typically recommended in the work-up of a child with global developmental delay, with MRI being preferable to CT. An EEG should be obtained when there is a clinical suspicion for seizure activity, but does not need to be done on a routine basis.

Children with global developmental delay are at risk for vision and hearing abnormalities. A full ophthalmologic evaluation with vision screening and dilated funduscopic examination may be indicated in some patients. Behavioral audiometry or brainstem auditory-evoked responses should be performed when feasible, especially in children with speech and language delay and/or autistic features. Transient-evoked otoacoustic emissions may be a suitable alternative when audiometry cannot be performed.

The child in this case presents with a history and physical exam very suggestive of fragile X syndrome. Thus, it would be reasonable to initiate his work-up by using the direct DNA-based test to detect a mutation in the *FMR1* gene and to determine the size of the CGG repeat. This test is considered to be 99% sensitive and 100% specific. It should confirm the diagnosis in this case. However, if testing for fragile X syndrome is negative, further work-up, as discussed above, should be performed. A genetics consultation may also be helpful. Given this child's speech and language delay, he should also undergo a hearing evaluation. A thorough developmental evaluation is also warranted.

Management   There are no specific treatments for fragile X syndrome at this time. Patients should be referred for appropriate developmental and/or psychological testing. Early interventional services, such as speech, occupational, and physical therapy, should be encouraged to maximize the abilities of an affected child. The help of a developmental pediatrician may be enlisted in the management of behavior problems, symptoms associated with attention deficit disorder, or autistic features. The patient should also be referred to a geneticist to aid in the diagnosis of other family members who may be carriers of or clinically affected by the mutation. Direct DNA testing is available for prenatal diagnosis through amniotic fluid cells as well as chorionic villus sampling.

References

Jones KL. *Smith's Recognizable Patterns of Human Malformation.* 5th ed. Philadelphia, Pa: WB Saunders; 1997:150–153.

Kleefstra T, Hamel BCJ. X-linked mental retardation: further lumping, splitting and emerging phenotypes. Clin Genet. 2005; 67:451–467.

Shevell M, Ashwal S, Donley D, et al. Practice parameter: evaluation of a child with global developmental delay. *Neurology.* 2003; 60:367–380.

Terracciano A, Chiurazzi P, Neri G. Fragile X syndrome. *Am J Med Genet C Semin Med Genet.* 2005;137C:32–37.

Visootsak J, Warren ST, Anido A, et al. Fragile X syndrome: an update and review for the primary pediatrician. *Clin Pediatr.* 2005;44:371–381.

You are contacted by the emergency room to see **a 13-year-old girl** who presents for complaints of being tired and weak for 3 weeks. Her symptoms worsen over the course of the day. The weakness has kept her from participating in volleyball practice after school recently. She has had difficulty eating and in order to chew her food, has to manually move her jaw up and down to crush food. There has been no choking or difficulty breathing. The pediatric intern tells you that she thinks the patient has had a stroke because her speech sounds funny. The patient's mother also says her eyelids have started to look more droopy than usual.

Physical Examination Vital Signs: Normal. General Examination: Unremarkable. Neurologic Examination: Mental Status: Alert. Language: She has normal naming, repetition, and comprehension but a hyponasal voice. Cranial Nerves: Her pupils are equal, round, and reactive to light. Her extraocular muscles are intact but there is fatigue on upgaze. Ptosis is noted bilaterally left greater than right. Facial sensation is intact. Her facial muscles are weak but move symmetrically. She cannot meet any resistance when opening her mouth. Her gag is present. The tongue is midline. Motor: She has normal bulk and tone. Neck flexor weakness is noted. Arm abduction is 4+/5 but the rest of her strength is 5/5 throughout. Coordination: There is no dysmetria. Sensory: No deficits are noted. Gait: There is no ataxia. Reflexes: 1+ throughout with bilateral plantar flexor responses.

Guide to Case Discussion

- Briefly summarize this case.
- Localize the examination findings.
- Give the most likely diagnosis and provide a differential diagnosis.
- Discuss an appropriate diagnostic work-up.
- Discuss the management of this patient.

Diagnosis Juvenile myasthenia gravis.

Discussion There are three recognized forms of myasthenia gravis in infants and children: transient neonatal myasthenia gravis, congenital myasthenia gravis, and juvenile myasthenia gravis (JMG). Transient neonatal myasthenia gravis occurs in 10% to 15% of infants born to myasthenic mothers and is caused by placental transfer of antiacetylcholine receptor antibodies. It resolves in the first few weeks to months of life. Congenital myasthenic syndromes are a heterogeneous group of diseases and are not autoimmune in origin. They are caused by presynaptic, synaptic, and postsynaptic defects in neuromuscular transmission. Congenital myasthenia gravis typically presents before 2 years of age with ptosis, ophthalmoplegia, hypotonia, feeding difficulty, or respiratory distress, but onset in later childhood or adolescence can occur.

JMG is an autoimmune disorder, much like that seen in adults. Ten percent to 20% of patients with autoimmune myasthenia gravis have the onset of symptoms before 20 years of age. Autoimmune myasthenia gravis is now believed to be caused by two different antibody-mediated processes. The majority of patients make antibody to the muscle acetylcholine receptor. However, there is a minority of patients who are "seronegative" and have autoantibodies against a muscle-specific tyrosine kinase (MuSK).

Summary The patient is a previously healthy 13-year-old girl who presents with a 3-week history of bulbar and generalized weakness. She is found to have ptosis, fatigue on upgaze, facial weakness, hyponasal voice, proximal muscle weakness, and hyporeflexia on neurologic examination.

Localization The distribution of this patient's weakness in addition to the absence of long tract signs suggests a disorder of the peripheral nervous system. The constellation of findings, including ptosis, ophthalmoplegia, facial weakness, hyponasal voice, and proximal weakness, are consistent with a disorder of the neuromuscular junction. That the weakness worsens over the course of the day (fatigability) further supports the diagnosis of a process involving the neuromuscular junction. Hyporeflexia is also suggestive of a motor unit disorder.

Differential Diagnosis Congenital myasthenia gravis must be differentiated from an autoimmune process in any child presenting with neuromuscular weakness. A detailed history should help clarify the onset of symptoms. The differential diagnosis should also include other disorders of neuromuscular transmission such as botulism and Lambert-Eaton myasthenic syndrome. Given the bulbar symptoms, motor neuron disease (Fazio-Londe disease, Kennedy disease), Guillain-Barré (Miller-Fisher variant), and a brainstem abnormality (meningitis, encephalitis, stroke, tumor) should be considered. Some congenital myopathies (centronuclear and myotubular myopathy) may present with facial weakness and ptosis, but this weakness is not typically fatigable. These diseases usually also have onset during infancy. In addition, mitochondrial disorders may present with a progressive ophthalmoplegia (Kearns-Sayre) and can be included in the differential diagnosis in a patient with ptosis and ophthalmoplegia.

Evaluation The diagnosis of myasthenia gravis can often be confirmed with an edrophonium (Tensilon) test. Edrophonium is a short-acting (5 minutes) acetylcholinesterase inhibitor that improves neuromuscular transmission. A test dose of 0.04 mg/kg may be given once intravenously. If there is no response after 1 minute, an additional 0.16 mg/kg may be given intravenously for a total of 0.2 mg/kg (maximum dose: 5 mg in patients weighing <34 kg; 10 mg in patients weighing ≥34 kg). Comparing results to the administration of a saline placebo might also be helpful. Resolution of ptosis and/or improvement in ophthalmoplegia are the most reliable end points. Atropine must be available at the bedside when performing this procedure because of the risk of bradycardia, asystole, and hypotension.

Diagnostic labs should include acetylcholine-receptor antibodies (binding, blocking, and modulating). If these antibodies are negative, testing for anti-MuSK antibodies might be useful, as they are detected in approximately 40% of seronegative patients. Myasthenia gravis can be associated with other autoimmune diseases; consequently, thyroid function tests, ANA, and an erythrocyte sedimentation rate might also be sent. A chest CT or MRI with and without contrast should be performed to evaluate for a thymoma.

If testing with edrophonium is not diagnostic, electrodiagnostic studies may be helpful. Repetitive nerve conduction studies are commonly used to assess neuromuscular transmission. A peripheral nerve is stimulated supramaximally and the compound muscle action potential is recorded. A decremental response of greater than 10% indicates abnormal neuromuscular transmission and supports the diagnosis. Single-fiber EMG is the most sensitive test for the diagnosis but is often difficult to perform, particularly in children. A concentric needle is used to record action potentials from individual muscle fibers. Prolonged jitter is the classic finding in myasthenia gravis.

Management Although this presentation is not a clear neurologic emergency, the patient has a several-week history of progressive weakness and is at risk of deterioration, warranting hospital admission for further work-up and initiation of therapy. She should be placed on a cardiorespiratory monitor and pulse oximeter. Negative inspiratory pressure should be checked on admission and regularly during the hospital stay to monitor her respiratory status. Given her facial weakness and difficulty chewing, aspiration precautions should be in place.

Treatment may be initiated with pyridostigmine, a long-acting (4 to 6 hours) cholinesterase inhibitor. Neostigmine is used less frequently because it only has a half-life of approximately 4 hours. The pyridostigmine dose must be titrated for the individual patient but is often enough to improve weakness in mild generalized or ocular cases. Corticosteroids are frequently added for immunosuppression in more severe and generalized cases, but must be used cautiously. They may cause acute but transient muscle weakness and neurologic deterioration within 3 weeks of starting. Consequently, patients are often hospitalized for observation when corticosteroids are initiated. The dose of steroids used varies but 1 to 2 mg/kg/day (maximum: 60 to 80 mg per day) of oral prednisone is commonly prescribed and weaned as tolerated after a response is seen. Improvement with steroids has been reported to be as high as 82% in pediatric series.

Later management of severe and generalized cases might include a thymectomy and/or other long-term immunosuppressants. The benefits of thymectomy have not been evaluated with controlled studies, but complete remission reportedly occurs in 11% to 75% with clinical improvement in 57% to 95% of patients in uncontrolled studies of seronegative and seropositive pediatric patients. However, the role of thymectomy in children and adolescents with pure ocular, seronegative, and anti-MuSK–positive myasthenia gravis is controversial. Immunosuppressants commonly used include azathioprine, cyclosporine, cyclophosphamide, and mycophenolate mofetil (CellCept).

Additional Questions

1. What is the appropriate treatment for myasthenic crisis?
2. What are the side effects of acetylcholinesterase inhibitors such as edrophonium and pyridostigmine?
3. What classes of drugs should myasthenia gravis patients be counseled to avoid and why?

References

Andrews PI. Autoimmune myasthenia gravis in childhood. *Semin Neurol.* 2004;24(1): 101–110.

Andrews PI, Sanders DB. Juvenile myasthenia gravis. In: Jones HR, De Vivo DC, Darras BT, eds. *Neuromuscular Disorders of Infancy, Childhood, and Adolescence: A Clinician's Approach.* Philadelphia, Pa: Butterworth-Heinemann; 2003:575–597.

Meriggioli MN, Sanders DB. Myasthenia gravis: diagnosis. *Semin Neurol.* 2004;24(1):31–39.

Siberry GK, Iannone R, eds. *The Harriet Lane Handbook.* 15th ed. St. Louis, Mo: Mosby; 2000.

A 9-month-old girl presents to your office for complaints of abnormal eye movements. One week prior to the visit, her parents noted the onset of jerky horizontal movements of her left eye. Then several days later, she started nodding her head intermittently. She has otherwise been well without fever, irritability, or other signs of illness. She is currently able to crawl, pull to a stand, babble, and wave bye-bye.

Physical Examination   General Examination: No dysmorphic facial features. There is occasional nodding of the head up and down. Neurologic Examination: Mental Status: Alert and playful. Cranial Nerves: The fundi are difficult to visualize. Her pupils are equal, round, and reactive to light. There is no afferent pupillary defect. She tracks objects in all directions and her visual fields appear to be full. Fine, intermittent, horizontal nystagmus is noted in the left eye. Her face is symmetric. Her palate elevates symmetrically and her tongue is midline without fasciculations. Motor: Normal tone with symmetric limb movement. She sits well without support and crawls. Coordination: There is no dysmetria grabbing for toys. Reflexes: 2+ throughout with bilateral plantar flexor responses.

Guide to Case Discussion

- Briefly summarize this case.
- Localize the examination findings.
- Give the most likely diagnosis and provide a differential diagnosis.
- Discuss an appropriate diagnostic work-up.
- Discuss the management of this patient.

Diagnosis Spasmus nutans.

Discussion Spasmus nutans (nodding spasms) is characterized by the clinical triad of nystagmus, titubation, and head tilt (torticollis). All three classic symptoms are not always present. It is an uncommon disorder, affecting approximately 3 in 1,000 infants. Spasmus nutans is typically seen in infants ages 4 to 8 months. However, it may be seen as early as 3 months and as late as 3 years of age.

The nystagmus is typically the first sign but it is often the head nodding that brings children to medical attention. The nystagmus may be monocular or binocular. If binocular, it is usually asymmetric or dysconjugate. The nystagmus is predominantly pendular, rapid, and horizontal, but oblique or vertical oscillations may be seen. Head movements may be side-to-side or up-and-down. Titubation is felt to be a compensatory mechanism to decrease the nystagmus. Head tilt is the least-common finding. The underlying pathophysiology of spasmus nutans is poorly understood.

Spasmus nutans is typically a transient, benign, self-limiting condition. Most children show significant improvement in their symptoms by 2 to 3 years of age. Although many cases resolve spontaneously with good visual acuity, residual amblyopia, strabismus, or nystagmus may occur.

Summary The patient is a developmentally normal 9-month-old girl who presents for evaluation of the subacute onset of monocular nystagmus and titubation. Her vision, as well as the remainder of her neurologic exam, appears to be normal.

Localization Monocular or binocular nystagmus as described in this patient may localize to several places in the central nervous system. Disorders involving the anterior visual pathway (retina, optic nerve, or chiasm) most commonly cause these symptoms. The upper midbrain or cerebellum could also potentially be involved. Titubation may be a compensatory mechanism to accommodate for nystagmus but can also occur in midline cerebellar disease.

Differential Diagnosis The diagnosis of spasmus nutans is one of exclusion. Transient monocular or binocular nystagmus with titubation and head tilt may be seen in other conditions. Most importantly, patients with structural abnormalities in the anterior visual pathway may present with these symptoms. Specifically, a tumor of the suprasellar region such as a chiasmatic and/or optic glioma should be ruled out.

The differential diagnosis also includes congenital nystagmus. However, congenital nystagmus typically begins at an earlier age (within the first 2 months of life). Titubation is much less common in congenital nystagmus, occurring in only 10% of patients, and is of smaller amplitude than that seen in spasmus nutans. In addition, in contrast to spasmus nutans, congenital nystagmus is associated with jerk and pendular eye movements that are conjugate and constant. Congenital retinal dystrophy and optic nerve hypoplasia may present in a similar fashion. Diseases causing cerebellar dysfunction, such as meningitis, encephalitis, head trauma, posterior fossa tumors, and medication ingestion, may cause nystagmus. Less commonly, patients with inborn errors of metabolism, such as Pelizaeus-Merzbacher disease, may demonstrate transient or intermittent nystagmus.

Evaluation The evaluation of a patient with spasmus nutans should begin with a complete, dilated eye exam performed by an ophthalmologist. The character of the nystagmus and visual acuity should be assessed. Examination of the fundus will rule out retinopathies as well as optic nerve abnormalities. Neuroimaging with a brain MRI with and without contrast is always indicated in these patients to evaluate for structural abnormalities, as discussed above.

Management After the work-up is complete, children with spasmus nutans should be followed regularly by an ophthalmologist. Additional intervention is not required.

Additional Questions

1. How would the approach to this patient be different if she also had a history of developmental regression?
2. What is Pelizaeus-Merzbacher disease?

References

Albright AL, Sclabassi RJ, Slamovits TL, et al. Spasmus nutans associated with optic gliomas in infants. *J Pediatr.* 1984;105:778–780.

Fenichel GM. *Clinical Pediatric Neurology: A Signs and Symptoms Approach.* 4th ed. Philadelphia, Pa: WB Saunders; 2001:117–147.

Good WV, Hou C, Carden SM. Transient, idiopathic nystagmus in infants. *Dev Med Child Neurol.* 2003;45(5):304–307.

Gottlob I, Zubcov AA, Wizov SS, et al. Head nodding is compensatory in spasmus nutans. *Ophthalmology.* 1992;99(7):1024–1031.

Victor M, Ropper AH. *Adam's and Victor's Principles of Neurology.* 7th ed. New York: McGraw-Hill; 2001:86–98.

Wright K, Spiegel P. *Pediatric Ophthalmology and Strabismus.* St. Louis, Mo: Mosby; 1999:140–148.

A community pediatrician calls the neurology referral line to discuss the work-up and management of **a 9-year-old, left-handed girl** with a 1-month history of headaches with occasional vomiting. Her headaches feel "like a drum beating." They occur primarily in the morning, but more recently have occurred intermittently throughout the day. The headaches may last up to 6 hours and are not exacerbated by bright lights or loud noises. She feels better when she lies down and goes to sleep. The pain is worse when she sneezes or coughs. She has tried acetaminophen and ibuprofen with minimal relief. She has not experienced any blurry vision, vision loss, or dizziness with the headaches. Over the last week there has been associated vomiting, particularly in the morning before she goes to school. As a result, her appetite and energy level have been somewhat decreased. There is no history of trauma, fever, diarrhea, or toxin exposure. There is no family history of migraines.

Physical Examination   Vital Signs: Normal. General Examination: There is no nuchal rigidity, papilledema, or photophobia. Neurologic Examination: Mental Status: Alert and oriented to person, place, and year. Language: She has normal comprehension, repetition, recall, and naming. Cranial Nerves: Her pupils are equal, round, and reactive to direct light and accommodation. She has normal visual fields. Her extraocular movements are full but there is nystagmus on left lateral gaze. Her face is symmetric with normal sensation. She has symmetric elevation of her palate and her tongue is midline. Motor: She has normal bulk and tone with 5/5 strength in all muscle groups. There is no pronator drift. Coordination: There is slight dysmetria on left finger-to-nose testing and decreased coordination with rapid alternating movements on the left. Heel-to-shin testing is normal bilaterally. Sensation: Normal light touch, temperature, and vibration throughout. Gait: Normal heel, toe, flat, and tandem gait. Reflexes: 2+ throughout with bilateral plantar flexor responses.

Guide to Case Discussion

- Briefly summarize this case.

- Localize the examination findings.

- Give the most likely diagnosis and provide a differential diagnosis.

- Discuss an appropriate diagnostic work-up.

- Discuss the management of this patient.

Diagnosis Juvenile pilocytic astrocytoma of the posterior fossa.

Discussion Brain tumors account for 20% of all pediatric malignancies and occur at an incidence of 2 to 4 in 100,000 children per year. Headache can be a presenting sign in up to 50% of pediatric brain tumors and is more common in posterior fossa than supratentorial tumors. However, the classic early morning headache and vomiting is present in only approximately 17% of patients. Concerning headache features that should prompt a diagnostic work-up include acute onset ("the worst headache of my life"), headache on exertion, early morning onset, progressively worsening headache, fever and/or systemic signs, meningismus, the presence of focal neurologic deficits, and pain that worsens with Valsalva maneuvers.

Juvenile pilocytic astrocytoma (JPA) is the most common glioma in childhood. It accounts for 10% of all pediatric tumors and 25% of all posterior fossa tumors. JPAs occur most commonly in the cerebellum. However, JPAs can exist in the hypothalamus/third ventricle, optic nerves, brainstem, cerebrum, and spinal cord. There is a strong correlation with neurofibromatosis type 1 when there is optic nerve involvement. Patients with cerebellar JPAs generally present early with signs of elevated intracranial pressure secondary to obstruction of the fourth ventricle in addition to appendicular ataxia from lateral cerebellar involvement.

JPAs are slow-growing, well-circumscribed, low-grade (fibrillary) tumors with both solid and cystic components. On brain MRI, they classically appear as a cystic lesion with a mural nodule compressing the fourth ventricle and one or both of the cerebellar hemispheres. They may also demonstrate diffuse heterogeneous enhancement. Glial fibrillary acidic protein (GFAP)–positive Rosenthal fibers are the histologic hallmark of these tumors.

Pilocytic astrocytomas usually have a good outcome with a recurrence rate of zero to 12% and a 5-year survival of greater than 90%. The extent of surgical resection carries the largest prognostic significance. It is achieved in two-thirds of cases and is required for cure. Additional predictors of good outcome include age and lack of brainstem involvement.

Summary The patient is a previously healthy 9-year-old girl who presents with a 1-month history of worsening intermittent headache and vomiting that are exacerbated by position change and Valsalva maneuvers. These features are concerning for hydrocephalus. Her neurologic exam is significant for left lateral gaze nystagmus, left dysmetria, and left dysdiadochokinesis.

Localization Left-sided dysmetria and dysdiadochokinesis localize to the left lateral cerebellum. Each lateral cerebellar hemisphere is responsible for fine motor control of the ipsilateral extremity. The classification of nystagmus is complex and often difficult to precisely localize. In general, it may have central or peripheral vestibular causes. The presence of cerebellar abnormalities in this patient points to a central etiology. Lesions of the flocculus or cerebellar hemisphere may be responsible.

This patient's symptoms of headache and vomiting suggest that early hydrocephalus may be developing. Because of the close proximity to the fourth ventricle, it is possible that a compressive cerebellar lesion could lead to noncommunicating hydrocephalus.

There are no findings on examination to suggest cortical or brainstem involvement in this patient. False localizing signs of ataxia include lesions of the cerebral peduncles/pons, frontopontine deficits related to hydrocephalus, disorders of the spinal cord, ataxia-hemiparesis syndromes (corona radiata/internal capsule lesions), and sensory ataxia involving the posterior columns, but lesions in these areas would not fit with this case.

Differential Diagnosis Given this child's presentation, the diagnosis of a posterior fossa tumor should be given first consideration. Most children with posterior fossa tumors present with symptoms of elevated intracranial pressure including progressive headache and recurrent vomiting. Irritability and lethargy may also be seen, especially in younger children. Cerebellar abnormalities are also the primary neurologic exam finding in these patients.

The most common pediatric posterior fossa tumors include medulloblastoma, ependymoma, brainstem glioma, and cerebellar astrocytoma. Medulloblastomas usually occur in the midline. They tend to cause obstructive hydrocephalus, in addition to truncal and gait ataxia, more than appendicular ataxia. Spinal drop metastases may also cause back pain and/or myelopathy. Ependymomas are less common than medulloblastomas and JPAs. They are slow-growing tumors and are more likely to present with nausea and vomiting from obstructive hydrocephalus and/or from their location around the emesis center on the floor of the fourth ventricle. They may also cause drop metastases along the spinal axis. Brainstem gliomas usually have a more varied presentation with multiple cranial neuropathies, long tract signs, and contralateral hemiparesis. Consequently, a JPA is highly likely in this patient.

Other rare posterior fossa lesions that should be considered are hemangioblastomas, meningiomas, sarcomas, chordomas, and metastatic disease.

Other disease processes also deserve consideration although they seem much less likely. Vascular lesions (arteriovenous malformation), posterior circulation territory cerebral infarction, infection (acute cerebellitis, encephalitis), postinfectious disorders (acute cerebellar ataxia, acute disseminated encephalomyelitis), autoimmune vasculitis (systemic lupus erythematosus), medications/toxins, trauma (cerebellar hemorrhage), and migraine headache disorder enter the broad differential of a child presenting with headache, vomiting, and cerebellar dysfunction.

Evaluation The first step in the management of this patient should include emergent neuroimaging with a head CT with and without contrast to rule out structural lesions that may be causing hydrocephalus. If the head CT reveals a posterior fossa tumor and/or hydrocephalus, further work-up for systemic and infectious diseases likely will be unnecessary. A follow-up brain MRI with and without gadolinium will be required to better document the extent of the lesion and to guide management decisions. JPAs rarely disseminate and a spinal MRI is not indicated if the diagnosis is relatively clear. She will require evaluation by oncology and neurosurgery. A formal ophthalmologic exam may also be helpful to assess for early signs of papilledema.

Management This patient requires hospitalization for further management. Her presentation is concerning for subacute hydrocephalus. She should be placed on a cardiorespiratory monitor and pulse oximeter. An intravenous line should be placed.

Close monitoring in the intensive care unit while her work-up is proceeding should be considered, depending on the degree of hydrocephalus present.

JPAs are low-grade lesions and are primarily managed with surgical resection. High-dose corticosteroids are usually given as first-line therapy prior to surgery to reduce surrounding edema. Gross total resection is curative in most cases and adjuvant treatment is unnecessary. Radiation therapy may actually increase the likelihood of a higher-grade malignancy if there is recurrence. Chemotherapy may be useful if there is subtotal resection or disseminated disease. In some cases, cerebrospinal fluid drainage or placement of a ventriculoperitoneal shunt is required to manage hydrocephalus. Given her cerebellar signs, physical and occupational therapy consults should be initiated early in her hospital course.

Additional Questions

1. What are the most common pediatric supratentorial brain tumors?
2. What other pediatric disease shares the same histopathologic finding of Rosenthal fibers?
3. Discuss the appropriate management of a patient with increased intracranial pressure.
4. What is posterior fossa syndrome?
5. How can you differentiate central versus peripheral nystagmus?

References

Brazis PW, Masdeu JC, Biller J. *Localization in Clinical Neurology*. 3rd ed. Philadelphia, Pa: Lippincott Williams & Wilkins; 1996:155–250.

Maher CO, Raffel C. Neurosurgical treatment of brain tumors in children. *Pediatr Clin North Am*. 2004;51(2):327–357.

Packer RJ. Brain tumors in children. *Arch Neurol*. 1999;56(4):421–425.

Packer RP, MacDonald TJ, Keating RA. Brain tumors. In: Maria BL, ed. *Current Management of Child Neurology*. 3rd ed. Hamilton, Ont: BC Decker; 2005:577–588.

Purdy RA, Kirby S. Headaches and brain tumors. *Neurol Clin*. 2004;22:39–53.

Ullrich NJ, Pomeroy SL. Pediatric brain tumors. *Neurol Clin*. 2003;21:897–913.

A 13-year-old boy is seen in your office on an urgent basis for complaints of lower-extremity weakness. The patient was in his usual state of good health until that morning when he noticed that his legs were weak when getting out of bed. His symptoms seem to be getting worse because now he is having difficulty walking. The patient does not have any medical problems. He had an upper respiratory tract infection like all of his friends about 2 weeks ago but he did not experience any fevers. He plays football but denies any recent trauma.

Physical Examination Vital Signs: Afebrile. General Examination: There is no nuchal rigidity or papilledema. Neurologic Examination: Mental Status: Alert. Language: He has fluent speech without dysarthria. Cranial Nerves: His pupils are equal, round, and reactive to light. His extraocular muscles are intact. His facial movements are symmetric and without weakness. There is a strong gag and his tongue is midline without fasciculations. Motor: He has normal bulk with mild hypotonia in the lower extremities. Strength in the upper extremities is 5/5 and there is no pronator drift. Lower-extremity strength is 3/5. Coordination: No dysmetria is noted. Sensory: Intact to light touch, temperature, vibration, and proprioception. Gait: Unable to walk unassisted. Reflexes: Absent in the lower extremities. Trace at the biceps and triceps. Bilateral plantar flexor responses are appreciated.

Guide to Case Discussion

- Briefly summarize this case.

- Localize the examination findings.

- Give the most likely diagnosis and provide a differential diagnosis.

- Discuss an appropriate diagnostic work-up.

- Discuss the management of this patient.

Diagnosis Guillain-Barré syndrome.

Discussion Guillain-Barré syndrome (GBS) or acute inflammatory demyelinating polyneuropathy (AIDP) is the most common cause of acute paralysis in childhood. It is an acquired, immune-mediated, demyelinating polyradiculoneuropathy. It is believed to be caused by humoral and cellular immune responses directed against Schwann cells and myelin proteins in the spinal nerve roots and peripheral nerves. Demyelination of peripheral nerves, as well as damage to the underlying axons, may occur.

Clinically, GBS usually presents as an ascending, symmetric paralysis in an otherwise healthy individual. There is an associated loss of deep tendon reflexes. Pain may be a prominent feature in more than half of affected patients. This may often lead to misdiagnosis, especially in young children who may be challenging to examine. Ataxia, distal paresthesias, and/or urinary retention may also be seen. Unilateral or bilateral peripheral seventh cranial nerve palsies can occur. Autonomic changes may include bradycardia, postural hypotension, and tachycardia. The course of symptoms may be very rapid, progressing over hours, or may occur more subacutely over days. Most children reach the nadir of neurologic dysfunction in 2 weeks. After weakness progresses, there is usually a stabilization or plateau phase, which may be of variable duration. This is followed by a recovery phase that may take weeks to months.

As many as two thirds of cases are associated with an antecedent fever or infection 2 to 6 weeks before the onset of neurologic symptoms. Frequently identified associated pathogens include EBV, CMV, hepatitis, varicella, *Mycoplasma pneumoniae*, and *Campylobacter jejuni*.

The clinical spectrum of acute peripheral nerve demyelinating diseases includes four variants with features similar to GBS: acute motor and sensory axonal neuropathy, acute motor axonal neuropathy, Miller-Fisher syndrome, and polyneuritis cranialis. Acute motor and sensory axonal neuropathy is clinically indistinguishable from GBS but involves motor and sensory deficits. It may have a more protracted recovery. There is severe degeneration of motor and sensory axons on histologic examination. Acute motor axonal neuropathy is most commonly seen in the Chinese population and is associated with *C. jejuni* infection. This is a distinct disorder that primarily affects motor axons, sparing peripheral sensory axons and dorsal spinal nerve roots.

Miller-Fisher syndrome involves a triad of ophthalmoparesis, ataxia, and areflexia. Increased levels of immunoglobulin IgM and IgG antibodies to the ganglioside GQ1b (a glycolipid expressed in the axolemma membrane) have been seen. Motor weakness usually does not occur. Polyneuritis cranialis is uncommon and results in bilateral facial neuropathy as well as other symptoms of GBS. It is associated with CMV.

The overall prognosis in children affected by GBS is excellent. The majority of pediatric patients will make a full recovery in 6 to 12 months. However, approximately 15% of children with GBS experience respiratory failure and require mechanical ventilation during the course of their illness.

Summary The patient is a previously healthy 13-year-old boy who presents with an acute, progressive, ascending paralysis in the setting of a recent viral illness.

His neurologic examination demonstrates proximal and distal lower-extremity weakness with areflexia and without apparent sensory abnormalities.

Localization The lower extremity weakness and areflexia in this case most likely localizes to the motor unit and, more specifically, to the peripheral nerve. The other primary consideration might be a central process involving the spinal cord. Although there is no comment in the vignette regarding a sensory level or sphincter tone, the sensory examination provided appears to be normal. There is no history of bowel/bladder incontinence or back pain that would be more suggestive of a spinal cord process. Also, the plantar responses are flexor and there are no long tract signs. Thus, a disorder of the peripheral nerves seems more likely.

Differential Diagnosis The differential diagnosis of GBS involves central nervous system, anterior horn cell, and neuromuscular junction disorders, in addition to other peripheral nerve and muscle diseases. (Table 11.1) The diagnosis of GBS can be especially challenging in very young children or infants who may not be able to articulate their complaints and who may not cooperate with a formal neurologic exam.

Neurologic emergencies such as GBS and acute spinal cord lesions should always be considered first in a child presenting with an ascending paralysis.

TABLE 11.1

Differential Diagnosis of Guillain-Barré Syndrome

Spinal Cord
  Demyelinating disease
  Tumor
  Trauma
  Infarction
  Epidural abscess

Anterior Horn Cell
  Poliomyelitis

Neuromuscular Junction
  Tick paralysis
  Myasthenia gravis
  Botulism

Peripheral Nerve
  Guillain-Barré syndrome and variants
  Chronic inflammatory demyelinating polyneuropathy
  Toxins

Muscle
  Myositis (inflammatory, infectious)
  Metabolic myopathies
  Periodic paralysis syndromes

Demyelinating disease (transverse myelitis, acute disseminated encephalomyelitis), a spinal cord tumor, spinal cord trauma, epidural abscess, or cord infarction may present all with similar features. They may be associated with acute/subacute progressive leg weakness, paresthesias, numbness, back pain, and areflexia. However, cord lesions are more likely than GBS to be associated with early sphincter dysfunction. It is important to know that a small number of patients with GBS have decreased urinary output and neurogenic bladder, but this is usually short-lived. Also, a sensory level would be specific for a spinal cord lesion.

Tick paralysis is also in the differential diagnosis of any child with an ascending paralysis. A thorough physical exam should rule out the presence of an engorged tick. The mechanism of action of the tick neurotoxin is not fully understood but it is believed to affect the distal peripheral nerve terminals or the neuromuscular junction. Neuromuscular disorders such as myasthenia gravis may present with weakness and areflexia. The onset of symptoms, pattern of weakness (ptosis, ophthalmoplegia, proximal weakness), and slower progression of weakness usually help differentiate myasthenia gravis.

Inflammatory myopathies, such as viral myositis, polymyositis, and dermatomyositis, may present with lower-extremity weakness and pain. The serum creatine kinase is elevated, whereas CSF and electrodiagnostic studies are normal. The broad differential diagnosis of acute weakness may also include other muscle diseases, such as metabolic myopathies (mitochondrial disorders, disorders of carbohydrate and glycogen metabolism), as well as the periodic paralysis syndromes. These disorders should produce more generalized weakness and can usually be differentiated by clinical presentation.

Several other disorders may be considered in young children. In this age group, GBS may present with ataxia as a consequence of muscle weakness that may appear to be either a sensory ataxia or cerebellar disease. A thorough neurologic exam should help rule out cerebellar etiologies. In addition, a pseudoencephalopathy with meningeal signs may be noted. Musculoskeletal abnormalities such as toxic synovitis or fractures may enter the differential if a child refuses to walk or experiences significant lower-extremity pain.

Poliomyelitis may cause an ascending paralysis but is usually in the setting of an acute illness and causes asymmetric weakness. It is rare in industrialized nations where vaccination is widespread. Finally, toxins such as heavy metals, glue sniffing, and fish toxins that affect the peripheral nerves should be considered.

Evaluation The evaluation of GBS begins with a thorough history and physical examination. The onset and time course of the progression of motor and sensory symptoms are of critical importance. In addition, any history of preceding viral illness is important to record.

A lumbar puncture should initially be performed to evaluate for CSF albuminocytologic dissociation and to rule out an infectious process. Typically, the protein is elevated (80 to 200 mg/dL) whereas the cell count is normal. However, the CSF protein may still be normal within the first week of symptoms. EMG and NCS can also be helpful in differentiating motor versus sensory nerve involvement. Classic nerve conduction abnormalities are consistent with a demyelinating process and include prolonged distal latencies, loss or prolongation of F-wave latencies, slowing of conduction velocity to less than two-thirds normal, and conduction block. EMG and NCS may also help with prognosis.

A spinal MRI with gadolinium is also often performed as a precautionary measure to rule out spinal cord pathology, particularly in atypical cases or in young children who may have difficulty providing a history or cooperating with a formal neurologic examination. Enhancement of nerve roots may be found but can also occur in other disorders. Pulmonary function should be assessed with negative inspiratory pressures (NIFs) and pulse oximetry.

In children with suspected Miller-Fischer variant, testing for the GQ1b antibodies may be done, and if present, supports the diagnosis. Serum antibody tests (IgM, IgG), CSF studies (antibodies, PCR), and/or stool cultures may also be done to evaluate for specific infections that may be involved such as EBV, CMV, or *Campylobacter jejuni*.

Management GBS should be recognized as a neurologic emergency. Any child presenting with suspected GBS should be admitted to the hospital for diagnostic testing and management. Assessment and stabilization of the airway, breathing, and cardiovascular status should be done immediately. There should be ongoing monitoring for autonomic instability. Patients with rapid progression of symptoms or respiratory compromise require close observation in the intensive care unit.

Treatment of GBS may involve administering IVIG or performing plasmapheresis. The mechanisms by which these therapies work are still not well understood. Intravenous immunoglobulin may act by binding pathologic antibodies or by decreasing B cell antibody production. Plasmapheresis may function to directly eliminate circulating autoantibodies. At this time, there are no prospective, randomized trials comparing these two therapies in children with GBS. It is thus thought that it is likely that the IVIG and plasmapheresis have similar efficacy at lowering morbidity by decreasing the course of the illness and speeding recovery time.

When a child is mildly affected and remains ambulatory, or in cases where neurologic symptoms have plateaued, therapeutic interventions may not be required. Optimal and/or standard protocols for the use of IVIG and plasmapheresis in children do not exist. IVIG may be more practical and less invasive, although it does involve administering a human blood product. The conventional total dose is 2 g/kg which may be given over 2 to 5 days. Side effects of IVIG are typically mild but can include an allergic reaction, anaphylaxis (particularly IgA-deficient individuals), headache, myalgias, fever, and aseptic meningitis. In refractory cases, both IVIG and plasmapheresis may be used. There is no role for the use of corticosteroids in the treatment of GBS.

GBS can be severely disabling and recovery can take months. Consequently, physical and occupational therapy should be instituted early in the disease course to promote mobility and strength building. In addition, as pain may be a significant symptom, involvement of a pain-management team may be helpful.

Additional Questions

1. What are F-waves on nerve conduction studies?
2. What animal model is used to study Guillain-Barré syndrome?
3. What is the mechanism by which CSF protein becomes elevated in patients with Guillain-Barré syndrome?
4. What is chronic inflammatory demyelinating polyradiculoneuropathy (CIDP)?

References

Fenichel GM. *Clinical Pediatric Neurology: A Signs and Symptoms Approach.* 4th ed. Philadelphia, Pa: WB Saunders; 2001:171–198.

Jones HR. Guillain-Barré syndrome: perspective with infants and children. *Semin Pediatr Neurol.* 2000;7(2):91–102.

Sater RA, Rostami A. Treatment of Guillain-Barré syndrome with intravenous immunoglobulin. *Neurology.* 1998;51(suppl 5):S9–S15.

Sladky JT. Guillain-Barré syndrome in children. *J Child Neurol.* 2004;19:191–200.

A **9-year-old girl** from El Salvador is brought to the emergency room for complaints of abnormal movements that began 1 month ago and are getting worse. Her parents are worried because she is very restless and often drops things. Her teacher has noted that she is having difficulty writing. She has also been very irritable and cries for no apparent reason. The patient was previously healthy and there is no family history of neurologic disease. She has lived in the United States for 3 months.

Physical Examination Vital Signs: Normal. General Examination: Unremarkable. Neurologic Examination: Mental Status: Alert but appears anxious and fidgety. Language: Fluent speech without dysarthria. Cranial Nerves: Her pupils are equal, round, and reactive to light. Her extraocular muscles are intact. There is no nystagmus. Her visual fields are full. Her facial movements are symmetric. Her gag is present and the tongue is midline. Motor: Normal bulk with mild diffuse hypotonia. Her strength is 5/5 throughout, but she seems to have trouble maintaining grip strength. Coordination: There is no dysmetria. Random jerky and writhing movements of the upper extremities and trunk are noted. Sensory: Normal temperature, light touch, and vibration. Gait: She ambulates independently without ataxia. Reflexes: 1+ throughout with bilateral plantar flexor responses.

Guide to Case Discussion

■ Briefly summarize this case.

■ Localize the examination findings.

■ Give the most likely diagnosis and provide a differential diagnosis.

■ Discuss an appropriate diagnostic work-up.

■ Discuss the management of this patient.

Diagnosis Sydenham chorea.

Discussion Sydenham chorea is the most commonly acquired chorea of childhood. It typically occurs several weeks to months after group A beta-hemolytic streptoccocal pharyngitis and is a major diagnostic criteria of rheumatic fever, a multisystem inflammatory condition associated with migratory polyarthritis, carditis, chorea, subcutaneous nodules, and erythema marginatum. Approximately one third of patients with Sydenham chorea have rheumatic heart disease. The peak incidence is between 7 and 12 years of age. There tends to be a female preponderance.

Children usually present with irritability or mood changes, developing restlessness and chorea over subsequent weeks to months. The neurologic exam may demonstrate chorea (random, purposeless, nonrhythmic jerking movements), athetosis (slow writhing movements of the upper extremities), hypotonia, and difficulty with grip ("milkmaid" hands). Motor impersistence may be seen with ocular fixation or tongue protrusion. The deep tendon reflexes can be pendular. Recent evidence suggests that Sydenham chorea may also be associated with other neuropsychiatric abnormalities such as obsessive-compulsive disorder (OCD) and attention deficit disorder (ADD).

The mechanism that causes chorea to develop after a streptococcal infection is poorly understood. However, patients with rheumatic chorea have been found to have antibasal ganglia antibodies to the caudate and subthalamic nuclei. This is thought to be caused by an abnormal immune response with antibodies cross-reacting with both streptococcal and basal ganglia proteins.

Sydenham chorea often spontaneously remits after 8 to 9 months. However, many patients may continue to have chorea for many years and as many as 20% of patients may have a recurrence several months after their initial episode.

Summary The patient is a previously healthy 9-year-old girl who presents with the subacute onset of restlessness, labile mood, upper extremity choreoathetosis, hypotonia, and difficulty maintaining grip strength.

Localization The labile mood and irritability are suggestive of a generalized encephalopathy that diffusely localizes to the cortex. Chorea most commonly localizes to the striatum but can also be caused by lesions of the subthalamic nucleus and ventral thalamic nucleus. Hypotonia is a nonspecific finding but is likely cerebral in origin, given this child's history and physical examination. Difficulty maintaining grip strength is probably a result of motor impersistence rather than weakness and is hard to specifically localize.

Differential Diagnosis Sydenham chorea is the most likely diagnosis in this case. It is the most common chorea of childhood. The patient also has a very typical presentation with the onset of mood changes followed by the development of a movement disorder. In addition, the diagnosis is supported by the fact that the patient is from an underdeveloped country and is at risk for rheumatic fever because she may not have received appropriate antibiotics for a streptococcal pharyngitis. There is also no family history of neurologic disease.

The differential diagnosis of the insidious onset of chorea in childhood is broad (Table 12.1). It includes hereditary disorders such as Huntington disease,

TABLE 12.1

Differential Diagnosis of Chorea in Childhood

Genetic/Metabolic Diseases
  Huntington disease
  Benign hereditary chorea
  Wilson disease
  Neuronal ceroid lipofuscinosis
  Fahr disease
  Gangliosidosis
  Glutaric aciduria
  Lesch-Nyhan disease
  Mitochondrial disorders
  Neuroacanthocytosis
  Pantothenate kinase-associated neurodegeneration
  Phenylketonuria
  Ataxia-telangiectasia

Paroxysmal Chorea
  Familial paroxysmal choreoathetosis
  Paroxysmal kinesigenic dyskinesia
  Paroxysmal nonkinesigenic dyskinesia

Structural Abnormalities
  Arterial venous malformation
  Trauma
  Tumor

Ischemia
  Cerebrovascular disease
  Hypoxia (postpump chorea)

Infection
  Bacterial Infection
    Group A beta-hemolytic streptococcal infection (Sydenham chorea)
    Lyme disease
    Tuberculosis
  Viral Infection/Encephalitis
    Epstein-Barr infection
    HIV
    Varicella

Autoimmune Disorders
  Anticardiolipin syndrome
  Behçet disease
  Systemic lupus erythematosus
  Sarcoidosis

(Continued)

TABLE 12.1

Differential Diagnosis of Chorea in Childhood (*continued*)

Medications
  Oral contraceptive pills
  Anticonvulsants
  Neuroleptic medications
  Levodopa
  Dopamine agonists
  Lithium
  Methylphenidate

Toxins
  Carbon monoxide
  Toluene
  Manganese

Endocrine/Metabolic
  Pregnancy (chorea gravidarum)
  Hyperthyroidism
  Addison's disease
  Hyper/hypoglycemia
  Hyper/hyponatremia
  Hypocalcemia
  Hypomagnesemia
  Hyper/hypoparathyroidism

Kernicterus

---

neuroacanthocytosis, benign hereditary chorea, ataxia-telangiectasia, and Wilson disease. Chorea may be seen with inborn errors of metabolism, such as glutaric aciduria, abetalipoproteinemia, Fahr disease, pantothenate kinase-associated neurodegeneration (Hallervorden-Spatz disease), phenylketonuria, mitochondrial disorders, and Lesch-Nyhan syndrome, in addition to many others. The paroxysmal choreas may also be a cause. Structural abnormalities of the basal ganglia caused by stroke, trauma, or tumor are important to consider.

Multiple bacterial and viral infections are associated with chorea in children, such as rheumatic fever, Lyme disease, herpes simplex virus encephalitis, HIV, and varicella. Vasculitis caused by sarcoidosis, systemic lupus erythematosus, and other autoimmune disorders must be considered. Medication (oral contraceptives, methylphenidate, anticonvulsants, antiemetics, levodopa, and dopa agonists) side effects are also in the differential diagnosis. Toxins such as carbon monoxide and manganese reportedly have caused chorea. Endocrine and metabolic abnormalities, such as hyperthyroidism, pregnancy (chorea gravidarum), hyper-/hypoparathyroidism, hypocalcemia, hypomagnesemia, hyper-/hypoglycemia, and hyper-/hyponatremia, also are associated with chorea.

Evaluation   A throat culture is typically done to verify an exposure to group A beta-hemolytic streptococci but is negative in the majority of patients with suspected Sydenham chorea. Antistreptolysin-O antibodies (ASO titers) are routinely obtained, but may not be significantly elevated except in an acute infection. Anti-DNAase B and antinicotinamide adenine dinucleotidase (anti-NADase) titers are of greater diagnostic value because they often stay elevated for a longer period of time. A brain MRI with and without gadolinium should be performed to rule out alternative diagnoses such as structural abnormalities, infectious etiologies, or metabolic disease. Neuroimaging is usually normal in Sydenham chorea but the caudate and putamen have been reported to be enlarged and hyperintense on T_2-weighted MRI in some cases.

Any patient with suspected Sydenham chorea should also undergo a thorough cardiac evaluation to rule out carditis. Cardiac auscultation must be performed to evaluate for a murmur. Referral to a cardiologist for an ECHO and ECG is appropriate. Input from an infectious disease specialist can also be helpful in confirming a diagnosis of rheumatic fever.

A work-up for an alternative diagnosis is required if there is a family history of chorea or if the initial work-up demonstrates no prior exposure to streptococcal infection. A lumbar puncture is often performed to exclude central nervous system infections or inflammation. Screening testing to rule out other conditions may be done by obtaining basic chemistries, liver function tests, CBC, erythrocyte sedimentation rate, calcium, magnesium, phosphorus, urine toxin screen, urine heavy metal screen, thyroid function tests, ANA, anticardiolipin antibody, HIV, and a urine pregnancy test in menstruating, sexually active females. Initial testing for an underlying metabolic or genetic disease might include plasma amino acids, urine organic acids, lactate/pyruvate, copper, ceruloplasmin, alpha-fetoprotein, and lysosomal enzymes. A formal ophthalmologic examination can be helpful in evaluating for Kayser-Fleischer rings associated with Wilson disease, as well as for optic nerve or retinal abnormalities that might suggest a metabolic disorder.

Management   When rheumatic fever is diagnosed, streptococcal pharyngitis must be eradicated. Penicillin is the antibiotic of choice. It may be given orally for 10 days or intramuscularly as a single dose. Secondary prevention of recurrent rheumatic fever is also necessary and requires long-term prophylactic treatment with oral penicillin, intramuscular penicillin, or oral sulfadiazine. When present, carditis and arthritis also must be treated accordingly.

Multiple medications have been used to control the chorea. Diazepam in nonsedating doses may be helpful. Valproic acid is frequently used as a first-line therapy because it has been shown to be effective and well-tolerated. Dopamine receptor blocking agents such as haloperidol and pimozide are typically a second-line therapy as they carry a risk of more serious side effects, such as extrapyramidal symptoms. More recently, oral prednisone and intravenous methylprednisolone have been tried with some success based on the rationale that Sydenham chorea is an immune-mediated process.

Management of the emotional and behavioral changes associated with Sydenham chorea is often challenging. Like chorea, these problems may linger for years. The patient's school must be informed. Often educational modifications need to be made to accommodate for the patient's emotional condition. Input from psychiatry can also be useful in these cases.

Additional Questions

1. What is pediatric autoimmune neuropsychiatric disorders associated with streptococcal infection (PANDAS)?

2. What are the clinical manifestations of Wilson disease?

3. What disorders are associated with basal ganglia calcification?

References

Barash J, Margalith D, Matitiau A. Corticosteroid treatment in patients with Sydenham's chorea. *Pediatr Neurol.* 2005;32:205–207.

Cardoso F. Chorea: nongenetic causes. *Curr Opin Neurol.* 2004;17:433–436.

Church AJ, Cardoso F, Dale RC, et al. Anti-basal ganglia antibodies in acute and persistent Sydenham's chorea. *Neurology.* 2002;59:227–231.

Dajani A, Taubert K, Ferrieri P, et al. Treatment of acute streptococcal pharyngitis and prevention of rheumatic fever: a statement for health professionals. Committee on Rheumatic Fever, Endocarditis, and Kawasaki Disease of the Council on Cardiovascular Disease in the Young, the American Heart Association. *Pediatrics.* 1995;96:758–764.

Daoud AS, Zaki M, Shakir R, et al. Effectiveness of sodium valproate in the treatment of Sydenham's chorea. *Neurology.* 1990;40:1140–1141.

Fernandez-Alvarez E, Aicardi J. *Movement Disorders in Children.* London, UK: Mac Keith Press; 2001:63–78.

Ikuta N, Hirata M, Sasabe F, et al. High-signal basal ganglia on T_1-weighted images in a patient with Sydenham's chorea. *Neuroradiology.* 1998;40(10):659–661.

Swedo SE, Leonard HL, Garvey M, et al. Pediatric autoimmune neuropsychiatric disorders associated with streptococcal infections: clinical description of the first 50 cases. *Am J Psychiatry.* 1998;155(2):264–271.

A healthy 2-year-old boy was brought to the emergency room after experiencing a new-onset seizure. The parents report that the child has had a decreased appetite with slight irritability for the last 12 hours. While taking a nap, he experienced the sudden onset of rhythmic jerking of the upper and lower extremities with his eyes rolling back into his head for approximately 1 minute. This prompted his parents to bring him to the emergency room where he experienced a second event. On review of developmental milestones, he walks and runs well, speaks in short phrases, and identifies body parts. An older sister experienced a similar seizure at 18 months of age.

Physical Examination Vital Signs: Temperature, 103°F. Mild tachypnea. General Examination: No dysmorphic facial features. No nuchal rigidity. Neurologic Examination: Mental Status: Sleepy but arousable. Cranial Nerves: His pupils are equal, round, and reactive to light. He tracks objects in all directions when awake. His face is symmetric. The tongue is midline. Motor: He has normal bulk and tone. He moves all four extremities against gravity. Coordination: He grabs objects without dysmetria. Gait: He has a normal toddler gait without ataxia. Reflexes: 2+ throughout with bilateral plantar flexor responses.

Guide to Case Discussion

  ▦ Briefly summarize this case.

  ▦ Localize the examination findings.

  ▦ Give the most likely diagnosis and provide a differential diagnosis.

  ▦ Discuss an appropriate diagnostic work-up.

  ▦ Discuss the management of this patient.

Diagnosis Complex febrile seizures.

Discussion Febrile seizures are very common, occurring in approximately 5% of children ages 6 months to 5 years. The peak incidence occurs at 18 months. Approximately 60% to 70% of febrile seizures are simple, whereas 30% to 40% are complex. By definition, simple febrile seizures are primary generalized seizures that last less than 15 minutes and do not recur within a 24-hour period. Complex febrile seizures are focal, last more than 15 minutes, or occur more than once within a 24-hour period. Febrile status epilepticus may also occur. There is a strong genetic predisposition for febrile seizures and 25% to 40% of children presenting with febrile seizures have a family history of febrile seizures.

Children younger than 12 months of age at the time of their first febrile seizure have a 50% chance of having more febrile seizures. Children older than 1 year of age who present with a first febrile seizure have a slightly lower risk (30%) of having additional febrile seizures. A family history of febrile seizures, low fever at the time of the seizure, and a short duration of illness prior to the seizure also predict a higher risk of febrile seizure recurrence.

The outcome for children with febrile seizures is excellent. It is generally agreed that febrile seizures are benign. They do not cause long-term neurologic deficits or intellectual deterioration. The risk of subsequent epilepsy after a febrile seizure is approximately 2% to 5%. Factors known to increase the risk of developing unprovoked seizures later in life include a family history of epilepsy, complex febrile seizures, and the presence of neurodevelopmental abnormalities.

Summary The patient is a healthy, developmentally normal 2-year-old boy who presents with two generalized seizures that have been provoked by a fever (complex febrile seizures). Although he is sleepy, his neurologic examination is normal. The family history is significant for febrile seizures.

Localization The patient experienced generalized seizures that localize to the cortex of both cerebral hemispheres. Although there are no localizing features on the neurologic examination, tachypnea suggests an underlying pneumonia, which could be the cause of the fever.

Differential Diagnosis Alternative diagnoses must be considered in any child presenting with a febrile seizure. First, children who are predisposed to having seizures or who have an underlying epilepsy may seize because the fever lowered their seizure threshold. Also, an underlying meningitis or encephalitis should be considered. In children with fever, focal seizures and/or focal neurologic deficits, HSV encephalitis should be recognized as a potentially treatable infection that must be ruled out.

Evaluation In the emergency room, an evaluation should be performed to identify the source of fever in any child who experiences a febrile seizure. A thorough history and physical examination should be done initially. A family history of febrile seizures or epilepsy should be noted.

The American Academy of Pediatrics has published guidelines for the evaluation of a first simple febrile seizure. Laboratory studies such as a CBC, serum electrolytes, calcium, magnesium, phosphorus, and glucose are not routinely recommended unless clinically indicated. Thus, any labs performed should be more directed at identifying a source of the fever, rather than the source of the seizure. For example, a CBC and/or blood culture may be useful in identifying bacteremia in a child younger than 2 years of age. In this case, the patient presents with tachypnea so a chest radiograph is indicated. Any child with nuchal rigidity, photophobia, mental status changes, lethargy, irritability, or a bulging fontanelle should promptly undergo a lumbar puncture to rule out meningitis and/or encephalitis. In addition, a lumbar puncture should be strongly considered in any child younger than 12 months of age with a febrile seizure because clinical signs of meningitis may be subtle in this age group. For the 12- to 18-month age group, similar recommendations apply. Thought must also be given to the possibility of a partially treated meningitis in a patient who has recently received antibiotics for another infection. Evidence-based medicine has not shown any benefit to performing either an EEG or neuroimaging after a first simple febrile seizure and these diagnostic tests are not routinely recommended for these patients.

Guidelines are less clear for children who present with complex febrile seizures, as in this case. Clinical judgement should be used in determining the work-up but a more aggressive evaluation is often pursued. Again, the possibility of HSV encephalitis must be considered in any child presenting with fever, focal seizures, and/or a focal neurologic deficit. Ruling this out necessitates a lumbar puncture with PCR testing for HSV. Neuroimaging may also be more strongly considered for a child with focal seizures, a focal neurologic examination, micro-/macrocephaly, a pre-existing neurologic deficit, developmental delay, a neurocutaneous syndrome, or suspected inborn error of metabolism, and when there is a question as to whether a seizure was truly febrile. According to evidence-based medicine, EEGs performed after complex febrile seizures do not help predict recurrent febrile seizures or the later development of epilepsy and are not routinely recommended.

Management Management begins with appropriate treatment for any infection identified in the initial work-up. Parents must also be educated with regards to febrile seizures, as well as general seizure management. Parental anxiety is often high in children with new-onset seizures (febrile or afebrile) and appropriate counseling might prevent unnecessary emergency room visits and diagnostic tests.

Although both phenobarbital and valproic acid are effective in preventing febrile seizure recurrences, placing children with febrile seizures (simple or complex) on long-term anticonvulsants is not routinely recommended because the risks of prophylactic treatment do not outweigh the benefits. Antipyretics are often recommended at the onset of illness, but it is important to recognize that there is no evidence to suggest that antipyretics prevent recurrent febrile seizures.

In clinical practice, rectal diazepam gel is often prescribed as abortive therapy for children with prolonged or recurrent febrile seizures. It can limit the duration of seizures and provide parents with a sense of control. It is absorbed rapidly and can easily be given by caregivers at home. Although diazepam can cause somnolence, ataxia, and respiratory depression, overall it is a safe and effective medication. Dosing is based on a patient's age and weight. Oral benzodiazepines (lorazepam, diazepam) and midazolam (buccal, intranasal) have been given as alternative abortive treatments in the acute management of febrile and afebrile seizures, but in most cases, the current availability and convenience of rectal diazepam suppositories in pediatric dosing units has made the use of other forms of benzodiazepines unnecessary.

Additional Questions

1. What is generalized epilepsy with febrile seizures plus (GEFS+)?
2. Which genes are involved in GEFS+? What is the function of these genes?
3. What is the suspected relationship between febrile seizures and mesial temporal sclerosis?
4. What are the general seizure management instructions that should be discussed with the parents of a child presenting with a new-onset seizure?

References

Camfield P, Camfield C, Kurlemann G. Febrile seizures. In: Roger J, Bureau M, Dravet C, et al., eds. *Epileptic Syndromes in Infancy, Childhood and Adolescence*. 3rd ed. Eastleigh, UK: John Libbey; 2002:145–152.

Committee on Quality Improvement, Subcommittee on Febrile Seizures. Practice parameter: long-term treatment of the child with simple febrile seizures. *Pediatrics*. 1999;103(6): 1307–1309.

Duchowny M. Febrile seizures. In: Wyllie E, ed. *The Treatment of Epilepsy: Principles and Practice*. 3rd ed. Philadelphia, Pa: Lippincott Williams & Wilkins; 2001:601–608.

Knudsen FU. Febrile seizures: treatment and prognosis. *Epilepsia*. 2000;41(1):2–9.

Provisional Committee on Quality Improvement, Subcommittee on Febrile Seizures. Practice parameter: the neurodiagnostic evaluation of the child with a first simple febrile seizure. *Pediatrics*. 1996;97(5):769–772.

Waruiru C, Appleton R. Febrile seizures: an update. *Arch Dis Child*. 2004;89:751–756.

You are contacted by the emergency room to see **an 18-month-old girl** brought in by her mother for evaluation of an abnormal gait after a minor fall with impact to the head. There was no loss of consciousness. Immediately after the fall the child appeared normal. However, over the ensuing days her mother noticed a limp and brought her to the emergency room when this did not improve. In addition, over the past weeks she has seen her pediatrician three times for recurrent emesis, which occurs shortly after eating. It is nonbilious in nature and does not appear associated with nausea. The pediatrician has diagnosed gastroesophageal reflux. The child has suffered a 3-pound weight loss with the emesis. Several weeks ago she had an upper respiratory infection associated with stridor and she still has somewhat stridulous respiration in sleep.

The child was born full term after an uneventful pregnancy. She had normal early milestones. At 1 year of age, she began walking well independently, but after a minor fall, she refused to walk and she crawled exclusively again for 1 month. Afterwards she resumed walking. The patient used independent words at age 1 year and has continued to acquire new words, but is still very difficult to understand. Her family history is unremarkable. There is no consanguinity.

Physical Examination Vital Signs: Normal. General Examination: Head circumference is 95%. Neurologic Examination: Mental Status: Alert. Language: Normal naming and comprehension for age but apparent dysarthria. Cranial Nerves: Her pupils are equal, round, and reactive to light. Her extraocular muscles are intact. Funduscopic examination reveals normal optic nerves. There is decreased facial movement. Her gag is present but decreased. The tongue is midline. Motor: She has normal bulk. Diffuse appendicular hypertonicity is noted with axial hypotonia. Formal muscle strength testing is limited by the patient's developmental age but there is decreased movement and strength for spontaneous tasks in the proximal lower and upper extremities with some asymmetry in the lower extremities with only antigravitational proximal strength on the right lower extremity. Coordination: She has dysmetria more on the right than the left. Sensory: No deficits are noted. Gait: Wide-based for age with circumduction in the right lower extremity. Reflexes: 3+ throughout with bilateral crossed adductor responses. Bilateral plantar extensor responses are appreciated.

Guide to Case Discussion

- Briefly summarize this case.

- Localize the examination findings.

- Give the most likely diagnosis and provide a differential diagnosis.

- Discuss an appropriate diagnostic work-up.

- Discuss the management of this patient.

Diagnosis Alexander disease.

Discussion Alexander disease is a rare leukodystrophy caused by a mutation in the glial fibrillary acidic protein (*GFAP*) gene on chromosome 17. Alexander disease follows an autosomal dominant inheritance pattern but is usually caused by a de novo sporadic mutation. It is characterized by extensive white matter abnormalities that primarily affect the frontal lobes.

Three primary clinical syndromes have been identified. The infantile form is most common and presents before the age of 2 years with megalencephaly with frontal bossing, bulbar dysfunction, seizures, spasticity, and motor delays with developmental regression. Hydrocephalus with aqueductal stenosis is seen in some patients. It is typically rapidly progressive, with death by the age of 10 years. The juvenile form occurs between 2 and 12 years. Bulbar symptoms with dysarthria and swallowing abnormalities are typically seen in addition to ataxia. Vomiting, megalencephaly, seizures, lower-extremity spasticity, and cognitive decline may also occur. Individuals with the juvenile form may live into their 40s. The adult form presents during adolescence or early adulthood with a variety of neurologic symptoms that can mimic multiple sclerosis. Palatal myoclonus may be present. Neuroimaging with infantile onset demonstrates primarily frontal white matter signal abnormalities with rostrocaudal progression, whereas later-onset disease tends to affect the brainstem and cerebellum more.

Rosenthal fibers are the pathologic marker of Alexander disease. Although they may occur in other disorders (pilocytic astrocytomas, multiple sclerosis plaques), they are abundant in the perivascular, subpial, and subependymal astrocytes in Alexander disease. Rosenthal fibers represent protein aggregates of GFAP, the main intermediate filament within astrocytes. The pathogenesis is suspected to be caused by the toxic effect of accumulated intermediate protein. Prior to the clinical availability of molecular genetic testing for causative mutations in the *GFAP* gene, the diagnosis was confirmed with these histologic findings.

Summary The patient is an 18-month-old girl with recurrent neurologic regression after minor falls, refractory emesis, and stridor. Her neurologic exam is notable for large head size, bulbar dysfunction, truncal hypotonia with extremity spasticity, asymmetric weakness (right worse than left), dysmetria (right worse than left), brisk reflexes with bilateral plantar extensor responses, and wide-based gait with right leg circumduction.

Localization The association of facial weakness, decreased gag, stridor, and the history of recurrent emesis suggest bulbar dysfunction and brainstem involvement.

The truncal hypotonia associated with appendicular spasticity suggests a disorder located in the central nervous system. Much like in children with cerebral palsy as a consequence of periventricular white matter injury, truncal hypotonia with appendicular spasticity suggests injury to the deep white matter in this child. The proximal weakness can be seen in central nervous system disorders. That she has extremity spasticity and brisk reflexes makes peripheral nervous system disorders unlikely. Her weakness is more prominent on the right than the left, suggesting an asymmetric process that is worse in the left hemisphere. Dysmetria and gait ataxia are a result of involvement of the cerebellar pathways. Brisk deep tendon reflexes and bilateral plantar extensor responses again denote a central process with involvement of the corticospinal tracts. Thus, the disorder affecting this child has caused diffuse abnormalities, presumably affecting the central white matter and brainstem.

Differential Diagnosis   The recurrent neurologic regression and diffuse involvement of the central nervous system in this child suggest a heritable disorder. However, although unlikely, structural lesions, such as primary central nervous system tumors of the posterior fossa, and inflammatory disorders of the brain, such as infection, a postinfectious process, or vasculitis, should be considered. Hydrocephalus may also enter the differential diagnosis given the history of frequent vomiting.

Heritable disorders that affect the central white matter and the brainstem include leukodystrophies such as Alexander disease, for which the history of refractory emesis, slow decline, and episodes of regression, as well as the physical exam findings are typical. Other leukodystrophies are less likely to cause prominent brainstem findings, but the differential can include Canavan disease, metachromatic leukodystrophy, adrenoleukodystrophy (in males), childhood ataxia with central nervous system hypomyelination (vanishing white matter disease), and megalencephalic leukoencephalopathy with subcortical cysts (MLC). Canavan disease and MLC in particular may be associated with megalencephaly. White matter injury with brainstem involvement can also be caused by inborn errors of metabolism, most predominantly mitochondrial disorders.

Evaluation   The child in this case should be admitted to the hospital for a thorough diagnostic work-up. Screening lab testing including basic chemistries, liver function tests, and a CBC should be done. An imaging study should immediately be performed to evaluate for the etiology of her neurologic exam abnormalities and progressive decline. Although a head CT might be useful to rule out diagnoses such as a posterior fossa mass or acute ischemic change, a brain MRI (with and without gadolinium) is necessary to evaluate the white matter and brainstem, helping to narrow the differential diagnosis. Magnetic resonance spectroscopy and diffusion tensor imaging may also be useful in evaluating leukodystrophies.

In Alexander disease, the brain MRI characteristically reveals (a) diffuse bilaterally, symmetric white matter signal abnormalities with a frontal predominance; (b) a periventricular rim of low signal intensity on T_2-weighted images and high signal intensity on T_1-weighted images; (c) signal abnormalities, swelling, or atrophy involving the basal ganglia and thalami; (d) brainstem signal abnormalities; and (e) contrast enhancement involving the frontal white matter, basal ganglia, thalami, and/or brainstem, among other structures. In contrast, adrenoleukodystrophy primarily affects the parietal and occipital lobes, progressing anteriorly. Metachromatic leukodystrophy, Krabbe disease, and Canavan disease have more diffuse white matter involvement.

Specific molecular genetic testing for Alexander disease is now clinically available. For a patient presenting with classic clinical and brain MRI findings, a focused work-up for a mutation in the *GFAP* gene may first be performed. If other leukodystrophies and/or inborn errors of metabolism are considered, a broadened screening work-up might include chromosomal analysis, thyroid function studies, vitamin B_{12} level, biotinidase, serum lactate/pyruvate, very-long-chain fatty acids, lysosomal enzymes, plasma amino acids, and urine organic acids.

Management   Alexander disease is a neurodegenerative, heritable disorder for which there is no current treatment. Management is based on preventing and treating complications, but the disorder is uniformly fatal. The complications that can be seen in Alexander disease are consistent with the parts of the central nervous system affected by the disorder and the mechanism of disease. Patients with Alexander disease suffer from progressive bulbar dysfunction. Recurrent emesis is a disabling and frequent symptom that responds only partially to antiemetics. Swallowing dysfunction often requires the need for gastrostomy tube support. Respiratory complications, including the stridor seen in this patient, sleep apnea, and respiratory failure are frequently seen. Thus, input from a gastroenterologist, nutritionist, and pulmonologist is eventually necessary.

Scoliosis has been known to be the sole physical exam finding in some patients and is present in many more severely involved patients. Referral to an orthopaedic surgeon is appropriate as scoliosis develops and progresses. Rosenthal fibers can accumulate within CSF spaces and result in hydrocephalus. Shunting may be required so neurosurgeons may become involved in a patient's care. Seizures are seen frequently in Alexander disease patients, especially in infantile presentations but are usually easily controlled with anticonvulsants.

Finally, genetic counseling is an important part of the approach to such patients. Prenatal testing is available. In cases of adult-onset Alexander disease, familial cases have been reported. Because there is little available information about genotype–phenotype correlations, prognosis cannot be made based on which mutation is seen in the *GFAP* gene.

Additional Questions

1. What are the clinical features of Canavan disease, adrenoleukodystrophy, metachromatic leukodystrophy, childhood ataxia with central nervous system hypomyelination (vanishing white matter disease), and megalencephalic leukoencephalopathy with subcortical cysts?

2. How are the above-mentioned leukodystrophies diagnosed?

3. What is the difference between megalencephaly and macrocephaly?

4. What other acquired, genetic, and metabolic disorders cause macrocephaly?

References

Brenner M, Johnson AB, Boespflug-Tanguy O, et al. Mutations in GFAP, encoding glial fibrillary acidic protein, are associated with Alexander disease. *Nat Genet.* 2001;27(1):117–120.

Gorospe JR. Alexander disease. 2004 (cited December 4, 2005). Available at: http://www.genetests.org. Last accessed January 16, 2006.

Li R, Johnson AB, Salomons G, et al. Glial fibrillary acidic protein mutations in infantile, juvenile and adult forms of Alexander disease. *Ann Neurol.* 2005;57(3):310–326.

Noetzel MJ. Diagnosing "undiagnosed" leukodystrophies: the role of molecular genetics. *Neurology.* 2004;62(6):847–848.

Schiffmann R, Boespflug-Tanguy O. An update on the leukodystrophies. *Curr Opin Neurol.* 2001;14(6):789–794.

Van der Knaap MS, Naidu S, Breiter SN, et al. Alexander disease: diagnosis with MR imaging. *AJNR Am J Neuroradiol.* 2001;22(3):541–552.

Van der Knaap MS, Salomons GS, Li R, et al. Unusual variants of Alexander's disease. *Ann Neurol.* 2005;57(3):327–338.

A **2-month-old girl** was referred to the emergency room for complaints of lethargy and floppiness. Her mother reports a very weak cry for 1 day. The child has been breast-feeding poorly for 2 days and has had very little oral intake today. There has been no fever, irritability, vomiting, diarrhea, or cough. She was previously healthy other than constipation for a week, which has not resolved with attempts to give added water by mouth. She was previously smiling, visually attentive, and starting to hold up her head.

Physical Examination Vital Signs: Afebrile. Mild tachycardia, breathing quietly. General Examination: She appears slightly dehydrated. There are no dysmorphic facial features. Neurologic Examination: Mental Status: The child appears drowsy but can easily be aroused. Cranial Nerves: Her pupils are equal, round, and reactive to light, but on prolonged observation, the pupils initially constrict then slowly dilate with light maintained on macula. She is initially visually attentive when aroused and tracks a face in all directions but fatigues quickly, appearing to become drowsy and visually inattentive. Her face has minimal movement on stimulation and she lacks tight eye closure. Immediately on arousal, her lids are symmetric and open, but ptosis develops after a brief period of observation. She has a poor suck and her gag is weak. The tongue is midline without fasciculations. Motor: There is normal bulk with moderate hypotonia that is most notable in the neck musculature. She has no head control on either pull-to-sit or on ventral suspension. The tone is slightly better in the legs, which flex in ventral suspension. She has symmetric but weak proximal limb movements barely against gravity and she appears stronger at the hips than at the shoulder girdle. Her toes and fingers move normally. Sensory: There is withdrawal and grimace to pain. Reflexes: 1+ throughout with bilateral plantar flexor responses.

Guide to Case Discussion

- Briefly summarize this case.

- Localize the examination findings.

- Give the most likely diagnosis and provide a differential diagnosis.

- Discuss an appropriate diagnostic work-up.

- Discuss the management of this patient.

Diagnosis Infantile botulism.

Discussion Infantile botulism typically occurs between birth and 1 year of age. It is caused by neurotoxins produced by *Clostridium botulinum*, an anaerobic, spore-forming rod. While various strains of *C. botulinum* produce different toxins (labeled A to G), the majority of cases of infantile botulism are caused by types A (more prevalent in the western United States) and B (relatively more prevalent in the eastern United States). Botulinum toxins produce symptoms by blocking the presynaptic release of acetylcholine at the neuromuscular junction. In toxin types A and B, this is thought to be irreversible, with recovery occurring with new axon sprouting and the formation on new motor endplates.

Immaturity and diet are age-dependent determinants of gut flora that make infants particularly susceptible to gut colonization with *C. botulinum*. The introduction of new foods into the diet and weaning from breast-feeding are implicated, but not proven, factors. Botulism spores are commonly found in samples of dust and soil but are present in multiple geographic areas where cases of infantile botulism are rare. There is a weak association of infantile botulism with residence in suburban areas where construction is ongoing. *C. botulinum* spores are common in honey and corn syrup samples, but in the United States, the incidence of botulism as a result of ingestion of these sweeteners has declined because of public awareness campaigns.

Clinically, infantile botulism often presents with constipation due to the neurotoxin's effects on gastrointestinal motility. Poor suck, weak cry, or decreased spontaneous motor movements may also occur early on. The infant is often thought to be lethargic as a result of a combination of ptosis, facial weakness, poor suck, and fatigue of extraocular movements causing poor visual tracking. As the disease progresses over hours to days, patients develop hypotonia and descending flaccid paralysis. Notably, after involvement of cranial nerve–innervated muscles, the shoulder girdle and neck are involved prior to lower extremities and hip girdle musculature involvement. In mild cases, leg movement may be nearly normal while shoulder girdle and neck muscles are very weak and hypotonic. Distal movement tends to be preserved. Ultimately, respiratory failure can occur. Because the weakness is variable, the infant does not appear to be in respiratory distress, even as respiratory failure occurs and carbon dioxide pressure (PCO_2) begins to rise. At this stage, the infant may be quite lethargic, but the apparent "central" effect is readily reversed once adequate respiratory support is provided.

Cranial neuropathies are nearly universal. The pupils may be dilated or sluggishly reactive, but fatigable pupils are a more specific finding. There is good initial constriction followed by gradual dilation even when light stimulus is maintained over the macula. Notably, testing for fatigable pupils requires that the lids be held open for a prolonged period, a task that is nearly impossible in an infant without facial weakness. Facial weakness is manifested by poor eye closure, poor mouth closure around a nipple, and poor movement with cry. Ptosis is common. The gag may be weak or absent, and with further progression, extraocular muscles become weak. The deep tendon reflexes may be normal or decreased. General fatigability is notable in that the exam may change from moment to moment. The infant examined on arousal from a nap may look relatively stronger, whereas the same infant kept awake for several minutes may become weaker with more evident findings.

Summary The patient is a 2-month-old, previously healthy, developmentally normal girl who presents with the subacute development of lethargy, floppiness, weak cry, poor feeding, and constipation in absence of other signs of illness. Her exam is remarkable for tachycardia, mild dehydration, fatigable pupils, intermittent ptosis, bulbar weakness (poor suck, facial weakness, weak gag), hypotonia (that is worse in the neck and shoulder girdle muscles), and proximal weakness (that is more prominent in the neck and shoulder girdle than the hip girdle muscles). Her weakness also appears to fluctuate during the examination.

Localization Localization in a hypotonic infant begins with consideration of central versus peripheral causes. The findings of hypotonia, bulbar, proximal weakness, and fatigability are highly suggestive of involvement of the peripheral nervous system. The next step is to determine what level of the motor unit is affected—the anterior horn cell, neuromuscular junction (NMJ), peripheral nerve, or muscle.

Given the constellation and progression of symptoms in this infant, a disorder of the NMJ seems most likely. Hypotonia, weakness, and hyporeflexia are not specific for a particular disorder. However, given the fatigability and autonomic abnormalities, this case is most easily explained by a disorder of the NMJ such as infantile botulism. Fatigable pupils localize to the muscles of pupillary constriction innervated by the third cranial nerve. Constipation can also be explained by the anticholinergic effects of botulism toxin on the parasympathetic nerves of the gastrointestinal tract (which are responsible for secretion and motility). At the NMJ, botulism toxin prevents the presynaptic release of acetylcholine.

The patient does not have cortical abnormalities such as encephalopathy, dysmorphic features, or seizures that would point to a central cause. Anterior horn cell disorders typically cause proximal weakness. Tongue fasciculations are also commonly seen. Bulbar involvement as seen in this infant is unusual for a peripheral nerve disorder, and the reflexes are depressed but present. The presence of autonomic symptoms also argues against a myopathy.

Differential Diagnosis At initial presentation, common disorders causing lethargy and hypotonia, such as sepsis, meningitis, or electrolyte abnormalities, must first be excluded. Inborn errors of metabolism can also be considered early in the broad differential diagnosis.

In the setting of a previously healthy, developmentally normal infant who presents with the subacute onset of a disorder of the NMJ, infantile botulism is the most likely diagnosis. However, other disorders of the NMJ should be considered. Congenital myasthenia gravis can present in infancy with hypotonia, bulbar, and generalized weakness, ptosis, respiratory distress, and feeding problems. Congenital myasthenia gravis is the only disorder other than infant botulism with striking fatigability of the weakness. An edrophonium test may be helpful in confirming the diagnosis in cases of suspected congenital myasthenia gravis, but is relatively contraindicated with suspected infantile botulism. Electrodiagnostic studies differentiate the two disorders but are relatively difficult to perform in young infants and are not completely specific. Congenital myasthenia gravis may be apparent at birth or shortly thereafter and is unlikely to cause relatively acute onset of progressive weakness in a previously healthy child. Organophosphate poisoning can present as acute weakness, but pupils are profoundly constricted. They are frequently used in pesticides and act as acetylcholinesterase inhibitors, causing overstimulation of the parasympathetic nervous system.

Anterior horn cell diseases such as spinal muscular atrophy (SMA) are also in the differential diagnosis but SMA typically causes proximal weakness, which is somewhat more evident in the hip girdle than in the shoulders. SMA may also cause tongue fasciculations in the denervated tongue muscle, which are relatively easy to observe. SMA does not cause autonomic findings. Poliomyelitis is unlikely in the United States because of widespread vaccination. Infantile poliomyelitis also causes a different clinical picture with recurrent diarrhea (rather than constipation), fever, aseptic meningitis, and weakness, which may be asymmetric.

Acute disorders of the peripheral nerve, such as Guillain-Barré syndrome, are rare in infancy, but can present with a similar clinical picture. However, Guillain-Barré usually causes an ascending, rather than a descending, paralysis. Similarly, tick paralysis can cause a rapid ascending paralysis and hyporeflexia, mimicking Guillain-Barré syndrome. The tick neurotoxin likely acts proximal to the NMJ in the distal nerve fibers.

Finally, muscle diseases, such as congenital myopathies, congenital muscular dystrophies, metabolic myopathies (acid maltase deficiency), and congenital myotonic dystrophy, must be considered. It would be unusual, though, for an infant with a primary muscle disorder to present acutely or subacutely after a period of normal development, making these diseases much less likely in this case.

Evaluation A work-up to rule out other treatable and/or life-threatening diagnoses may be necessary until the diagnosis of botulism is established. Screening testing for other conditions can be considered and might include routine labs (CBC, chemistries, calcium, magnesium, phosphorus, liver function tests, thyroid function tests, creatine kinase, blood culture, urinalysis, urine culture), metabolic testing (plasma amino acids, urine organic acids, lactate-pyruvate, ammonia level), and brain and/or spine neuroimaging, as well as a lumbar puncture.

In clinical cases with typical findings of infant botulism, however, it is highly desirable to avoid invasive and/or fatiguing procedures such as lumbar puncture or neuroimaging because they might abruptly precipitate clinical deterioration. A Tensilon test should *not* be performed when there is a strong suspicion of infant botulism. Monitoring of respiratory function is essential, usually with arterial or capillary blood gas determination. The lack of appearance of respiratory distress is typical as respiratory failure progresses.

Identification of botulism organisms or toxins in the stool confirms the diagnosis. However, constipation associated with this condition may make the collection of normal passed stool difficult. Saline "minienemas" are sometimes effective in collection of a sample for lab testing but more often, stool testing must wait until the infant is fed and recovers some gut motility. Stool is generally tested for toxins using a bioassay (injection into mice, along with various antitoxins to determine botulism type). Testing is expensive and generally available only in state lab facilities. It takes a minimum of 24 hours for results, so treatment is often started without available results. Serum testing for exposure to botulism is much less sensitive and not generally recommended.

Electrodiagnostic studies may support the diagnosis of infantile botulism but often produce nonspecific findings. In addition, adequate studies are difficult to perform. Nerve conduction velocities are typically normal. With repetitive stimulation at high frequency (20 Hz and 50 Hz), an incremental response may be seen (increase in the compound muscle action potential amplitude) and is consistent with a presynaptic NMJ defect. EMG typically shows brief small amplitude potentials (BSAPs), which are nonspecific. There may also be evidence of acute denervation with increased insertional activity, but these findings are not specific for botulism and may be seen in axonal neuropathies or myopathies. Single-fiber EMG may show increased jitter or blocking in cases with mild to moderate weakness.

Management Airway protection is always the first step in management of an infant or child presenting with progressive weakness and bulbar dysfunction, regardless of the cause. This infant should be placed on a cardiorespiratory monitor and pulse oximeter immediately. Admission to the intensive care unit for close observation of her respiratory status should be considered. Depending on the progression of the disease, respiratory support and intubation might be required. Until the diagnosis is clear, patients presenting with botulism are often treated for presumed sepsis. Broad-spectrum antibiotics are undesirable and may abruptly worsen the condition by lysis of large numbers of *C. botulinum* in the gut with a resultant surge in toxin exposure. In addition, aminoglycosides have neuromuscular blocking action and can exacerbate a patient's condition.

Because of bulbar dysfunction, patients generally require feedings by nasogastric tube. Gut motility generally improves with establishment of nasogastric feeding. A rare patient requires parenteral nutrition because of severe dysmotility. Autonomic dysfunction may also cause urinary retention requiring intermittent catheterization.

Treatment of infantile botulism with human botulism immune globulin (BabyBIG) is approved by the FDA and represents a significant advancement in the management of this disorder. BabyBIG is made from the pooled plasma of adults immunized with botulism toxoid and contains high titers of antibodies that neutralize type A and B toxins. The use of BabyBIG decreases the length of hospital stay, the need for mechanical ventilation, and duration of tube feedings. A single dose of 50 mg/kg should be given intravenously as soon as possible after presentation, preferably within the first 3 days of hospitalization in any infant with a classic presentation.

Additional Questions

1. What is the prognosis in infantile botulism?
2. What is the pattern of recovery of strength in infantile botulism?

References

Crawford TO. Infantile botulism. In: Jones HR, De Vivo DC, Darras BT, eds. *Neuromuscular Disorders of Infancy, Childhood, and Adolescence: A Clinician's Approach.* Philadelphia, Pa: Butterworth-Heinemann; 2003:547–554.

Fenichel GM. *Clinical Pediatric Neurology: A Signs and Symptoms Approach.* 4th ed. Philadelphia, Pa: WB Saunders; 2001:149–169.

Fox CK, Keet CA, Strober JB. Recent advances in infantile botulism. *Pediatr Neurol.* 2005;32:149–154.

Mitchell WG, Tseng-Ong L. Catastrophic presentation of infantile botulism may obscure or delay diagnosis. *Pediatrics.* 2005;116(3):e426–e438.

Thompson JA, Filloux FM, Van Orman CB, et al. Infant botulism in the age of botulism immune globulin. *Neurology.* 2005;64:2029–2032.

A 6-year-old boy presents for evaluation of incoordination and gait abnormalities. He was born at full term by normal vaginal delivery with a birth weight of 8 pounds. He has a history of mild cognitive and speech delay but met all motor milestones on time. His current symptoms started approximately 2 years ago and have been progressive. He is now having difficulty walking and falls frequently. He has been unable to participate in sports or gym class. His writing is also becoming shaky. He had multiple episodes of acute otitis media as a young child and more recently has had two hospitalizations for pneumonia. There is no family history of neurologic disease.

Physical Examination General Examination: Normal with the exception of dilated blood vessels on the sclera. Neurologic Examination: Mental Status: Alert and cooperative. Language: He speaks in full sentences with mild dysarthria. Cranial Nerves: His pupils are equal, round, and reactive to light. He has a difficult time tracking with smooth pursuits. His face is symmetric. The tongue is midline without fasciculations. Motor: He has normal bulk and tone with 5/5 strength throughout. Coordination: There is significant dysmetria on finger-to-nose testing bilaterally. Sensory: Normal light touch, temperature, vibration, and proprioception. Gait: Mild truncal ataxia is noted while sitting. He has a wide-based ataxic gait and is unable to tandem walk. Reflexes: 1+ throughout with bilateral plantar flexor responses.

Guide to Case Discussion

- Briefly summarize this case.
- Localize the examination findings.
- Give the most likely diagnosis and provide a differential diagnosis.
- Discuss an appropriate diagnostic work-up.
- Discuss the management of this patient.

Diagnosis Ataxia-telangiectasia

Discussion Ataxia-telangiectasia (AT) is a progressive ataxia of childhood with an incidence of 1 in 40,000 to 1 in 100,000 individuals. Cardinal features of AT include ataxia, telangiectasias, immunodeficiency, an increased risk of malignancies, and cellular sensitivity to ionizing radiation. AT is caused by a mutation in the *ATM* gene on chromosome 11q and has an autosomal recessive inheritance pattern. The *ATM* gene codes for a protein with serine/threonine kinase activity which is activated by oxidative stress or damage. Defective or absent ATM protein may lead to difficulty repairing breaks in DNA. It is also felt to be important in suppressing tumorigenesis in T-cell lines. However, much of the pathogenesis of this disorder is poorly understood.

Truncal ataxia and unsteady gait are the first symptoms, typically noted by 3 years of age. By 10 years of age, most children will demonstrate the full constellation of neurologic symptoms, including prominent gait, limb, and truncal ataxia in addition to intention tremor, dysarthria, and dysphagia. Most children are wheelchair-bound by the age of 12 years. Other abnormal movements, such as choreoathetosis and dystonia, are common as the disease progresses. Abnormal eye movements are also characteristic of AT and develop early. Oculomotor apraxia of voluntary gaze with limited upgaze and abnormal smooth pursuits are most common. Dorsal column involvement with impaired vibration and proprioception, as well as a primary axonal peripheral neuropathy, can also develop with time. Cognition is usually preserved.

The presence of telangiectasias or small, dilated blood vessels may significantly aid in the diagnosis. They arise between the ages of 3 and 6 years, after the onset of ataxia, making the diagnosis more challenging in the younger age group. Telangiectasias are most prominent on the sclera, earlobes, and bridge of the nose. Hypertrichosis of the forearms and gray hairs may also occur.

Immunodeficiencies occur in the majority of patients, with severe immunocompromise seen in one third of patients. Sinopulmonary infections such as sinusitis, bronchitis, and pneumonia are most common. Patients with AT are also susceptible to malignancies and approximately one third of affected individuals will develop a malignancy during their lifetime. Lymphoreticular cancers such as leukemia and lymphoma occur most frequently in children. Other malignancies such as breast, stomach, ovarian, liver, and basal cell cancers develop in older patients.

The brain MRI in AT demonstrates cerebellar and vermian atrophy. Pathologically, there is significant cerebellar degeneration with striking loss of Purkinje cells, granular cells, and vermian neurons. Afferent and efferent pathways in the medulla, pons, and spinal cord may also be affected.

Life expectancy in AT varies. Some patients may live into their 60s but many affected individuals succumb to infection, malignancy, or respiratory failure earlier in life.

Summary The patient is a 6-year-old boy with a history of mild cognitive and speech delay as well as frequent sinopulmonary infections who presents with a chronic, progressive ataxia. His neurologic exam is remarkable for abnormal smooth pursuits, dysarthria, and dysmetria in addition to truncal and gait ataxia. Telangiectasias are also present on the sclera making a diagnosis of AT highly likely.

Localization This child's symptoms of abnormal smooth pursuits, dysarthria, dysmetria, and truncal/gait ataxia are likely caused by a pan-cerebellar process.

Differential Diagnosis Disorders of ataxia in childhood have chronic, intermittent, and acute presentations. The patient in this case demonstrates a chronic and progressive disease course. The presence of telangiectasias in addition to cerebellar signs are specific for the diagnosis of AT. However, in younger children who have not developed telangiectasias, the diagnosis may be less clear and other etiologies need to be ruled out.

Acquired disorders causing a slowly progressive ataxia are more common than rare genetic diseases. For example, a slow-growing posterior fossa tumor or hydrocephalus may present with cerebellar signs. Additional symptoms such as headache, lethargy, and vomiting are usually also present and are not seen in the patient in this vignette. Demyelinating diseases such as acute disseminated encephalomyelitis and multiple sclerosis can be considered but usually present as discrete attacks of neurologic symptoms, which may include ataxia. An infectious process such as meningitis or encephalitis would be associated with fever, headache, and photophobia. Opsoclonus-myoclonus syndrome may be the heralding feature of neuroblastoma and must be considered in any young child presenting with worsening ataxia. Trauma, conversion reactions, and chronic exposure to toxins (medications, heavy metals) may also manifest with ataxia. Congenital structural abnormalities of the posterior fossa often present with ataxia but cerebellar signs are apparent very early and are not consistent with the patient in this case.

When considering inherited causes of chronic ataxia, the differential diagnosis is broad. Table 16.1 summarizes this differential but several disorders deserve discussion.

Ataxia with oculomotor apraxia (AOA) may closely resemble AT or Friedreich ataxia. AOA1 is caused by a mutation in the *APTX* gene on chromosome 9p13, whereas AOA2 maps to chromosome 9q34. Clinical features include progressive ataxia, oculomotor apraxia, and areflexia as a result of an axonal neuropathy. Onset is later than in AT, however, and patients do not have immunodeficiency or telangiectasias.

The spinocerebellar ataxias are a large, heterogeneous group of disorders with an autosomal dominant inheritance pattern. Most cases present in adulthood but cases of childhood and adolescent onset have been reported. Affected individuals display a variety of symptoms including progressive ataxia, dysarthria, extrapyramidal symptoms, ophthalmoplegia, retinal abnormalities, dorsal column dysfunction, deafness, and peripheral neuropathy. Dentatorubral-pallidoluysian atrophy (DRPLA) may also present with ataxia or other abnormal movements in childhood.

Friedreich ataxia is an autosomal recessive disorder clinically characterized by gait and limb ataxia in addition to dorsal column abnormalities, areflexia, and plantar extensor responses. Cardiomyopathy, arrhythmias, diabetes mellitus, optic atrophy, and sensorineural hearing loss also frequently occur. Onset is later than that of AT, usually around the time of puberty. A mutation in the *FRDA* gene on chromosome 9 is responsible.

Ataxia with vitamin E deficiency (AVED) is caused by mutations in the alpha-tocopherol transfer protein (*TTPA*) gene on chromosome 8q. Although clinically very similar to Friedreich ataxia, the progression of AVED is slower and peripheral neuropathy is less prominent. Cardiac abnormalities rarely occur. Serum vitamin E levels are invariably low and are diagnostic. AVED is an especially important consideration in the differential diagnosis as it is treatable with high doses of vitamin E.

In addition, a wide variety of metabolic diseases are associated with progressive ataxia and are always included in the differential diagnosis of chronic ataxia

TABLE 16.1

Differential Diagnosis of Chronic, Progressive Ataxia in Childhood

Acquired Conditions
  Brain tumors
    Posterior fossa tumor
    Supratentorial tumor
  Hydrocephalus
  Demyelinating disease
    Acute disseminated
      encephalomyelitis
    Multiple sclerosis
  Infection
    Meningitis
    Encephalitis/cerebellitis
  Opsoclonus-myoclonus syndrome
  Conversion reaction
  Trauma
  Toxins

Congenital Structural Abnormalities
  Arnold-Chiari malformation
  Joubert syndrome
  Dandy-Walker malformation
  Dysgenesis of cerebellum/vermis
  Basilar impression

Inherited Ataxias
  Friedreich ataxia
  Ataxia-telangiectasia
  Spinocerebellar ataxias (SCA 1-17)
  Dentatorubral-pallidoluysian atrophy
  Ataxia with oculomotor apraxia
    (1 and 2)
  Ataxia with vitamin E deficiency

Inborn Errors of Metabolism
  Mitochondrial disorders
    Neurogenic atrophy, ataxia,
      retinitis pigmentosa (NARP)
    Mitochondrial encephalomyopathy
      with lactic acidosis and
      stroke-like episodes (MELAS)
    Myoclonic epilepsy associated
      with ragged red fibers (MERRF)
    Leigh disease
    Kearns-Sayre syndrome
  Peroxisomal disorders
    Refsum disease
    Adrenoleukodystrophy
  Leukodystrophies
    Alexander disease
    Canavan disease
    Pelizaeus-Merzbacher disease
    Childhood ataxia with central
      hypomyelination
  Lysosomal storage diseases
    Krabbe disease
    Metachromatic leukodystrophy
    Niemann-Pick type C
  Other
    Abetalipoproteinemia
    Congenital disorders of
      glycosylation

Genetic syndromes
  Rett syndrome
  Angelman syndrome

of childhood. They may initially be difficult to clinically discern from the hereditary ataxias discussed above. Age of onset, other organ involvement, family history, developmental history, MRI/magnetic resonance (MR) spectroscopy and results of initial metabolic screening tests may help distinguish individual diseases. Briefly, mitochondrial disorders, peroxisomal disorders, leukodystrophies, and lysosomal storage diseases, among others deserve consideration. Intermittent ataxias may be caused by urea cycle defects, aminoacidurias, and mitochondrial diseases, but are not relevant to this case. Finally, genetic syndromes such as Rett and Angelman syndromes often manifest with ataxia in addition to other neurologic abnormalities.

Evaluation   Several methodologies may be used to support and to confirm the diagnosis of AT. Screening tests may be easily performed but more extensive molecular genetic testing is best done under the supervision of a geneticist.

Even if the diagnosis of AT is relatively certain, any child presenting with a chronic ataxia should undergo neuroimaging with a brain MRI to rule out other pathologies. MR spectroscopy may also be helpful in discerning metabolic disorders, such as mitochondrial disease. Next, the initial screening evaluation of a child with AT includes measurement of the serum alpha-fetoprotein (AFP) level. AFP is elevated in the majority of patients but may be falsely negative in children younger than 2 years of age. Serum carcinoembryonic antigen may also be elevated. Serum immunoglobulins are typically sent. Significant deficiencies in immunoglobulins IgE, IgA, and IgG_2 are often noted and are responsible for the susceptibility to sinopulmonary infections. In addition, a high resolution karyotype may be helpful. Translocations between chromosomes 7 and 14 frequently occur in AT.

AT cells are highly radiosensitive and this may also be used to confirm the clinical diagnosis. The in vitro colony survival assay (CSA) assesses the viability of lymphoblastoid cell lines after exposure to ionizing radiation and has been validated for the diagnosis of AT. Immunoblotting to determine the presence or absence of the ATM protein in affected cells is the most reliable means of diagnosis, with the majority of patients having no ATM protein. ATM kinase activity can also be assessed with immunoblotting and supports the diagnosis when diminished. Sequencing of the *ATM* gene is also currently available on a clinical basis.

In a child with a chronic ataxia whose diagnosis is less clear at presentation, a screening work-up should begin with a brain MRI and MR spectroscopy. Neuroimaging rules out structural abnormalities and may point to a specific category of disease. Additional testing screens for other organ involvement, as well as metabolic and genetic abnormalities, might include a basic chemistry panel, CBC, liver function tests, urine heavy metal screen, thyroid function tests, urine organic acids, plasma amino acids, lactate/pyruvate battery (mitochondrial disorders), mitochondrial DNA studies, high-resolution karyotype, vitamin E level, vitamin B_{12} level, phytanic acid (Refsum disease), cholesterol/triglycerides (abetalipoproteinemia), transferrin isoelectric focusing (congenital disorders of glycosylation), lysosomal enzymes, and very-long-chain fatty acids (peroxisomal disorders). EMG and NCS can also be useful in assessing the presence and/or extent of peripheral neuropathy. In addition, a baseline ophthalmologic examination is helpful in the evaluation of a patient with a suspected genetic or metabolic disease. Findings such as optic atrophy or retinitis pigmentosa may provide clues to a diagnosis. As the differential diagnosis narrows, more refined diagnostic tests, such as molecular genetic testing for specific disorders, becomes necessary.

Management Currently, there are no specific therapies for patients with AT. Management involves a multidisciplinary team of specialists familiar with the disorder and its complications. Management of the neurologic complications are symptomatic at this time.

Patients have many rehabilitative needs and must be followed by physical, occupational, and speech therapists. Adaptive equipment becomes necessary as mobility decreases. Special attention needs to be paid to nutritional status as eating becomes more challenging. Nasogastric and subsequent gastrostomy tube feedings are inevitable. Input from a gastroenterologist and nutritionist is typically required.

Patients with AT also need to be monitored closely for their immunodeficiency and require aggressive treatment of infections. An immunologist and pulmonologist often need to be involved. Early diagnosis is also important because of the high risk of malignancies. Monitoring by a hematologist-oncologist may also be required.

Unnecessary ionizing radiation should be avoided. Although of no proven benefit, treatment with antioxidants, such as vitamin E, alpha-lipoic acid, and folic acid, is sometimes recommended to protect against chromosomal breaks. Finally, any child presenting with AT should be evaluated by a geneticist to aid in counseling with the family.

References

Miller VS. Ataxia-telangiectasia. In: Roach ES, Miller VS, eds. *Neurocutaneous Disorders*. Cambridge: Cambridge University Press; 2004:112–116.

Nance MA. Genetic testing in inherited ataxias. *Semin Pediatr Neurol.* 2003;10(3):223–231.

Parker CC, Evans OB. Metabolic disorders causing childhood ataxia. *Semin Pediatr Neurol.* 2003;10(3):193–199.

Perlman S, Becker-Catania S, Gatti RA. Ataxia-telangiectasia: diagnosis and treatment. *Semin Pediatr Neurol.* 2003;10(3):173–182.

Rosa AL, Ashizawa T. Genetic ataxia. Neurol Clin. 2002;20:727–757.

Vedanarayanan VV. Mitochondrial disorders and ataxia. *Semin Pediatr Neurol.* 2003;10(3): 200–209.

A healthy, 3-year-old boy is brought to your office because of concerns about a language delay. The patient was born at full-term by spontaneous vaginal delivery to a 32-year-old G_3P_2 mom. The pregnancy was uncomplicated and his birth weight was 7 pounds. He crawled at 8 months and walked at 13 months. His mother became concerned when he was 2 years old because he was not yet saying any words. Now he has a vocabulary of 30 words but he does not make phrases. He also does not play very well with his older brothers; rather, he prefers to play alone. His mother reports that he enjoys lining up his toy dinosaurs and cars. However, he is very active and will run around the dining room table for minutes at a time unless she stops him.

Physical Examination General Examination: There are no dysmorphic facial features. Neurologic Examination: Mental Status: Alert but makes poor eye contract. The child is uncooperative with the examination and shows little interest in toys used to try to get his attention. Language: He appears to understand a few basic commands given by his mother and says "ball" but no other words. Cranial Nerves: His pupils are equal, round, and reactive to light. His extraocular muscles are intact. His face is symmetric and his tongue is midline. Motor: Normal bulk with a mild diffuse hypotonia. He has symmetric limb movements against gravity but formal motor testing is not possible. Coordination: No dysmetria is noted. Gait: He has a normal toddler gait. Reflexes: 2+ throughout with bilateral plantar flexor responses.

Guide to Case Discussion

- Briefly summarize this case.
- Localize the examination findings.
- Give the most likely diagnosis and provide a differential diagnosis.
- Discuss an appropriate diagnostic work-up.
- Discuss the management of this patient.

Diagnosis   Autistic spectrum disorder.

Discussion   Autistic spectrum disorder (ASD) describes a highly variable group of developmental disabilities seen in early childhood. Autism and pervasive developmental delay (PDD) are characterized by deficits in social and communication skills, as well as behavior. If symptoms are recognized early, children may be diagnosed between the ages of 2 and 3 years. ASD is believed to affect as many as 1 in 500 children. There is a strong male predominance, with a male-to-female ratio of approximately 3:1 to 4:1. Genetics also plays an important role as the sibling recurrence risk is reported to be 3% to 7%.

The diagnostic criteria for autism are defined in the *Diagnostic and Statistical Manual of Mental Disorders* (DSM-IV-TR). There must be a delay in social interaction, language as used in social communication, or imaginative play before 3 years of age. Dysfunction in other realms must also be noted. Impairments in social interaction can include difficulty with nonverbal behaviors (making eye contact, interpreting facial expressions), failure to develop age-appropriate peer relationships, lack of sharing interests (does not point out objects of interest), and lack of social reciprocity. Communication difficulties can include a delay in the development of spoken language, inability to maintain a conversation (when speech is developed), repetitive speech, and lack of make-believe play. Restricted interests involve fixation on certain toys or objects, such as cars, trucks, trains, books, and dinosaurs. Repetitive behaviors, such as hand flapping, running in circles, rocking, and spinning, are considered to be self-stimulatory motor stereotypies and occur in 37% to 95% of children with an ASD. A history of regression in language and social skills, typically between 18 and 24 months, is reported in as many as one third of children with autism. It is often difficult, however, to determine if development was truly normal before this time in many cases. ASD subtypes include Asperger syndrome, Rett syndrome, childhood disintegrative disorder (CDD), atypical autism and PDD-not otherwise specified (NOS).

Other comorbid conditions exist with ASD. Mental retardation is an associated condition and an IQ of less than 70 is seen in 70% of individuals with ASD. Also, approximately 30% of children with autism have epilepsy. All seizure types have been reported.

Summary   The patient is a healthy 3-year-old boy who presents with a speech and language delay, impaired social skills, restricted interests, and repetitive behaviors. Expressive more than receptive language skills appear to be impaired. His neurologic exam is nonfocal but he makes poor eye contact and is uninterested in his environment.

Localization   The language delay, socialization difficulties, restricted interests, and repetitive behaviors seen in ASD likely reflect a diffuse cortical process. His neurologic exam demonstrates a mild hypotonia which is a non-specific finding in children with developmental delays and is likely cortical in origin. There are no additional neurologic exam findings to suggest a disorder of the motor unit.

Differential Diagnosis   Autistic spectrum disorders are heterogeneous. Characterization of the subtype of a child's autism, however, is important in order to provide appropriate interventions. Thus, autism should be first be differentiated from other related spectrum disorders. Asperger syndrome is regarded as a form of high-functioning autism. Affected children have no speech or language impairments, although they do experience social impairments and behavioral abnormalities (restricted interests, repetitive behaviors). They also have near-normal or normal intelligence.

CDD represents approximately 5% of ASD patients. Normal development occurs until the onset of symptoms between 2 and 10 years of age. Unexplained catastrophic global regression occurs in these children with or without epilepsy. CDD differs from autism in that regression occurs later (usually between 3 and 6 years of age) and the regression is much more profound. Epileptic encephalopathies, genetic disorders, and inborn errors of metabolism may be responsible for symptoms in this population. The prognosis for CDD is much worse than for autism. PDD-NOS describes children with some, but not all, features of autism.

Autism must also be differentiated from Landau-Kleffner syndrome (LKS) as both conditions may be associated with language regression. Although the pathophysiology is poorly understood, children with LKS develop an acquired epileptic aphasia or verbal agnosia. Language regression typically occurs after 3 years of age, whereas in autism, it occurs between 18 and 24 months of age. Intelligence is preserved in LKS and affected children do not develop the social impairments or behavioral abnormalities that are seen in autism. EEGs show epileptiform activity in cortical temporoparietal language areas in addition to electrical status epilepticus during slow sleep (ESES). Most children with LKS have epilepsy that is easily controlled with anticonvulsants.

The possibility of an underlying genetic disease must also be considered. Fragile X syndrome, tuberous sclerosis complex, Rett syndrome, and duplication of chromosome 15q (Angelman and Prader-Willi syndromes) are the syndromes most highly associated with ASD. Specific genetic testing is currently clinically available for these syndromes. Each of these disorders also has characteristic clinical features that may facilitate the determination of a genetic disorder as the underlying etiology for a given child's ASD. A variety of other genetic syndromes and inborn errors of metabolism have also been associated with ASD.

Finally, although mental retardation can occur in the setting of an ASD, some children with mental retardation may be misdiagnosed as having autism because of profound impairment of speech and language skills. Psychiatric disorders such as childhood schizophrenia, mood disorders, bipolar disorder, and neglect can mimic ASD when mutism or social avoidance occur.

Evaluation Early recognition of an ASD is important. An initial evaluation of a child with a suspected ASD should begin with a thorough birth history, medical history, developmental history, and physical examination. A family history of ASD, mental retardation, epilepsy, or genetic syndromes is highly relevant.

Practice parameters for the screening and diagnosis of autism have been published. The responsibility of screening for autism and other developmental disabilities initially lies with the pediatrician and is to be done at well-child checkups. Several standardized screening tools for ASD are available. Referral for further evaluation by a developmental specialist should be done for any child who is not babbling by 12 months, not gesturing (waving, pointing) by 12 months, not using a single word by 16 months, or not making two-word phrases by 24 months. Any regression of language or social skills also demands immediate referral.

Laboratory investigations in any child with suspected autism or developmental delay should include audiology and lead screening.

A more in-depth evaluation is necessary if a child fails the pediatrician's screening evaluations and is suspected to have autism. Further work-up allows autism to be differentiated from other developmental disorders. Children with autism and mental retardation, dysmorphic features, and/or a family history of mental retardation should have a high-resolution karyotype and DNA analysis for fragile X syndrome performed. It is likely that less than 5% of children presenting with autism have an inborn error of metabolism. Consequently, routine screening for metabolic diseases is not recommended unless associated clinical or physical findings such as episodic lethargy, cyclic vomiting, coarse or dysmorphic features, early onset epilepsy, or mental retardation are present.

There is insufficient evidence to support recommending a routine EEG in every child presenting with autism. However, in children with suspected seizures or a history of developmental regression (especially toddlers and preschoolers) an EEG containing an adequate sampling of slow-wave sleep is indicated to help rule out LKS, epilepsy, and subclinical seizure activity. This may require a routine or an overnight video EEG. Neuroimaging is not indicated in the work-up of a child with suspected autism but no additional neurologic abnormalities, even when macrocephaly is present. Circumstances such as the development of focal seizures may necessitate obtaining a brain MRI to rule out structural abnormalities. In addition, there is no evidence-based support for performing alternative diagnostic testing, such as heavy metal analysis in hair, celiac antibodies, food and environmental allergy testing, vitamin levels, or immunologic studies.

Finally, the diagnosis of a child with autism should be made by a clinician familiar with this condition. Appropriate diagnostic instruments for observing autistic behaviors and parental interviews should be used. A speech and language evaluation, as well as a cognitive and adaptive behavior evaluation, are also required. Additional developmental testing also may be necessary if delays in other areas are noted.

Management Management of a child with autism involves a multidisciplinary approach. The team might include psychologists, psychiatrists, neurologists, developmental pediatricians, audiologists, therapists (speech, occupational, physical), and educators. The primary goal is to maximize an autistic child's social and academic potential. Early diagnosis and interventional therapies may improve long-term outcome.

The wide variety of behavioral abnormalities associated with ASD may be particularly challenging to manage. Appropriate pharmacologic treatment may be required for aggressive or self-injurious behavior, self-stimulatory behaviors, hyperactivity, attentional deficits, and sleep disorders. These medications are best prescribed by a psychiatrist familiar with the treatment of children with ASD.

Additional Questions

1. Describe the clinical features and specific genetic mutations associated with fragile X syndrome, tuberous sclerosis complex, Rett syndrome, Angelman syndrome, and Prader-Willi syndrome.

2. What is the relationship between autism and head size?

References

American Psychiatry Association. *Diagnostic and Statistical Manual of Mental Disorders.* 4th ed. Text rev. Washington, DC: American Psychiatry Association; 1994.

Che MG, Memon S, Hung PC. Neurologic treatment strategies in autism: an overview of medical intervention strategies. *Semin Pediatr Neurol.* 2004;11:229–235.

Filipek PA, Accardo PJ, Ashwal S, et al. Practice parameter: screening and diagnosis of autism. *Neurology.* 2000;55(4):468–479.

Spence SJ, Sharifi P, Wiznitzer M. Autism spectrum disorder: screening, diagnosis and medical evaluation. *Semin Pediatr Neurol.* 2004;11:186–195.

Spence SJ. The genetics of autism. *Semin Pediatr Neurol.* 2004;11:196–205.

Tuchman R, Rapin I. Epilepsy in autism. *Lancet Neurol.* 2002;1:352–358.

References

A community pediatrician contacts you to discuss the management of **an 18-month-old girl** who is currently in his office. The patient has been a healthy, developmentally normal child but the mother is worried because over the last week the girl has had increasing difficulty walking and has developed tremulousness of her arms and hands. She has also been irritable, with difficulty sleeping. The child is in daycare and frequently has a cold, but there has been no recent fever or other illness. She has a healthy 3-year-old brother.

Physical Examination Vital Signs: Afebrile. She has a normal head circumference. General Examination: She does not have dysmorphic facial features, hepatosplenomegaly, or birth marks. Neurologic Examination: Mental Status: The patient is slightly agitated and difficult to console. Cranial Nerves: Her pupils are equal, round, and reactive to light. She tracks objects in all directions, but on close observation, she has rapid, conjugate jerks of her eyes in all directions. Her face is symmetric. Her gag is present and her tongue is midline without fasciculations. Motor: She has normal bulk and tone. She has symmetric extremity movements and is not weak. Coordination: Tremulousness of both upper extremities is noted in addition to truncal ataxia. Gait: She has an ataxic gait and needs help to walk. Reflexes: 2+ throughout with bilateral plantar flexor responses.

Guide to Case Discussion

- Briefly summarize this case.

- Localize the examination findings.

- Give the most likely diagnosis and provide a differential diagnosis.

- Discuss an appropriate diagnostic work-up.

- Discuss the management of this patient.

Diagnosis Opsoclonus-myoclonus syndrome.

Discussion Opsoclonus-myoclonus syndrome (OMS) or "dancing-eye syndrome," is a rare, serious, immune-mediated neurologic disorder that usually presents in children 6 months to 3 years of age. OMS can also present in older children and adults. The immunopathologic mechanism involved is poorly understood and no consistent causative autoantibodies have been identified in childhood cases. Both B-cell– and T-cell–mediated mechanisms may be involved. OMS is associated with neuroblastoma in approximately 50% of cases, likely representing a paraneoplastic syndrome. It can also occur with ganglioneuroblastoma. It is presumed that the immune response directed at the tumor cross reacts with tissues of the cerebellum. Postviral, postvaccine, and idiopathic etiologies account for other cases.

OMS occurs in approximately 1% to 2% of children with neuroblastoma. Neuroblastoma associated with OMS has a better long-term prognosis than neuroblastoma without the neurologic syndrome. Tumor pathology is usually low-grade (stage I or II) with favorable histologic features and is not associated with amplification of the *N-myc* gene. Metastases are rare.

Clinically, OMS is characterized by irritability, tremor, ataxia, loss of developmental milestones, opsoclonus, and myoclonus. Opsoclonus is described as chaotic, conjugate, rapid, irregular jerks of the eyes in all directions (horizontal, vertical, and diagonal). Irritability and sleep disturbance may be the first symptoms and can be extreme. Behavioral changes are soon followed by a progressive movement disorder. Affected children are at first tremulous and uncoordinated, but within days may become so ataxic that they cannot sit or walk. Opsoclonus may begin simultaneously or shortly after the onset of other symptoms. Myoclonic jerks of the face, trunk, extremities, or whole body also may occur. Frank motor, cognitive, and language regression are frequently seen as the syndrome evolves. OMS symptomatology may be either nonrelapsing or relapsing. Relapse occurs most often with viral infections.

Children with neuroblastoma presenting with OMS have an excellent survival rate. However, the prognosis of neurologic sequelae associated with OMS is guarded. Without treatment, severe cognitive and motor impairments occur. Even with treatment, affected children are at significant risk of ongoing developmental disabilities. Recent research with serial developmental testing has suggested that OMS sometimes results in a progressive encephalopathy. Opsoclonus usually eventually resolves but smooth pursuit abnormalities and hypometric saccades may persist for years after treatment.

Summary The patient is a previously healthy, developmentally normal 18-month-old girl who presents with the subacute onset of irritability and abnormal chaotic, conjugate eye movements (opsoclonus) in addition to tremulousness with truncal and gait ataxia.

Localization Irritability in a young child is a nonspecific finding but typically denotes a generalized illness that may or may not involve the central nervous system. Opsoclonus may localize to the cerebellum or to the brainstem (especially the midbrain). Tremulousness, as well as truncal and gait ataxia, localize to the midline cerebellum.

Differential Diagnosis When a patient presents with fully developed OMS, the diagnosis is straightforward. The finding of opsoclonus is unusual in other neurologic disorders of childhood. However, making the diagnosis may be more challenging when opsoclonus is subtle or intermittent.

The differential diagnosis of a young child presenting with the subacute onset of irritability and cerebellar signs includes toxic ingestion, central nervous system infections (meningitis, encephalitis), acute cerebellar ataxia, acute disseminated encephalomyelitis (ADEM), head trauma, hydrocephalus, and posterior fossa tumors. Inborn errors of metabolism, such as mitochondrial diseases, urea cycle disorders, and aminoacidopathies, can present with intermittent ataxia and abnormal eye movements. An inborn error of metabolism is a less likely consideration in this patient as she has been developmentally normal and her neurologic problems have not been intermittent. Myoclonic epilepsies and myoclonic status epilepticus may also present with myoclonus and ataxia but are also lower on the differential diagnosis in this case.

Evaluation The patient in the vignette needs to be immediately brought to the hospital and admitted for a diagnostic work-up. Any child presenting with suspected OMS needs a very thorough evaluation to search for an underlying neuroblastoma. The urine should be screened for catecholamines (HMA, VMA, dopamine). However, negative urine catecholamine studies do not rule out neuroblastoma because tumors may be small and/or nonsecreting. MRI and/or CT scanning of the chest and abdomen should be performed but may miss small tumors. In these cases, more sensitive radiologic studies may be required. Scintigraphic testing with the radioisotope metaiodobenzylguanidine (MIBG) may be helpful. MIBG acts as an analogue of norepinephrine. It is taken up and stored in neural crest tumors. Octreotide, an analogue of somatostatin, may also be useful in identifying small lesions. If these tests are initially negative, follow-up repeat studies may also be recommended several weeks to months later to insure that a tumor has not become evident with time. While idiopathic cases are reported, it is a diagnosis of exclusion and missing the diagnosis of a neuroblastoma may have a significant impact on a patient's outcome. Patients also need to be evaluated by ophthalmology to confirm the presence of opsoclonus and to rule out other ophthalmologic abnormalities.

If the diagnosis is less clear, additional testing may be warranted. An EEG may help rule out epileptic myoclonus. A lumbar puncture may help rule out an infectious or parainfectious process if a neuroblastoma is not identified. However, OMS patients may acutely demonstrate a mild pleocytosis. In addition, a brain MRI with and without contrast should be performed to rule out brainstem and/or cerebellar structural lesions.

Management Patients with OMS and neuroblastoma obviously need to be followed and managed by an oncologist. Tumor removal has a variable effect and may not correlate with resolution of symptoms. Affected children should also be monitored regularly by an ophthalmologist.

A variety of immunosuppressant treatments are available for OMS. Treatment with adrenocorticotropic hormone (ACTH) is standard and can often abolish symptoms. ACTH may need to be continued for months or even years. Tapering the dose needs to be done very carefully to prevent relapses. Oral prednisone has also been used and its efficacy compared to ACTH is controversial. Other agents, including propranolol, diazepam, cyclophosphamide, and azathioprine, have been tried but have had limited success. Finally, intravenous immunoglobulin and plasmapheresis reportedly have been useful in some patients. Rituximab, a humanized monoclonal antibody against B cells, is being tested in children who have not responded to steroids.

Because developmental and cognitive abilities may be significantly impaired as a result of OMS, developmental and, when applicable, neuropsychological testing should be performed. Early interventional services with speech, occupational, and physical therapy should be instituted as early as possible as recovery from OMS is often a prolonged process.

Additional Questions

1. What are the four most common posterior fossa tumors presenting in childhood?
2. What tumors and autoantibodies are associated with OMS in adults?

References

Brazis PW, Masdeu JC, Biller J. *Localization in Clinical Neurology*. 3rd ed. Philadelphia, Pa: Lippincott Williams & Wilkins; 1996:155–250.

Fernandez-Alvarez E, Aicardi J. *Movement Disorders in Children*. London, UK: Mac Keith Press; 2001:170–191.

Matthay KK, Blaes F, Hero B, et al. Opsoclonus myoclonus syndrome in neuroblastoma: a report from a workshop on the dancing eyes syndrome at the advances in neuroblastoma meeting in Genoa, Italy, 2004. *Cancer Lett*. 2005;228:275–282.

Mitchell WG, Brumm VL, Azen CG, et al. Longitudinal neurodevelopmental evaluation of children with opsoclonus-ataxia. *Pediatrics*. 2005;116(4):901–907.

Mitchell WG, Davalos-Gonzalez Y, Brumm VL, et al. Opsoclonus-ataxia caused by childhood neuroblastoma: developmental and neurologic sequelae. *Pediatrics*. 2002;109(1):86–98.

Pranzatelli MR, Tate ED, Travelstead AL, et al. Immunologic and clinical responses to rituximab in a child with opsoclonus-myoclonus syndrome. *Pediatrics*. 2005;115(1):e115–e119.

A 3-month-old boy is referred to your office for evaluation of large head size. His head circumference was 98% at birth but now is even higher. He was born at full-term by vaginal delivery in Mexico. His mother did not receive prenatal care but she denies any infections during the pregnancy. The baby is now smiling and making eye contact but has not rolled over. He breast-feeds well but has been gaining weight poorly and is now falling off his growth curve. The mother tells you that she also has an appointment with the cardiologist next week because the pediatrician heard a heart murmur.

Physical Examination Vital Signs: Mild tachypnea. His head circumference is greater than the 98% at birth. General Examination: Small 3-month-old boy with no dysmorphic facial features. His anterior fontanelle is open and full. A loud murmur is heard on auscultation. There is no hepatosplenomegaly. Neurologic Examination: Mental Status: Alert. Cranial Nerves: His pupils are equal, round, and reactive to light. He tracks objects in all directions. His face is symmetric. The tongue is midline. Motor: There is normal bulk and tone. He has a symmetric Moro reflex and moves all four extremities against gravity. Sensory: He responds to tactile stimulation throughout. Reflexes: 2+ throughout. His plantar responses are equivocal.

Guide to Case Discussion

▨ Briefly summarize this case.

▨ Localize the examination findings.

▨ Give the most likely diagnosis and provide a differential diagnosis.

▨ Discuss an appropriate diagnostic work-up.

▨ Discuss the management of this patient.

Diagnosis   Vein of Galen malformation.

Discussion   Vein of Galen malformations (VOGMs) are rare central nervous system arteriovenous malformations (AVMs) found primarily in young children. There is a male predominance. VOGMs occur in the midline choroidal fissure and consist of multiple feeding arteries. The anterior and posterior choroidal arteries, as well as the anterior and posterior cerebral arteries, are most commonly involved, draining into a large venous pouch. The malformation then drains into the superior sagittal sinus and typically does not communicate with the deep venous system of the brain.

A variety of presentations may be seen, largely depending on the size of the malformation. A VOGM may be diagnosed antenatally as a midline cystic structure on ultrasonograph. Large shunts may cause a vascular steal syndrome, depriving the developing brain of its critical blood supply, which results in significant brain atrophy. Neonatally, shunting of blood from the arterial to the venous system from the VOGM elevates the preload on the right side of the heart and results in high-output congestive heart failure. In severe cases, rapid deterioration with multiorgan system failure can occur. Older infants (1 month to 2 years of age) may experience hydrocephalus. There are two proposed mechanisms leading to hydrocephalus. It may result from direct compression by the dilated vein of Galen on the aqueduct of Sylvius, or by elevation of intracranial venous pressure, leading to diminished CSF absorption. Children older than 1 year may present with macrocephaly and dilated facial and cervical veins. Dilated veins occur with progressive obliteration of the straight sinus and jugular veins. Intracranial hemorrhage and seizures have been reported but are rare.

Damage to the brain is likely multifactorial. Four possible mechanisms have been identified: vascular steal phenomenon, perfusion failure as a consequence of congestive heart failure, venous thrombosis, and atrophy of adjacent structures caused by compression.

Prognosis varies by size of the lesion, age at presentation, and angioarchitecture. Neonates with large VOGMs and congestive heart failure tend to have the highest morbidity and mortality. Children presenting beyond the neonatal period may have a better developmental outcome.

Summary   The patient is a 3-month-old full-term infant who presents with progressive macrocephaly and failure to thrive. His general exam is remarkable for tachypnea, a full fontanelle, and a heart murmur. His neurologic exam and development appear to be normal.

Localization   Macrocephaly localizes to the compartments of the skull and may be caused by abnormalities in the ventricular system, brain, subdural/subarachnoid space, and skull. In this case, the presence of a full fontanelle is suggestive of ventricular dilatation and hydrocephalus. This patient's neurologic examination is nonfocal. Tachypnea with a heart murmur is concerning for a degree of congestive heart failure.

Differential Diagnosis   The differential diagnosis of an infant with macrocephaly is broad but can be broken down by involvement in the different compartments of the skull (Table 19.1). Macrocephaly is defined as a head circumference greater than

TABLE 19.1

Causes of Macrocephaly

Hydrocephalus
  Communicating
    Meningitis/encephalitis
    Intracranial hemorrhage
    Meningeal malignancy
  Noncommunicating
    Aqueductal stenosis
    Arnold-Chiari malformation
    Dandy-Walker malformation
    Intracranial tumor
    Vein of Galen malformation

Megalencephaly
  Anatomic
    Neurofibromatosis type 1
    Tuberous sclerosis complex
    Sotos syndrome
    Achondroplasia
  Metabolic
    Leukodystrophies
    Lysosomal storage diseases

Subdural and Subarachnoid Space Abnormalities
  Hematoma
  Empyema
  Benign enlargement of subarachnoid space

Thickened Skull
  Anemia
  Osteogenesis imperfecta
  Osteopetrosis
  Rickets

two standard deviations above the mean for age and gender. The normal rate of head growth during infancy is 2 cm per month in the first 3 months, 1 cm per month for the next 3 months, then 0.5 cm per month until 1 year of age.

Obstruction of the flow of CSF through the ventricular system may produce macrocephaly as a consequence of hydrocephalus. Noncommunicating hydrocephalus may be caused by aqueductal stenosis, Dandy-Walker malformation, Arnold-Chiari malformation, VOGMs, and neoplasms. Communicating hydrocephalus may result from infection or inflammatory processes in addition to intracranial hemorrhage.

Macrocephaly may also be caused by megalencephaly (enlarged brain). Megalencephaly also has multiple causes that are usually divided into anatomic and metabolic etiologies. Anatomic abnormalities include neurocutaneous diseases (tuberous sclerosis complex, neurofibromatosis type 1) and genetic syndromes (Sotos syndrome, achondroplasia), among others. Metabolic storage diseases such as leukodystrophies (Alexander disease, Canavan disease), and lysosomal storage diseases (Tay-Sachs disease, mucopolysaccharidoses) may also result in megalencephaly.

Enlargement of the subdural/subarachnoid space by a hematoma (subdural), empyema, or benign enlargement of the subarachnoid space may also cause enlarged head size. Finally, a thick skull may contribute to a large head size and can be caused by bone disorders such as anemia (sickle cell anemia, thalassemia) and skeletal dysplasias (rickets, osteopetrosis, osteogenesis imperfecta).

The patient in this case has increasing head size in addition to a full fontanelle, which is concerning for hydrocephalus. Congestive heart failure in addition to these findings is highly suggestive of a VOGM as the underlying etiology. Once a VOGM is suspected, it must be differentiated from an AVM that drains into the vein of Galen. The distinction is important as AVMs have a worse prognosis.

Evaluation   The evaluation of this patient should begin with immediate neuroimaging. Although a head CT could be obtained quickly, a brain MRI and magnetic resonance (MR) angiogram would best define the basic anatomy of the lesion. A catheter angiogram would subsequently be required prior to or at the time of embolization for a more detailed evaluation of vessel involvement.

The patient should also be evaluated by neurosurgery for management of hydrocephalus. Ventriculoperitoneal shunts are sometimes required. Cardiology should be consulted for management of the associated congestive heart failure. An ECHO, ECG, and chest radiograph are indicated.

Management   Correction of a VOGM is primarily managed by an interventional neuroradiologist. Embolization of the VOGM is the preferred procedure, but is a high risk procedure. It is technically easier if performed after the patient is 5 to 6 months of age. Infants may be managed medically until that time. Larger lesions might require several procedures. Surgical closure of the shunt carries a very high mortality rate and is usually not performed. As mentioned above, some patients require a ventriculoperitoneal shunt to manage hydrocephalus.

The patient in this vignette also requires ongoing monitoring by a cardiologist. Nutritional support might also be required given his failure to thrive. There is a risk of developmental disabilities and an evaluation for early interventional services is warranted.

Additional Questions

1. What is the differential diagnosis of microcephaly?
2. What is the average head circumference of a newborn infant?
3. What are the radiographic features of Dandy-Walker malformation?

References

Ashwal S. Congenital structural defects. In: Swaiman KS, Ashwal S, eds. *Pediatric Neurology: Principles and Practice*. 3rd ed. St. Louis, Mo: Mosby; 1999:234–300.

Bhattacharya JJ, Thammaroj J. Vein of Galen malformations. *J Neurol Neurosurg Psychiatry*. 2003;74(suppl 1):i42–i44.

Brunelle F. Arteriovenous malformation of the vein of Galen in children. *Pediatr Radiol.* 1997;27:501–513.

Brunelle F. Brain vascular malformations in the fetus: diagnosis and prognosis. *Childs Nerv Syst.* 2003;19:524–528.

Fenichel GM. *Clinical Pediatric Neurology: A Signs and Symptoms Approach.* 4th ed. Philadelphia, Pa: WB Saunders; 2001:353–370.

Fullerton HJ, Aminoff AR, Ferriero DM, et al. Neurodevelopmental outcome after endovascular treatment of vein of Galen malformations. *Neurology.* 2003;61:1386–1390.

You are consulted by the pediatric service to see **a 5-day-old female infant** who presented to her first visit with her pediatrician with lethargy and hypotonia. She was immediately referred for hospital admission. The mother reports a normal, healthy pregnancy with very active fetal movements. The birth weight was 7 pounds. The infant has been mostly sleeping since birth, but at times she is more alert and active. She has been feeding poorly because of her sleepiness. During sleep, the parents also have seen frequent myoclonic jerks. There is a family history of a paternal uncle with spinal muscular atrophy. There is no history of consanguinity.

Physical Examination Vital Signs: Normal. General Examination: Her anterior fontanelle is flat. There are no dysmorphic facial features. She has no hepatosplenomegaly. Neurologic Examination: Mental Status: She is sleeping and unarousable. She moves but does not open her eyes to external stimuli. Cranial Nerves: Her pupils are equal, round, and reactive to light. Her facial movements are symmetric. Oculocephalic, corneal, and gag reflexes are present. The tongue is midline without fasciculations. Motor: She has normal bulk with marked truncal and appendicular hypotonia. The infant moves her extremities symmetrically against gravity with deep pain stimuli. Reflexes: 2+ throughout. Bilateral plantar extensor responses are present.

Guide to Case Discussion

- Briefly summarize this case.
- Localize the examination findings.
- Give the most likely diagnosis and provide a differential diagnosis.
- Discuss an appropriate diagnostic work-up.
- Discuss the management of this patient.

Diagnosis   Nonketotic hyperglycinemia.

Discussion   Nonketotic hyperglycinemia (NKH), or glycine encephalopathy, is an inborn error of glycine metabolism resulting in the abnormal accumulation of glycine. The accumulation of glycine in the brain causes the neurologic manifestations of this disorder. Glycine is a neurotransmitter with inhibitory functions in the brainstem and spinal cord, but excitatory action in the cerebral cortex.

Three clinical syndromes of glycine encephalopathy are described: (a) an infantile form with apnea, seizures, and developmental delay; (b) a mild episodic form with attacks of delirium, choreoathetosis, behavior change, and vertical gaze palsy precipitated by stress or infection; (c) a late-onset form with mental retardation, choreoathetosis, optic atrophy, and spastic paraparesis. The classic neonatal form presents in the first few days of life with progressive encephalopathy resulting in apnea, hypotonia, and myoclonic seizures. Apnea is caused by glycine's effect on the brainstem, whereas seizures are caused by the excitatory effects of glycine on cortical neurons. Hiccups may prove a clue to the diagnosis. The atypical forms usually present after 6 months of age; they retain residual enzyme activity, which results in the clinical heterogeneity of milder symptoms and later presentation.

There also are reported cases of transient glycine encephalopathy. These newborns present clinically as if they have NKH and have biochemical features similar to those of NKH, but the symptoms and hyperglycinemia resolve spontaneously. Often there are few or no long-term neurologic complications.

NKH is an autosomal recessive disorder of the glycine cleavage enzyme system (GCS), which converts glycine to carbon dioxide, ammonia, and hydroxymethyltetrahydrofolic acid. The GCS complex is comprised of four proteins: P protein (pyridoxal phosphate-dependent glycine decarboxylase), H protein (lipoic acid-containing protein), T protein (tetrahydrofolate-requiring enzyme), and L protein (lipoamide dehydrogenase). These proteins are located on the inner mitochondrial membrane in tissues of the liver, kidney, and brain. P protein (*GLDC* gene) mutations account for 80% of NKH cases. T protein (*AMT* gene) mutations account for 10% to 15% of NKH cases. H protein (*GCSH* gene) mutations are very rare. L protein defects usually present as a variant form of branched-chain amino acidemia.

MRI of the brain may show cerebral dysgenesis in up to one third of affected infants. Agenesis of the corpus callosum, hydrocephalus, immature gyral pattern, and retrocerebellar cysts also have been described. Increased signal in areas of myelinated white matter may be seen on diffusion-weighted imaging. Magnetic resonance (MR) spectroscopy may demonstrate an elevated glycine level. A variety of EEG findings have been reported, including discontinuous and burst suppression patterns.

The prognosis in NKH is guarded. Severely affected infants may die early in their disease course. Children with milder forms may have a better developmental outcome, with some patients eventually walking and communicating. However, the majority experience moderate to severe psychomotor retardation and ongoing seizures.

Summary   The patient is a 5-day-old full-term female infant born without complications who presents with encephalopathy, hypotonia, and myoclonic seizures.

Her exam is significant for marked lethargy, extreme hypotonia without weakness, and bilateral extensor plantar responses.

Localization The presence of encephalopathy suggests a diffuse disorder of the central nervous system. Myoclonic seizures are a form of generalized epilepsy and localize to the bilateral cerebral cortex.

Hypotonia in infancy and childhood has central and peripheral causes. In this case, a central etiology is most likely. The presence of encephalopathy and seizures first suggests a central cause. In addition, there are no signs of a disorder affecting the motor unit. For example, proximal weakness and/or tongue fasciculations might suggest a disorder of the anterior horn cell (spinal muscular atrophy). The patient is hypotonic but not weak, which also helps exclude myopathies and neuromuscular junction disorders. In addition, deep tendon reflexes are present, which argues against a peripheral neuropathy. Note should also be made of the fact that the infant has bilateral plantar extensor responses. Although this may suggest involvement of the corticospinal tracts, it is also a normal newborn finding and is of uncertain significance in this case.

Differential Diagnosis The patient's young age at presentation in addition to the symptoms of lethargy, hypotonia, and seizures are highly suggestive of an inborn error of metabolism. However, acquired disorders are much more common than metabolic diseases and should be ruled out first. These include infection (sepsis, meningitis, encephalitis), hypoxic-ischemic encephalopathy with seizures, intracranial hemorrhage, neonatal stroke, head trauma, and medication toxicity (Table 20.1).

Once acquired etiologies are excluded, the broad differential diagnosis of inborn errors of metabolism causing neonatal encephalopathy, hypotonia, and seizures must be considered. Typically, these symptoms are produced by the accumulation of small-molecule metabolites, insufficient amounts of a necessary enzymatic pathway product, or abnormal transport of certain molecules. The pregnancy is often unremarkable and affected infants are typically normal at birth. Lethargy, seizures, vomiting, poor feeding, and irritability begin hours to days after birth. In general terms, aminoacidopathies, organic acidurias, urea cycle disorders, peroxisomal disorders, fatty acid oxidation defects, and mitochondrial disorders should be considered. When seizures are also a prominent feature, NKH, pyridoxine-dependent seizures, folinic acid-responsive seizures, sulfite oxidase deficiency, molybdenum cofactor deficiency, and glucose transporter 1 (GLUT1) defects enter the differential diagnosis. Seizures may even begin in utero in these conditions, and are suggested in the case presented above by the history of very active fetal movements.

A thorough physical examination, family history, screening metabolic work-up, specialized metabolic/genetic testing, and neuroimaging with brain MRI and MR spectroscopy may be required to narrow the differential diagnosis. The presence of abnormal smells that accompany many inborn errors of metabolism might also be significant. Laboratory findings suggestive of an underlying metabolic disease include persistent metabolic acidosis with an anion gap (especially higher than 20 mEq/L), elevated lactate, hyperammonemia, and hypoglycemia.

Persistent metabolic acidosis may be caused by organic acidurias, mitochondrial respiratory chain abnormalities, or disorders of pyruvate metabolism.

TABLE 20.1

Differential Diagnosis of Acute Neonatal Encephalopathy

Acquired
  Infection (sepsis, meningitis, encephalitis)
  Hypoxic-ischemic encephalopathy
  Cerebral hemorrhage
  Stroke
  Trauma
  Drug toxicity

Inborn Errors of Metabolism
  Aminoacidurias
  Organic acidurias
  Urea cycle disorders
  Mitochondrial disorders
  Fatty acid oxidation defects
  Peroxisomal disorders

Disorders with Prominent Seizure Activity
  Nonketotic hyperglycinemia
  Pyridoxine-dependent seizures
  Folinic acid-responsive seizures
  Sulfite oxidase deficiency
  Molybdenum cofactor deficiency
  Glucose transporter deficiency disorders

Organic acidurias such as methylmalonic aciduria, propionic aciduria, and isovaleric aciduria can cause an elevated serum glycine level but can be differentiated from NKH by the presence of ketosis and by measurement of urine organic acids (which are both normal in NKH). Most amino acid disorders do not cause an acute neonatal encephalopathy. The neonatal presentation of maple syrup urine disease, however, is an exception. In these cases, the urine may smell sweet because of the presence of ketoacids. A variety of mitochondrial respiratory chain disorders may present with profound encephalopathy in addition to serum and CSF lactic acidosis. Disorders of pyruvate metabolism (pyruvate dehydrogenase and pyruvate carboxylase deficiency) must also be considered with this clinical and laboratory picture.

Hyperammonemia as seen with urea cycle defects can also result in encephalopathy and seizures secondary to cerebral edema and the neurotoxic effects of ammonia. The most common urea cycle disorder, ornithine transcarbamylase (OTC) deficiency (X-linked), presents shortly after birth and is usually fatal in males. Heterozygous females present later with intermittent episodes of lethargy, vomiting, and ataxia. Seizures are less prominent. A secondary hyperammonemia may also be seen in organic acidurias and fatty acid oxidation defects.

Hypoglycemia is commonly seen in sepsis, prematurity, and maternal diabetes mellitus but when presenting with metabolic acidosis, it is suggestive of an organic aciduria or disorder of gluconeogenesis (glycogen storage disease type 1). Fatty acid oxidation defects like short-chain acylcoenzyme A (acyl-CoA) dehydrogenase deficiency can also present with hypoglycemia in infancy. Disorders of peroxisome biogenesis (Zellweger syndrome, neonatal adrenoleukodystrophy, infantile Refsum syndrome) can be considered but are a less likely cause of neonatal encephalopathy. Laboratory findings include abnormal very-long-chain fatty acids. Urine organic acids, as well as the acylcarnitine profile, are expected to be normal in these cases.

Several inborn errors of metabolism may present with acute encephalopathy in addition to intractable seizures and deserve special mention. The diagnosis of pyridoxine-dependent seizures and folinic acid-responsive seizures can be excluded as they respond to intravenous pyridoxine or folinic acid, respectively. Sulfite oxidase and molybdenum cofactor deficiency are autosomal recessive disorders that demonstrate poor feeding, intractable seizures, axial hypotonia, and extremity hypertonicity in the first few days to weeks of life. Routine metabolic tests do not detect these disorders and special testing for elevated urine S-sulfocysteine and thiosulfate must be performed. GLUT1-deficiency syndrome may present with a similar clinical picture. A low CSF glucose, low CSF lactate, and normal serum glucose are characteristic of this disease.

Finally, other disorders should be considered when a patient is found to have elevated glycine levels. Valproic acid and D-glyceric acidemia can also present with secondary hyperglycinemia as a result of a decrease in liver GCS activity.

Evaluation The patient's evaluation should begin with a thorough history of the mother's pregnancy, the child's birth, feeding history, and family history. It is important to know if fetal movements were normal, whether the mother had any infections during the pregnancy, whether the mother used any drugs during the pregnancy, and whether there was vaginal bleeding or any additional complications. Increased fetal movements, as in this case, may be indicative of in utero seizure activity. It is relevant to know whether the child had any difficulties with feeding or breathing after birth. Many metabolic diseases present after the introduction of protein or glucose feeds so a detailed history of the onset of symptoms and the infant's diet must be obtained. Noting any family history of consanguinity and/or unexplained infant death is also very important. Abnormal smells might be relevant.

At the time of presentation, the patient should have a screening work-up performed to evaluate for the most common acquired disorders. This screening work-up should include basic chemistries (to rule out acidosis and anion gap), blood gas, CBC, glucose, liver function tests, creatine kinase, urinalysis, blood culture, and urine culture. A noncontrast head CT also needs to be done, followed by a lumbar puncture for cell count, glucose, protein, bacterial culture, and HSV PCR. Given the presence of seizures, an EEG is warranted early in her evaluation.

Finally, testing for inborn errors of metabolism in an infant with encephalopathy should be initiated by obtaining plasma amino acids, urine organic acids, a lactate/pyruvate battery, and an ammonia level. Additional tests can include urine analysis for ketones and reducing substances in addition to serum carnitine, acylcarnitine profile, and very-long-chain fatty acids. CSF lactate and glycine can also be measured as part of the initial work-up when there are strong suspicions of an inborn error of metabolism. A brain MRI and MR spectroscopy are further recommended and may help point to a type of metabolic disease. The diagnosis of pyridoxine-dependent seizures is evaluated by giving 100 mg of pyridoxine intravenously during an EEG. Epileptiform activity should resolve while or shortly after the dose is given.

NKH should be suspected in individuals with elevated urine, serum, and CSF glycine. However, the urine and serum glycine levels may often not be elevated and therefore, simultaneous CSF and plasma glycine levels are needed. An abnormal CSF-to-plasma glycine ratio of >0.08 is consistent with NKH (the normal ratio is <0.02). Once NKH is strongly suspected, confirmatory biochemical, quantitative amino acid analysis, and molecular genetic testing should be done. Biochemical enzyme assays of GCS activity obtained on liver biopsy are available on a research basis only. The specific protein deficiency (P, T, or H) also can be identified on liver tissue but, again, is not clinically available. Molecular genetic testing by sequence analysis of the *GLDC*, *GCSH*, and *ATM* genes is clinically available and confirms the diagnosis in a majority of patients.

Management   The patient in this case needs to be admitted to the hospital immediately. Close observation in an intensive care unit should be considered given the degree of encephalopathy. She should be placed on a cardiorespiratory monitor and a pulse oximeter. Intubation should be performed for airway protection. As the initial work-up proceeds, she should be placed on empiric broad-spectrum antibiotic coverage and acyclovir until the diagnosis is clearer. Given that she appears to be having seizures, it is reasonable to load her with phenobarbital and place her on a maintenance dose (although, ideally, this should happen after her EEG).

In general, infants with suspected inborn errors of metabolism should be taken off of enteral feeds; instead, intravenous fluids of 10% dextrose with appropriate electrolytes should be provided. If there are concerns for a fatty acid oxidation defect, intravenous interlipids should not be given. Other complications, such as hypoglycemia and metabolic acidosis, should be aggressively medically managed. Management strategies may then be tailored as the work-up points toward a specific diagnosis.

Currently, there is no effective treatment available for NKH. Sodium benzoate has been used to normalize serum glycine but does not normalize CSF glycine levels; high doses, however, can lower CSF glycine levels. It might be useful for episodes of lethargy and seizures in the milder forms of NKH. Sodium benzoate has not been shown to change outcome in the classic severe neonatal form.

Traditional anticonvulsants such as phenobarbital and phenytoin may not be effective at seizure control in these patients. Benzodiazepines and sodium benzoate appear to be more effective antiepileptic agents. Valproic acid is contraindicated as it can cause secondary hyperglycinemia by decreasing liver GCS activity. Antagonism of the NMDA glutamate receptor, which is stimulated by glycine, also has been attempted without success with dextromethorphan, ketamine, felbamate, and lamotrigine.

Supportive care for the patient and counseling for the family plays a large role in caring for these patients. Genetic counseling is recommended for parents and family members. As both parents are carriers, each new child has a 25% chance of being affected, a 50% chance of being a carrier, and a 25% chance of being neither affected nor a carrier. Prenatal molecular genetic testing of extracted fetal DNA or chorionic villus sampling is available and can be offered to the parents.

Additional Questions

1. What is the difference between a neonatal EEG and a routine 18-lead EEG?

2. What is the appropriate treatment for status epilepticus in a newborn?

3. Which pathogens commonly cause neonatal meningitis?

References

Applegarth DA, Toone JR. Nonketotic hyperglycinemia (glycine encephalopathy): laboratory diagnosis. *Mol Genet Metab.* 2001;74(1-2):139–146.

Baxter P. Pyridoxine-dependent and pyridoxine-responsive seizures. *Dev Med Child Neurol.* 2001;43:416–420.

Clarke JTR. *A Clinical Guide to Inherited Metabolic Diseases.* 2nd ed. Cambridge, UK: Cambridge University Press; 2002:18–64.

Ellaway CJ, Wilcken B, Christodoulou J. Clinical approach to inborn errors of metabolism presenting in the newborn period. *J Paediatr Child Health.* 2002;38:511–517.

Hoover-Fong JE, Shah S, Van Hove JLK, et al. Natural history of nonketotic hyperglycinemia in 65 patients. *Neurology.* 2004;63:1847–1853.

Pascual JM, Wang D, Lecumberri B, et al. GLUT1 deficiency and other glucose transporter diseases. *Eur J Endocrinol.* 2004;150(5):627–633.

Shah DK, Tingay DG, Fink AM, et al. Magnetic resonance imaging in neonatal nonketotic hyperglycinemia. *Pediatr Neurol.* 2005;33:50–52.

Tada K, Kure S. Non-ketotic hyperglycinaemia: molecular lesion, diagnosis and pathophysiology. *J Inherit Metab Dis.* 1993;16(4):691–703.

Van Hove JLK, Kerckhove KV, Hennermann JB, et al. Benzoate treatment and the glycine index in nonketotic hyperglycinemia. *J Inherit Metab Dis.* 2005;28:651–663.

A 13-year-old girl presents to the office for complaints of a new-onset movement disorder. For the last 3 months, she has had episodes of repetitive stiffening, contraction, and rotation of her left hand, arm, and leg that occasionally generalize. Occasionally there is facial involvement with grimacing, torsion of the tongue, and guttural sounds. The episodes last approximately 1 to 2 minutes and then resolve spontaneously. The events happen most often when she begins a movement after resting, like getting up from a chair. There has been an increase in frequency and they now occur 5 to 10 times each day. She has never had an impairment of consciousness, incontinence, tongue biting, or cyanosis with the spells. She was born at full-term by cesarean section without complications. Her growth and development are normal. She is an honor roll student. There is no family history of epilepsy, migraines, tics, or other movement disorders.

Physical Examination General Examination: Normal. No abnormal movements are noted during the exam. Neurologic Examination: Mental Status: Alert and cooperative. Cranial Nerves: The pupils are equal, round, and reactive to light. Her extraocular muscles are intact. Her face is symmetric. The tongue is midline without fasciculations. Motor: Normal bulk and tone with 5/5 strength throughout. Coordination: No dysmetria, tremor, dystonia, or choreoathetosis noted. Sensory: Normal light touch, temperature, and vibration. Gait: Normal heel, toe, flat, and tandem gait. Reflexes: 2+ throughout with bilateral plantar flexor responses.

Guide to Case Discussion

- Briefly summarize this case.

- Localize the examination findings.

- Give the most likely diagnosis and provide a differential diagnosis.

- Discuss an appropriate diagnostic work-up.

- Discuss the management of this patient.

Diagnosis   Paroxysmal kinesigenic dyskinesia.

Discussion   The paroxysmal dyskinesias are a heterogeneous group of involuntary, hyperkinetic movement disorders of unclear etiology. They are characterized by sudden attacks of choreoathetoid or dystonic movements without associated loss of consciousness. An aura or warning, such as paresthesias or dizziness, may precede the dyskinesias in some patients. The neurologic exam is normal between attacks.

This group of disorders is typically classified into paroxysmal kinesigenic and paroxysmal nonkinesigenic dyskinesias. A third form of the disease is known as the intermediate type or paroxysmal exertion-induced dyskinesia. It is unclear whether paroxysmal dyskinesia occurring during sleep (paroxysmal hypnogenic dyskinesia) is a distinct clinical entity. Abnormal dystonic and choreoathetoid movements in sleep may be confused with autosomal dominant nocturnal frontal lobe epilepsy. The term *dyskinesia* is used because the abnormal movements are usually complex with components of dystonia, chorea, athetosis, and ballismus. Cases may be primary or secondary in etiology. Associated neurologic conditions include epilepsy, benign rolandic epilepsy with writer's cramp, and hemiplegic migraine.

In individuals with paroxysmal kinesigenic dyskinesia, episodes of dystonia, choreoathetosis, and ballismus are precipitated by sudden voluntary movements. For example, they may begin when a patient rises from a chair after resting. Other triggers include excitement, anxiety, and stress. Movements are usually unilateral or asymmetric but more generalized movements can also occur. The extremities, face, neck, and trunk may be involved. Most attacks last several seconds but almost always last less than 5 minutes. Attacks typically occur multiple times daily, with some patients experiencing symptoms up to 100 times per day. When dyskinesias occur frequently, they may be very disruptive and impair quality of life. Onset is usually in childhood between the ages of 6 and 16 years. There is a male predominance. Most cases are associated with autosomal dominant familial inheritance but autosomal recessive and sporadic cases are not uncommon. Candidate genes lie on chromosome 16.

Paroxysmal nonkinesigenic dyskinesia is also characterized by transient attacks of dystonia, choreoathetosis or ballismus. In contrast to paroxysmal kinesigenic dyskinesia, this disorder is precipitated by ingestion of alcohol or caffeinated beverages. Stress, fatigue, and movement are less likely to serve as triggers. Onset typically occurs in infancy or early childhood. Movements more commonly affect the face and neck with dysarthria and dysphagia frequently seen. Attacks may last 10 to 15 minutes or persist for hours at a time. The attacks occur less frequently than the kinesigenic form, however, with no more than four per day, and sometimes none for several weeks. The causative gene has been mapped to chromosome 2q and inheritance is autosomal dominant.

Reports of paroxysmal exertion-induced dyskinesia are more rare. Onset is between the ages of 2 and 30 years. These cases are most often sporadic. Dyskinesias usually occur after prolonged periods of strenuous exercise, like running. Attacks last several minutes but may occur for as long as 30 minutes. The episodes are relatively infrequent and usually do not happen more than once per day. The legs are most frequently involved, but there may be spread of abnormal movements to the upper body.

The anatomic basis and underlying pathophysiology of these complex movement disorders are poorly understood. Many hypotheses have been put forth to try to explain their etiology. Some researchers have proposed that a subcortical epilepsy involving the basal ganglia or thalamic nuclei may be responsible. Theories of an underlying causative somatosensory abnormality also exist. The possibility of abnormal basal ganglia neural networks with an imbalance between excitatory and inhibitory inputs has been proposed. Finally, recent research has suggested that paroxysmal dyskinesias are caused by a channelopathy. This theory is supported by their similarity to other paroxysmal ion channel-related disorders such as epilepsy, migraine, and episodic ataxia.

Summary   The patient is a healthy, developmentally normal adolescent girl who presents with brief episodes of dystonic facial and body movements that are initiated by movement. The neurologic exam is normal.

Localization   The patient's neurologic exam is normal and there are no localizing features. However, the presence of a paroxysmal movement disorder is suggestive of a disease process affecting the basal ganglia.

Differential Diagnosis   The presentation of paroxysmal kinesigenic dyskinesia is very characteristic and when a history of episodes of complex involuntary movements precipitated by sudden movement is elicited, the diagnosis is almost certain. However, the diagnosis of a primary kinesigenic dyskinesia is one of exclusion, as many secondary causes are known. Other paroxysmal movement disorders and conditions may also mimic this condition (Table 21.1).

A variety of secondary causes of paroxysmal dyskinesias (kinesigenic and nonkinesigenic forms) have been reported, including medication toxicity, endocrinopathies, metabolic disturbances, cerebral ischemia, traumatic brain injury, vascular abnormalities, and inborn errors of metabolism. Table 21.1 outlines these secondary causes.

Other paroxysmal disorders should also be excluded. The possibility of an underlying seizure disorder should be considered. In contrast to paroxysmal dyskinesias, seizures commonly involve more organized, rhythmic jerking of the body and impair consciousness. A postictal state usually occurs. Migraines also can cause transient neurologic deficits or abnormalities (hemiplegic migraine) but also are usually associated with significant headache, nausea, vomiting, and photophobia.

The episodic ataxias types 1 and 2 (EA1, EA2) also may be confused with the paroxysmal dyskinesias. The episodic ataxias manifest primarily with ataxia and gait abnormalities. However, like the paroxysmal dyskinesias, they are not associated with a loss of consciousness, may be provoked by movement, stress, or alcohol, and respond to acetazolamide. EA1 is caused by a mutation in a potassium channel gene on chromosome 12p. Brief episodes of ataxia are caused by startle and exercise, but myokymia is also characteristic of this disease. The ataxic movements in EA2 are precipitated by stress and exercise but not by startle. They occur less frequently but last longer than ataxic episodes in EA1. A pathologic mutation on chromosome 19p has been identified and causes an abnormality of a subunit in the voltage-gated calcium channel.

In young children, alternative diagnoses, such as motor tics, stereotypies, shuddering attacks, spasmus nutans, benign myoclonus, benign paroxysmal torticollis of infancy, benign paroxysmal tonic upgaze, transient idiopathic dystonia of infancy, and alternating hemiplegia of childhood, deserve consideration. In adolescents,

---

TABLE 21.1

Paroxysmal Dyskinesias in Childhood

Primary
 Paroxysmal kinesigenic dyskinesia
 Paroxysmal nonkinesigenic dyskinesia
 Paroxysmal exertion-induced dyskinesia
 Paroxysmal hypnogenic dyskinesia

Secondary
 Medications
   Phenytoin
   Gabapentin
 Infection
   Encephalitis
   Postinfectious disorders
 Endocrine disorders
   Hyperthyroidism
   Hypoparathyroidism
   Pseudohypoparathyroidism
 Metabolic disturbance
   Hypocalcemia
   Hyper-/hypoglycemia
   Kernicterus
 Traumatic brain injury
 Ischemic
   Perinatal hypoxic ischemic encephalopathy
   Transient ischemic attacks
   Cerebral infarction
   Cerebral hemorrhage
 Vascular
   Vasculitis
   Arteriovenous malformations
 Inborn errors of metabolism
   Hartnup disease
   Pyruvate decarboxylase deficiency
   Nonketotic hyperglycinemia

---

psychogenic disturbances may present with paroxysmal movement disorders. Finally, other causes of dystonia and chorea in childhood, such as idiopathic torsion dystonia, Wilson disease, and Sydenham chorea, may enter the differential diagnosis. However, these disorders manifest with different symptomatology and abnormal movements are not paroxysmal.

Evaluation   The diagnostic evaluation of a child with a suspected paroxysmal dyskinesia should be thorough. This is a rare syndrome and as the pathophysiology of these disorders is poorly understood, other more common disorders in the differential diagnosis should be ruled out before a definitive diagnosis is given.

Neuroimaging with a brain MRI with and without contrast is essential to rule out intracranial pathology involving the basal ganglia, such as a tumor, arteriovenous malformation, infectious process, demyelinating disease, vasculitis, or inborn error of metabolism. A brain magnetic resonance (MR) spectroscopy may also be helpful in investigating metabolic diseases, such as a mitochondrial disorder that might show a lactate peak. A routine or video EEG is also indicated to rule out the possibility of seizure activity. A dilated ophthalmologic exam is necessary to evaluate for Wilson disease, optic atrophy, retinitis pigmentosa, and other ophthalmologic abnormalities.

General screening laboratory investigations should include a CBC, basic chemistry panel, liver function tests, calcium, magnesium, phosphorus, copper, ceruloplasmin, creatine kinase, ANA, erythrocyte sedimentation rate, antistreptolysin-O titer, and anti-DNAase B antibody. Endocrine testing should include thyroid function tests, parathyroid hormone, and a cortisol level. Initial screening for inborn errors of metabolism should include a lactate/pyruvate battery, plasma amino acids, urine organic acids, ammonia level, very-long-chain fatty acids, and a vitamin E level.

Management   Pharmacologic management of paroxysmal dyskinesias is not standardized. With time, some patients experience a significant decrease in or resolution of the episodes of dyskinesia. Others continue to be frequently affected.

Paroxysmal kinesigenic dyskinesias respond well, and often dramatically, to common anticonvulsants. Phenytoin, carbamazepine, oxcarbazepine, primidone, phenobarbital, valproic acid, lamotrigine, and clonazepam have all been reported to work in select cases. Levodopa, acetazolamide, tetrabenazine, flunarizine, and trihexyphenidyl also have been tried with success. Similarly, paroxysmal nonkinesigenic dyskinesia has responded to a variety of pharmacologic agents, including valproic acid, gabapentin, clonazepam, haloperidol, and acetazolamide. However, the nonkinesigenic form of the disease is often more refractory to treatment. Cases of paroxysmal exertion-induced dyskinesia have been successfully treated with levodopa, trihexyphenidyl, and carbamazepine.

References

Fernandez-Alvarez E, Aicardi J. *Movement Disorders in Children.* London, UK: Mac Keith Press; 2001:152–169.

Lotze T, Jankovic J. Paroxysmal kinesigenic dyskinesias. *Semin Pediatr Neurol.* 2003;10(1):68–79.

Margari L, Presicci A, Ventura P, et al. Channelopathy: hypothesis of a common physiologic mechanism in different forms of paroxysmal dyskinesia. *Pediatr Neurol.* 2005;32:229–235.

A healthy 6-month-old female infant is referred for evaluation with a 2-week history of new-onset spells. The spells are described as brief episodes of her head falling forward with flexion at the waist and abduction of the arms. They occur in clusters on awakening that last for several minutes. The spells are occurring with increasing frequency and sometimes she cries afterwards. The parents have also noted that during this time the infant has stopped smiling, decreased her babbling, and is less interested in toys than previously. She was born at full term by normal spontaneous vaginal delivery to a 27-year-old G_2P_1 mother. The pregnancy, birth, and neonatal period were unremarkable. Her growth and development prior to her presentation has been normal.

Physical Examination General Examination: There are no dysmorphic facial features or birthmarks. Neurologic Examination: Mental Status: Alert. She does not smile spontaneously or responsively. Language: No babbling or cooing is noted. Cranial Nerves: II through XII are intact. Motor: She has normal bulk and tone. She moves all four extremities equally against gravity. Coordination: She has little interest in grabbing or playing with toys but there is no dysmetria. Reflexes: 2+ throughout with bilateral plantar flexor responses.

Guide to Case Discussion

- Briefly summarize this case.
- Localize the examination findings.
- Give the most likely diagnosis and provide a differential diagnosis.
- Discuss an appropriate diagnostic work-up.
- Discuss the management of this patient.

Diagnosis Infantile spasms (West syndrome).

Discussion Infantile spasms characterize a unique seizure disorder that occurs almost exclusively in infants younger than 1 year of age. The incidence of infantile spasms peaks at 3 to 7 months of age. They typically occur in clusters and are most common shortly after an affected infant awakens. Spasms are described as brief tonic contractions of the limbs and axial musculature. They may involve flexor, extensor, or mixed flexor-extensor musculature. Flexion spasms are most common and involve head drops and flexion of all four extremities with the arms moving up or out. Extensor spasms appear more like a Moro reflex with neck/lower extremity extension and arm extension/abduction. Hemispasms can also occur and suggest a focal etiology. It is not unusual for infants with spasms to experience plateauing or regression of developmental milestones prior to or at the onset of infantile spasms.

An underlying etiology can be determined in 60% to 90% of patients with infantile spasms. A variety of prenatal, perinatal, and postnatal causes are identified in these symptomatic cases (Table 22.1). Cortical migrational abnormalities, genetic syndromes, neurocutaneous syndromes, and inborn errors of metabolism are commonly found. Cortical damage from ischemia, infection, or trauma are also frequently seen. Tuberous sclerosis complex is a major cause of infantile spasms and may account for as many as 25% of cases. A minority of infants have idiopathic infantile spasms when no etiology is identified after a thorough diagnostic work-up.

Summary The patient is a healthy 6-month-old female infant who presents with developmental regression and new-onset spells, the description of which is consistent with a diagnosis of infantile spasms. Her neurologic exam is normal.

Localization Infantile spasms denote a generalized epileptic encephalopathy and, thus, localize to cortical and subcortical regions of both hemispheres. A loss of developmental milestones also implies a bihemispheric cortical disturbance. However, even though the encephalopathy is diffuse, the seizures in infantile spasms can sometimes result from a focal cortical lesion.

Differential Diagnosis The differential diagnosis of infantile spasms includes nonepileptic events such as colic, gastroesophageal reflux, Sandifer syndrome, hyperekplexia, and behavioral events such as masturbation or breath-holding spells. These diagnoses can usually be excluded by taking a thorough history. Benign myoclonus of infancy can also be considered. Infants with this syndrome are developmentally normal and have episodes of myoclonus with a normal ictal and interictal EEG.

Infantile spasms must also be differentiated from other seizure disorders that occur in infancy, including benign myoclonic epilepsy in infancy and severe myoclonic epilepsy in infancy (Dravet syndrome). Benign myoclonic epilepsy in infancy is a distinct form of idiopathic generalized epilepsy that is characterized by myoclonic seizures in infants 6 months to 2 years of age. This epilepsy may be genetically based. The interictal EEG is usually normal but myoclonic jerks may be associated with generalized polyspike and slow-wave discharges. Severe myoclonic epilepsy in infancy occurs in the first year of life in previously

TABLE 22.1

Etiologies of Infantile Spasms

Cerebral Malformations
  Lissencephaly
  Polymicrogyria
  Schizencephaly
  Focal cortical dysplasia

Genetic Syndromes
  Aicardi syndrome
  Down syndrome
  Williams syndrome

Neurocutaneous Diseases
  Tuberous sclerosis complex
  Neurofibromatosis type 1
  Incontinentia pigmenti
  Sturge-Weber syndrome

Hypoxic-Ischemic Disease
  Prenatal
  Postnatal

Infection
  Prenatal meningitis/encephalitis
  Postnatal meningitis/encephalitis

Inborn Errors of Metabolism
  Pyridoxine-dependent seizures
  Maple syrup urine disease
  Phenylketonuria
  Biotinidase deficiency
  Mitochondrial disorders
  Nonketotic hyperglycinemia

Trauma

normal children. It is a progressive epileptic encephalopathy with several stages of evolution. Early infantile clonic febrile seizures, myoclonic seizures, atypical absence, and complex focal seizures occur. The EEG may be normal initially, but then deteriorates to show background slowing as well as generalized polyspike and slow-wave discharges. Thus, the clinical symptomatology, as well as the EEG, can help to differentiate these syndromes from infantile spasms.

Evaluation A thorough physical examination should initially be performed to evaluate for evidence of obvious genetic syndromes or metabolic disease. Special attention should be paid to the skin examination and may require a Wood lamp examination of fair skin to rule out tuberous sclerosis complex.

The evaluation of an infant with infantile spasms begins with an EEG. Early in the course, the EEG may be normal but usually evolves to show hypsarrhythmia. Hypsarrhythmia describes an interictal pattern of chaotic, poorly organized, high-amplitude, intermixed slow waves and multifocal epileptiform activity.

The work-up of a child with infantile spasms also includes neuroimaging with an MRI to rule out structural abnormalities. Magnetic resonance (MR) spectroscopy may be helpful to evaluate for metabolic disease. A basic metabolic work-up including plasma amino acids, urine organic acids, lactate/pyruvate, and ammonia level should be done if a metabolic disorder is suspected or if the cause is not determined through history, physical examination, or neuroimaging. Any dysmorphic child should have a high-resolution karyotype performed and should be referred for evaluation by a geneticist. Additional genetic or metabolic testing also may be necessary, depending on the individual case. An ophthalmology evaluation may help rule out metabolic, genetic, or infectious disease.

Management The best treatment for infantile spasms is still controversial. The goal of treatment is to stop the seizures, resolve EEG abnormalities, and improve the encephalopathy. The approach may be different for symptomatic and idiopathic cases. Adrenocorticotropic hormone (ACTH) and vigabatrin are the most effective drugs. A wide range of ACTH doses and treatment regimens has been used. ACTH at doses of 50 to 150 international units (IU) per meter squared per day (20 to 80 IU) is typically used for no longer than 6 to 8 weeks. Although not FDA approved in the United States, vigabatrin has been particularly helpful for children with infantile spasms and tuberous sclerosis complex. Alternative therapies include oral steroids, topiramate, valproic acid, zonisamide, and the benzodiazepines (nitrazepam, clonazepam). A challenge with 100 mg of intravenous pyridoxine should be considered in infants without an obvious etiology for their seizures to rule out pyridoxine-dependent seizures. Epilepsy surgery may also be beneficial for patients with resectable brain lesions.

Children with infantile spasms are at risk for psychomotor retardation either before or after the onset of spasms and affected patients should be evaluated by a developmental specialist during the course of their disease. They should be referred for early interventional services, including physical, occupational, and speech therapy when appropriate.

Additional Questions

1. What is the prognosis for children with infantile spasms?
2. What are the side effects of high-dose steroids such as ACTH? Of vigabatrin? Of intravenous pyridoxine?
3. Describe the ictal EEG pattern of infantile spasms.
4. What is Aicardi syndrome?

References

Baxter P. Pyridoxine-dependent and pyridoxine-responsive seizures. *Dev Med Child Neurol.* 2001;43(6):416–420.

Dulac O, Plouin P, Schlumberger E. Infantile spasms. In: Wyllie E, ed. *The Treatment of Epilepsy: Principles and Practice.* 3rd ed. Philadelphia, Pa: Lippincott Williams & Wilkins; 2001:415–452.

Dulac O, Tuxhorn I. Infantile spasms and West syndrome. In: Roger J, Bureau M, Dravet C, et al., eds. *Epileptic Syndromes in Infancy, Childhood and Adolescence*. 3rd ed. Eastleigh, UK: John Libbey; 2002:47–63.

Elterman RD, Shields WD, Mansfield KA, et al. Randomized trial of vigabatrin in patients with infantile spasms. *Neurology*. 2001;57(8):1416–1421.

Panayiotopoulos CP. *A Clinical Guide to Epileptic Syndromes and Their Treatment*. Oxfordshire, UK: Bladon Medical; 2002:36–39.

A previously healthy 5-month-old girl presents to the emergency room for evaluation of fevers and lethargy. The patient was in her usual state of health until 7 days ago when she began having fevers up to 104°F. She was seen by the pediatrician 2 days after her fevers began and was diagnosed with a viral syndrome. Over the last 2 days she has become less energetic and playful. Her oral intake has also decreased. Over the last day her parents have noticed episodes of unresponsiveness, body stiffening, and left-sided jerking lasting up to 1 minute. There are no known sick contacts but she is in daycare.

Physical Examination Vital Signs: Tachycardic and febrile. General Examination: Ill-appearing, nondysmorphic 5-month-old girl. Her anterior fontanelle is full but not bulging. Her general exam is otherwise unremarkable. Neurologic Examination: Mental Status: She is irritable and lethargic but can be aroused. Cranial Nerves: Her pupils are equal, round, and reactive to light. Her extraocular movements appear intact without gaze preference. Her face is symmetric. Her tongue is midline. Motor: She has normal bulk and tone. She withdraws her extremities purposefully with antigravity strength to minimal pain stimuli. Coordination: No abnormal movements are noted. Reflexes: 2+ symmetrically with bilateral plantar extensor responses.

Guide to Case Discussion

- Briefly summarize this case.
- Localize the examination findings.
- Give the most likely diagnosis and provide a differential diagnosis.
- Discuss an appropriate diagnostic work-up.
- Discuss the management of this patient.

Diagnosis Herpes simplex virus encephalitis.

Discussion HSV is the most common cause of encephalitis in children older than 6 months of age and adults. It accounts for 10% to 20% of all encephalitic viral infections in the United States. The incidence is 1 in 250,000 individuals per year. There is no seasonal or gender variability.

HSV encephalitis has a bimodal distribution of onset, with one-third of cases occurring in persons younger than 20 years of age and one-half occurring in persons older than 50 years of age. Two strains of HSV may be responsible. HSV-1 occurs most commonly with oropharyngeal lesions. HSV-2 is more often seen with genital infections. As such, HSV-2 is typically vertically transmitted during the neonatal period, causing 70% of cases of neonatal HSV encephalitis. Encephalitis caused by HSV-1 tends to occur in the older age groups but may also be seen in newborns. In children older than 1 month of age, infection of the CNS can result in several clinical syndromes, including herpes encephalitis, aseptic herpes meningitis, and recurrent aseptic meningitis. Some series have a relapse rate of 5% to 26%. There is also a well-described associated postviral immune-mediated encephalomyelitis. This is a proinflammatory process with normal CSF studies.

Most infections in children are presumed to be primary. In infants and older children, there may be no clear history of orofacial lesions. The initial infection with oropharyngeal HSV-1 may be silent, establishing latency in the trigeminal sensory ganglion via axoplasmic transport of the virus. Reactivation can occur with retrograde transport. However, the precise pathway of HSV into the CNS in humans is still unclear. One proposed mechanism is that primary infection spreads via the olfactory bulbs in the nose and the olfactory pathway to the orbitofrontal and medial temporal lobes. Another theory is that reactivated virus spreads to the CNS via tentorial nerves to the anterior and medial cranial fossas.

When HSV affects the CNS, it usually results in an acute, necrotizing process. However, it also can present as a diffuse, nonfocal process. Patients can have a prodrome of fever, headache, malaise, and nausea, which is followed by an acute or subacute encephalopathy with symptoms of lethargy, confusion, and delirium. Headaches, seizures, and focal neurologic deficits commonly occur. On neurologic examination, findings can include encephalopathy, cranial nerve deficits, and focal weakness. HSV encephalitis is a neurologic emergency. If untreated, mortality can reach 70%.

Summary The patient is a previously healthy 5-month-old girl who presents with 1 week of fever, lethargy, and left focal seizures. Her examination demonstrates tachycardia, fever, and a full fontanelle, in addition to altered mental status and bilateral plantar extensor responses.

Localization Lethargy is a nonspecific sign and usually indicates diffuse cerebral dysfunction. Bilateral plantar extensor responses localize to the corticospinal tracts and given her lethargy, are most likely a result of the process involving her cortex. Her left focal seizures localize to the right cortex.

Differential Diagnosis Many processes can account for this patient's signs and symptoms. Although both noninfectious and infectious etiologies can be entertained, the presence of fever, lethargy, and a full fontanelle is most consistent with an acute

CNS infection. Focal neurologic signs, such as focal seizures in this clinical setting, are suggestive of HSV encephalitis.

Possible infectious etiologies in the differential diagnosis include viral encephalitis, bacterial meningitis, fungal infection, and tuberculosis meningitis. Common viral pathogens include HSV, Enterovirus, arboviruses (West Nile virus, Japanese B encephalitis, Eastern and Western equine viruses), human herpes virus 6 (HHV6), cytomegalovirus, Epstein-Barr virus, and adenoviruses, among others. Arboviruses account for 10% of the encephalitis cases reported in the United States. Bacterial causes in this age group include *Haemophilus influenzae*, *Neisseria meningitidis*, and *Streptococcus pneumoniae*. *Mycobacterium tuberculosis* can also present in this age group, but is uncommon. Tuberculosis represents fewer than 5% of cases of bacterial meningitis in children. Fungal pathogens can include *Candida*, *Cryptococcus*, coccidioidomycosis, histoplasmosis, and aspergillosis.

The finding of a focal seizure should also prompt consideration of a brain abscess, empyema, or neurocysticercosis. Nonviral causes of aseptic meningitis such as irritation of the meninges by blood or drugs, autoimmune vasculitis, leukemia, and Kawasaki syndrome, can also be considered but are much less likely.

Although not supported by the presence of fever, traumatic brain injury, hemorrhage, or ischemic infarct could also be considered. A metabolic encephalopathy such as hypoglycemia or electrolyte imbalance might explain the lethargy and could be associated with focal seizures. Acute demyelinating encephalomyelitis can also present with seizures, as well as signs of encephalitis. The seizure semiology should preclude simple febrile seizures. A CNS tumor can cause a seizure and increased intracranial pressure can cause lethargy but would not present with a febrile illness.

Evaluation This child presents with a presumptive CNS infection and seizures. Her initial work-up in the emergency room should include laboratory testing with a CBC, blood culture, urinalysis, urine culture, basic chemistry panel, and liver function tests. A head CT with and without contrast should be performed to evaluate for intracranial abnormalities prior to a lumbar puncture, after which a lumbar puncture should be performed with CSF analysis, including cell count, glucose, protein, bacterial culture, and HSV PCR testing. The presence of HSV DNA in the CSF by HSV PCR has a sensitivity of 98% and a specificity of 94%. Prior to the advent of PCR, brain biopsy was the gold standard. The highest yield by PCR CSF analysis occurs 48 hours to 1 week after the onset of symptoms. False-negative results can occur if CSF is obtained very early in the course of the illness. The CSF profile of HSV encephalitis is typical of viral meningoencephalitis with a lymphocytic pleocytosis, increased protein, and normal glucose. There may be xanthochromia or the presence of red cells.

Additional neuroimaging with a brain MRI with and without contrast is also warranted. The brain MRI is abnormal in most cases. The herpes virus tends to affect the temporal lobes and abnormalities may include edema and necrosis. High signal is present on T_2-weighted images in the medial and inferior temporal lobes. Diffusion-weighted imaging abnormalities also can be seen and are indicative of acute ischemic change from an associated vasculitis.

Once she is stable, this child requires an EEG to evaluate for epileptiform activity. EEG abnormalities in HSV encephalitis include nonspecific spike and slow-wave activity in the first week, followed by paroxysmal sharp or triphasic waves with temporal predominance. Some patients develop periodic lateralizing epileptiform discharges (PLEDs) at 2 to 3 Hz, which originate from the temporal lobes. Although these are not specific for the diagnosis, in the appropriate clinical setting, they are highly suggestive of HSV encephalitis.

Management The patient in this case presents as a neurologic emergency. Her history of persistent high fevers, lethargy, and focal seizures signifies a serious CNS infection. She should be placed immediately on a cardiorespiratory monitor and pulse oximeter. An intravenous line should be placed and labs drawn. Her work-up should be performed quickly and she should be treated presumptively with intravenous antibiotics at meningitic doses, as well as with acyclovir, until her diagnosis is clear. For children older than 1 month of age with suspected bacterial meningitis, empiric coverage with a third-generation cephalosporin (ceftriaxone, cefotaxime) must be combined with vancomycin because of the high rate of *Streptococcus pneumoniae* resistance to penicillin.

When the diagnosis of HSV encephalitis is confirmed or strongly suspected based on clinical or radiographic features, the standard of care is intravenous acyclovir at 10 mg/kg every 8 hours for 21 days. Because prompt use of acyclovir decreases morbidity and mortality, acyclovir therapy should be instigated as soon as HSV encephalitis is suspected. Factors that influence outcome include age at diagnosis, duration of encephalitis, viral load, and initial level of consciousness. Reassessment of CSF for persistent HSV with PCR analysis is suggested upon completion of the antiviral course.

General nutritional and fluid support is important. Seizures should also be aggressively managed. Acute therapy might include benzodiazepines for status epilepticus. In this age group, loading with phenobarbital intravenously and then starting a maintenance dose is appropriate. Long-term care and neurologic rehabilitation might be necessary.

Additional Questions

1. What are other causes of PLEDs on EEG?
2. What are the most common causes of bacterial meningitis in newborns?

References

Boivin G. Diagnosis of herpes virus infections of the central nervous system. *Herpes.* 2004;11(suppl 2):48A–56A.

Bonthius DJ, Karacay B. Meningitis and encephalitis in children: an update. *Neurol Clin.* 2002;20:1013–1038.

De Tiege X, Rozenberg F, Des Portes V, et al. Herpes simplex encephalitis relapses in children. *Neurology.* 2003;61:241–243.

Fenichel GM. *Clinical Pediatric Neurology: A Signs and Symptoms Approach.* 4th ed. Philadelphia, Pa: WB Saunders; 2001:47–76.

Kennedy PGE. Viral encephalitis: causes, differential diagnosis, and management. *J Neurol Neurosurg Psychiatry.* 2004;75(suppl 1):i10–i15.

Kimberlin D. Herpes simplex virus, meningitis and encephalitis in neonates. *Herpes.* 2004;11(suppl 2):65A–76A.

Tyler KL. Herpes simplex virus infections of the central nervous system: encephalitis and meningitis, including Mollaret's. *Herpes.* 2004;11(suppl 2):57A–64A.

Whitley RJ, Kimberlin DW. Herpes simplex encephalitis: children and adolescents. *Semin Pediatr Infect Dis.* 2005;16(1):17–23.

A 5-year-old boy is brought to your office because his mother has noted that he has difficulty with activities that other children in his kindergarten class can do well. The patient sat up at 10 months and began to walk independently at 18 months. He is now unable to stand or hop on one foot. His mother complains that he runs very awkwardly and fatigues easily. He also has difficulty walking up stairs. In addition, he seems to be behind his peers in learning the alphabet, colors, and numbers. He was a full-term infant and his mother did not experience any pregnancy complications. There is no family history of neurologic disease.

Physical Examination General Examination: There is a mild spinal lordosis and tightness of the heel cords. Neurologic Examination: Mental Status: Alert. Language: He speaks in full sentences. Cranial Nerves: His pupils are equal, round, and reactive to light. His extraocular muscles are intact. His face is symmetric without weakness. His palate elevates symmetrically and his tongue is midline without fasciculations. Motor: He has mildly enlarged calves and mild diffuse hypotonia. Formal testing is difficult given his age but demonstrates lower more than upper extremity proximal weakness. When lying on the examination table, he has trouble flexing his neck against gravity. He places one hand on his knee to stabilize himself when arising from the floor. Coordination: There is no dysmetria. Sensory: No deficits are noted. Gait: He has a mildly waddling gait with toe walking and lordosis. Reflexes: 1+ throughout with bilateral plantar flexor responses.

Guide to Case Discussion

- Briefly summarize this case.

- Localize the examination findings.

- Give the most likely diagnosis and provide a differential diagnosis.

- Discuss an appropriate diagnostic work-up.

- Discuss the management of this patient.

Diagnosis   Duchenne muscular dystrophy.

Discussion   Duchenne muscular dystrophy (DMD) is the most common and severe form of childhood muscular dystrophy; it is seen in approximately 1 in 3,300 live male births. It is an X-linked, recessive neurologic disorder characterized by muscle degeneration. DMD is caused by a mutation in the dystrophin gene on chromosome Xp21. The dystrophin gene is prone to spontaneous mutations because of its large size. Two thirds of cases are familial and one third of cases arise from a new mutation. Deletions in the dystrophin gene account for the majority of mutations but duplications and point mutations also occur. Becker muscular dystrophy (BMD) is a milder, more slowly progressive form of the disease and is much less common.

Dystrophin is a critical protein in the muscle dystrophin-glycoprotein complex (DGC). Disruptions in other components of the DGC are found in other forms of muscular dystrophy. The DGC connects intracellular actin to the basal lamina in the extracellular matrix and functions to stabilize the sarcolemma through muscle contraction and relaxation. Dystrophin is expressed in skeletal muscle, smooth muscle, cardiac muscle, and brain. In muscle, it localizes to the cytoplasmic side of the plasma membrane of muscle fibers. Little or absent dystrophin is identified in cases of DMD, whereas BMD is associated with dystrophin of abnormal size and/or quantity.

A spectrum of clinical presentations is seen in children with hereditary dystrophinopathies. Boys with DMD may exhibit mild gross motor developmental delays in the first 2 years of life. The average age of walking is 18 months. Weakness and gait abnormalities (frequent falls, toe walking) are usually apparent by 3 years of age. Weakness is proximal more than distal and affects the legs before the arms. Between the ages of 3 and 6 years other features develop, such as lumbar lordosis, waddling gait, and Gower's sign. Calf hypertrophy develops as muscle fibers are replaced with fat and connective tissue. Leg pain may be common during this time. Although mental retardation is rare in this population, nonprogressive cognitive dysfunction associated with DMD may become apparent as affected children enter school. The cognitive impairment may be explained by the expression of abnormal dystrophin in brain tissue.

Between the ages of 6 and 12 years, tasks such as climbing stairs and arising from a sitting position become increasingly more difficult. Deep tendon reflexes are lost during this time but ankle jerks may be preserved well into the late stages of the disease. Contractures of the heel cords, iliotibial bands, and hips develop and are followed by the appearance of contractures in upper-extremity joints. Most children become confined to a wheelchair by the age of 12 years. Kyphoscoliosis and impaired pulmonary function soon follow. Cardiomyopathy is inevitable. Congestive heart failure and arrhythmias typically develop during the teenage years but might not cause symptoms until later stages of the disease. Most patients die between their late teen years and mid-20s. Respiratory failure or progressive cardiomyopathy are the usual culprits.

BMD has the same pathogenesis as DMD but manifests with milder symptoms and slower disease progression. The primary clinical difference between DMD and BMD is defined by the time at which independent ambulation is lost. Boys with BMD present between the ages of 5 and 15 years. They become wheelchair-bound after the age of 16 years. They typically survive into their 30s or 40s. Intermediate forms of DMD/BMD also exist. This group becomes wheelchair-bound between the ages of 12 and 16 years.

Although the dystrophinopathies almost exclusively affect males, females can experience mild to severe symptoms. The degree of severity is the result of random X chromosome inactivation (lyonization) in affected cells. Female carriers are usually asymptomatic but may have an elevated serum CK or mild calf hypertrophy. Some carriers may manifest more significant proximal weakness, as well as other symptoms of DMD/BMD-like cardiomyopathy.

Summary The patient is a healthy 5-year-old boy who presents with progressive proximal weakness, fatigability, and mild cognitive delay. His general exam demonstrates lordosis and tight heel cords, and his neurologic exam shows proximal more than distal weakness, Gower's sign, hypotonia, calf hypertrophy, hyporeflexia, and an abnormal gait (waddling, toe walking).

Localization Progressive proximal weakness appears to be this boy's primary neurologic problem. It is the cause of his difficulties with tasks such as hopping, climbing stairs, and rising from the floor without support. It also explains his lordosis, which is caused by weakness of pelvic girdle, abdominal, and back musculature. Tight heel cords and toe walking are caused by weakness of the more distal anterior tibial and peroneal musculature. Proximal weakness is usually caused by disorders of the motor unit. Thus, diseases affecting the anterior horn cell, peripheral nerve, neuromuscular junction, and muscle must be considered. However, given his presentation, a disease of the muscle seems most likely. Calf hypertrophy is relatively specific for a myopathic process, in particular DMD. Mild cognitive delay is suggestive of a global cortical process and is likely related to the patient's underlying disorder.

Differential Diagnosis The differential diagnosis of a child with progressive proximal weakness is broad and, as discussed above, includes diseases of the anterior horn cell, peripheral nerve, neuromuscular junction, and muscle. Myopathies, however, are the most common culprit.

Spinal muscular atrophy (SMA) is a motor neuron disease caused by a mutation in the survival motor neuron gene on chromosome 5. Inheritance follows an autosomal recessive pattern. SMA III presents after 18 months with proximal weakness and gait abnormalities (lordosis, waddling). Weakness may progress to involve more distal musculature. A fine action tremor is often present. Reflexes are depressed or absent. The CK may be normal or mildly increased (two to four times the upper limit of normal). Bulbar dysfunction and tongue fasciculations are sometimes present and may help distinguish SMA from other neuromuscular disorders. Intelligence is usually normal. Juvenile-onset variants of GM_2 gangliosidosis (Tay-Sachs disease) can also mimic the clinical features of later onset SMA.

Peripheral neuropathies tend to affect distal more than proximal musculature and would be unlikely to explain the symptoms seen in this case. They are not associated with muscle hypertrophy.

Neuromuscular junction diseases such as immune-mediated juvenile myasthenia gravis should also be considered. Limb-girdle myasthenia gravis in particular may present with progressive proximal weakness without oculomotor or bulbar dysfunction. Weakness may not be fluctuating as in typical juvenile myasthenia gravis. Deep tendon reflexes are usually present but can be depressed. Children are usually older than 10 years of age at onset, however.

A variety of acquired and inherited muscle diseases are also in the differential diagnosis of a child with proximal weakness. Acquired causes include inflammatory myositis (dermatomyositis, polymyositis) and infectious myositis. This child has not had any signs of illness or other organ involvement to suggest these systemic disorders. Endocrinopathies as seen with hypo-/hyperthyroidism, hypo-/hyperparathyroidism, and hypo-/hyperadrenalism can also cause a proximal myopathy, but would again be associated with additional systemic features.

Congenital myopathies usually manifest at birth with poor feeding, respiratory difficulties, and weakness. They may be associated with minor dysmorphic features not present in this patient. Congenital muscular dystrophies are a heterogeneous group of disorders that resemble congenital myopathies but, again, tend to present at younger ages. Metabolic myopathies (mitochondrial cytopathies, glycogen storage diseases) can present in childhood with proximal muscle weakness and deserve consideration. Acid maltase deficiency may even cause mild calf hypertrophy. CK values are only minimally increased in these disorders though.

Finally, the limb-girdle muscular dystrophies enter into the differential diagnosis. Limb-girdle muscular dystrophies are a related group of disorders that also are caused by disturbances in the DGC. The clinical presentation may be similar to that of DMD/BMD but cognition is usually not affected, cardiomyopathy is rare, and there is little calf hypertrophy.

Bethlem myopathy is a form of progressive limb-girdle muscular dystrophy associated with mutations in the collagen type VI gene on chromosome 21. It is transmitted by autosomal dominant inheritance. Mild proximal weakness and motor delays are common features, developing most often before 2 years of age. Contractures at the elbows, ankles, and interphalangeal joints also occur. Autosomal recessive limb-girdle muscular dystrophies (LGMD-2A, 2B, 2C, 2D, 2E, 2F) may present with slowly progressive proximal weakness, with or without facial involvement, during childhood. Pelvic or shoulder girdle musculature may be affected first. Although the presentation of DMD is relatively characteristic, the limb-girdle muscular dystrophies may be difficult to clinically differentiate from the milder BMD. These dystrophies are best distinguished by genetic testing and by immunostaining on muscle biopsy.

Evaluation The evaluation of a patient with proximal weakness should begin with measurement of the serum CK level. A markedly elevated CK level in addition to classic physical examination findings, is highly suggestive of the diagnosis of DMD. In the early phases of the disease, CK levels are usually ten times the upper limit of normal in DMD and five times the upper limit of normal in BMD.

In appropriate patients, DNA testing using PCR methods may be performed as the next step to detect a deletion or duplication in the dystrophin gene on chromosome Xp21. This test is positive in approximately 90% of patients with DMD/BMD. The availability of specific genetic testing in this disorder has significantly decreased the need for more invasive tests such as electrodiagnostic studies and muscle biopsy. However, if this test is negative, a muscle biopsy is typically performed for immunostaining or Western blot analysis for the dystrophin protein. The muscle biopsy in DMD typically shows dystrophic changes such as variation in fiber size, areas of necrosis and regeneration, hyalinization, deposition of fat, and connective tissue. Further evaluation for point mutations is challenging because of the large size of the dystrophin gene but is now clinically available.

If atypical features are present, further evaluation with EMG and NCS may be warranted prior to performing a muscle biopsy. EMG in DMD demonstrates myopathic changes (short-duration, low-amplitude, polyphasic recruited potentials; increased insertional activity; positive sharp waves; and complex repetitive discharges). NCSs usually show normal motor and sensory conduction velocities in early childhood.

Management   At the time of diagnosis, patients should be referred to a geneticist. Evaluation of family members who may be disease carriers, especially female relatives of childbearing age, is important. Genetic counseling should also be provided.

The long-term management of DMD is primarily supportive. Affected children need to be followed closely for anticipated complications. Regular monitoring by a cardiologist is required as cardiomyopathy develops at later stages. As the disease progresses, a pulmonologist should become involved in the patient's care and oversee measurement of pulmonary function tests. Scoliosis usually begins 1 to 2 years after a child has been wheelchair bound and management by an orthopaedic surgeon is required. Scoliosis surgery may help improve respiratory capacity and sitting posture. A rehabilitation specialist can be helpful in the management of contractures and can aid in prescribing appropriate adaptive equipment. Ongoing physical therapy is essential for maintaining flexibility and mobility.

The use of corticosteroids in children with DMD can slow the rate of disease progression and stabilize muscle strength. The cellular mechanisms by which steroids improve muscle strength are incompletely understood and many theories have been proposed. Although there has been little consensus on the appropriate steroid regimen in these patients, recent practice parameters have been published.

Prednisone prescribed at 0.75 mg/kg/day improves muscle strength and pulmonary function in boys with DMD. If side effects occur, lower doses (with a minimum of 0.3 mg/kg/day) can still be helpful but may produce a less-robust response. Every-other-day dosing of prednisone has not proven to have the same benefits as daily dosing. The primary side effects noted in clinical trials have been the development of weight gain and cushingoid facies 6 to 18 months after the initiation of treatment. Other known side effects of corticosteroids, such as hypertension, diabetes mellitus, osteoporosis, compression fractures, cataracts, behavior problems, and gastrointestinal bleeding, are uncommon. The risks and benefits of steroid therapy must be discussed thoroughly with the family. Excessive weight gain from steroid use may limit the physical benefits and may require decrease of the prednisone dosage. There are no standard recommendations on when to begin steroid treatment, but most clinicians will begin steroids in children older than 5 years of age when a decline in motor function has been noted. If tolerated, steroids may be continued indefinitely until a patient becomes confined to a wheelchair.

Deflazacort is a synthetic corticosteroid that is not approved for use by the FDA in the United States. It is widely used in Europe and Canada. Doses of 0.9 mg/kg/day have been used most commonly with similar efficacy. The side effects of deflazacort seem to be similar to those of prednisone but asymptomatic cataracts may be more common.

Other treatment strategies for DMD are currently under investigation. In the future, gene therapy, cell therapy with myogenic-cell transplant into abnormal tissue, and other pharmacologic therapies may be available.

References

Darras BT, Menache CC, Kunkel LM. Dystrophinopathies. In: Jones HR, De Vivo DC, Darras BT, eds. *Neuromuscular Disorders of Infancy, Childhood, and Adolescence: A Clinician's Approach.* Philadelphia, Pa: Butterworth-Heinemann; 2003:649–699.

Fenichel GM. *Clinical Pediatric Neurology: A Signs and Symptoms Approach.* 4th ed. Philadelphia, Pa: WB Saunders; 2001:171–198.

Mathews KD. Muscular dystrophy overview: genetics and diagnosis. *Neurol Clin.* 2003;21: 795–816.

Moxley RT, Ashwal S, Pandya S, et al. Practice parameter: corticosteroid treatment of Duchenne dystrophy. *Neurology.* 2005;64:13–20.

Prior TW, Bridgeman SJ. Experience and strategy for the molecular testing of Duchenne muscular dystrophy. *J Mol Diagn.* 2005;7:317–326.

Skuk D, Vilquin JT, Tremblay JP. Experimental and therapeutic approaches to muscular dystrophies. *Curr Opin Neurol.* 2002;15:563–569.

A 17-year-old boy presents to the office for concerns regarding declining academic performance. Over the last year, his grades have fallen from As and Bs to Cs and Ds, even in his favorite subjects. His parents are worried because he will soon be applying for college. His teachers are concerned about his motivation. They report that he sits in the back of the room and is often found sleeping in class. The patient asserts that he always does his homework but feels like he is having trouble with his concentration and memory. The patient is sometimes moody but overall his family has not noted a change in his behavior. He has a good appetite and enjoys going to the movies with friends, as well as playing video games. However, he recently decided to stop playing on the school basketball team. He is otherwise healthy, although approximately 6 months ago he saw a cardiologist after several suspected syncopal episodes that occurred while he was arguing with his younger brother.

Physical Examination   Vital Signs: Blood pressure 120/74 mm Hg, pulse 68 beats/min. General Examination: Normal. Neurologic Examination: Mental Status: Alert and cooperative with appropriate affect. Language: Fluent without dysarthria. Cranial Nerves: His pupils are equal, round, and reactive to light. His extraocular muscles are intact. There are no visual field deficits. His face is symmetric. His tongue is midline. Motor: He has normal bulk and tone with 5/5 strength throughout. Coordination: No dysmetria or tremor is noted. Sensory: He has normal light touch, temperature, and vibration. Reflexes: 2+ throughout with bilateral plantar flexor responses.

Guide to Case Discussion

■ Briefly summarize this case.

■ Localize the examination findings.

■ Give the most likely diagnosis and provide a differential diagnosis.

■ Discuss an appropriate diagnostic work-up.

■ Discuss the management of this patient.

Diagnosis Narcolepsy.

Discussion Narcolepsy is a chronic intrinsic sleep disorder characterized by the four core symptoms of excessive daytime sleepiness, cataplexy, sleep paralysis, and hypnagogic hallucinations. An abnormal intrusion of rapid eye movement (REM) sleep into wakefulness underlies these phenomena. All patients experience excessive daytime sleepiness and up to 80% of affected individuals have some degree of cataplexy. However, only 10% will demonstrate the full tetrad of classic symptoms. The onset of narcolepsy typically occurs around the time of puberty in childhood forms of the disease. Symptoms may be more severe and more refractory to treatment than the adult-onset form.

Chronic daytime sleepiness is characteristic of narcolepsy and is superimposed on sleep attacks. General daytime sleepiness develops subacutely over weeks to months and occurs despite adequate nocturnal sleep. Sleep attacks are characterized by the sudden onset of brief naps and may occur at any time, such as while eating or talking.

Cataplexy is a unique manifestation of narcolepsy. It is described as sudden and brief attacks of loss of muscle tone without impairment of consciousness. Cataplexy may be mild with weakness of facial or neck musculature, or generalized with more dramatic loss of complete postural tone causing falls to the ground. Cataplexy is precipitated by emotions such as laughter, surprise, or anger. It may be a presenting symptom.

Sleep paralysis is characterized by a transient inability to move or speak when transitioning between sleep and wakefulness, lasting up to several minutes long. Hypnagogic hallucinations occur at the onset of sleep and consist of auditory, visual, or tactile vivid dreamlike experiences. These episodes may be very frightening.

Children with narcolepsy are at risk for comorbid psychosocial challenges, which underscores the importance of early recognition and treatment of this condition. Affected children may become embarrassed about their symptoms, which may lead to social withdrawal. They may experience disciplining in school for sleeping in class, tardiness, suspected laziness, or performing poorly on assignments. A secondary depression may also occur.

The pathogenesis of narcolepsy was recently linked to a deficiency in the newly discovered neuropeptides, hypocretins (also known as orexins). Hypocretins, located in the lateral hypothalamus, play an important role in maintaining wakefulness. An absence of CSF hypocretin is found in most narcoleptic patients with cataplexy. The genetic markers HLA-DR2 and DQB1*0602 are associated with the disorder.

Summary The patient is a healthy 17-year-old boy who presents with multiple symptoms, including declining school performance, excessive daytime sleepiness, social withdrawal, poor concentration and memory, in addition to possible syncopal episodes (which appear provoked). His neurologic exam is normal.

Localization The patient's symptoms are relatively nonspecific but could all be explained with a diagnosis of narcolepsy. Anatomically, the symptoms of narcolepsy are related to abnormalities in the hypocretin pathways subserving the sleep–wake cycle, including the locus ceruleus and the tuberomammillary nuclei of the hypothalamus, as well as the dorsal and median raphe nuclei. Dopaminergic, cholinergic, noradrenergic, and serotonergic networks may also be involved. The suspected syncopal episodes are precipitated by anger and likely represent cataplexy. The patient in this vignette has a normal neurologic exam.

Differential Diagnosis A wide variety of disorders can be considered in the differential diagnosis of narcolepsy. More common causes of excessive daytime sleepiness in an adolescent should first be considered, including poor sleep hygiene, depression, and illegal drug or alcohol dependency. Medical causes such as hypothyroidism, head injury, lesions of the diencephalon or mesencephalon, and encephalopathy associated with toxic, metabolic, or hypoxic-ischemic causes, must also be excluded. Genetic disorders like myotonic dystrophy and Prader-Willi syndrome also are highly associated with excessive sleepiness.

Intrinsic sleep disorders responsible for excessive daytime sleepiness include obstructive sleep apnea, periodic limb movement, restless leg syndrome, Kleine-Levin syndrome, idiopathic hypersomnia, and posttraumatic hypersomnia, in addition to narcolepsy. Some children overcompensate for their sleepiness with motor hyperactivity and fidgeting, which can lead to the diagnosis of attention deficit hyperactivity disorder. Learning disabilities are also considered under some circumstances.

Sleep attacks and cataplexy are often mistaken for other paroxysmal disorders of childhood. Lapses of attention may lead to suspicions of absence epilepsy. Loss of postural tone can mimic seizure activity, syncopal episodes, and even periodic paralysis.

Evaluation The diagnosis of narcolepsy in childhood and adolescence first requires a detailed review of the patient's sleep patterns and sleep hygiene. Maintenance of a sleep diary for several weeks may be helpful in making the diagnosis. Then a thorough review of the child's medical, social, family, psychological, and academic history should be performed. Inquiries into the use of illegal drugs, alcohol, and tobacco must be made. Any school or family psychosocial stressors should be identified. The signs and symptoms of depression should also be discussed.

Screening labs, including a CBC, basic chemistries, liver function tests, thyroid function tests, and urine toxicology screen, may be helpful in excluding medical causes. A history of syncopal-like spells may prompt performing an ECG to rule out arrhythmias, as well as evaluation of blood pressure in sitting, standing, and supine positions to rule out orthostatic hypotension. A routine or video EEG also might be helpful in excluding an underlying seizure disorder. Neuroimaging is not typically indicated in the work-up of narcolepsy, but might be useful in atypical cases or if structural etiologies are being considered.

Once the diagnosis of narcolepsy is clinically suspected, further specific diagnostic testing is indicated. Nocturnal polysomnography is used to evaluate the possible diagnosis of narcolepsy but is also a tool to exclude other sleep disorders such as obstructive sleep apnea, restless leg syndrome, periodic limb movements, and Kleine-Levin syndrome. A multiple sleep latency test (MSLT) is performed the day following the sleep study. During this test, the patient is provided four or five nap opportunities over a 2-hour period. The time from the beginning of the nap until the onset of the first stage of sleep is objectively measured; then the stages of sleep are monitored for 15 minutes, after which the patient is woken up. Pathologic sleep-onset REM periods occur within 15 minutes of sleep onset. The occurrence of two or more of these episodes during the MSLT is diagnostic of narcolepsy. It should be noted that sleep lab testing is often more difficult and less standardized in children than in adults.

Management The management of narcolepsy in childhood requires a dynamic approach. Pharmacotherapy is required in most cases. Stimulant medications are the mainstay of treatment for excessive daytime sleepiness. Low doses are used initially and titrated to maximize alertness during daytime hours. Methylphenidate, dextroamphetamine, and methamphetamine have most commonly been used. Modafinil has also been shown to be effective and is usually well tolerated. Its precise mechanism of action is unknown. Pemoline is a stimulant medication that is pharmacologically distinct from amphetamines but its use is often avoided because of idiosyncratic lethal liver toxicity. Tricyclic antidepressants and fluoxetine have been beneficial in the treatment of cataplexy, sleep paralysis, and hypnagogic hallucinations. Regularly scheduled daytime naps are also recommended and may be refreshing for narcoleptics.

Psychosocial and academic issues must also be addressed in these patients. Children with narcolepsy are at risk for a concomitant depression and should be monitored for symptoms. Driving safety must also be discussed with affected adolescents and their parents. Teenagers with narcolepsy should be counseled to avoid the use of illegal drugs and alcohol that may exacerbate their symptoms. The importance of compliance with sleep hygiene recommendations, nap schedules, and pharmacologic treatment should be stressed. Proper treatment may improve cognitive skills, such as memory and concentration. However, academic performance should be closely monitored and special educational accommodations sometimes need to be made.

Additional Questions

1. What are the common side effects of stimulant medications?
2. What is Kleine-Levin syndrome?

References

Capp PK, Pearl PL, Lewin D. Pediatric sleep disorders. *Prim Care*. 2005;32:549–562.

Dyken ME, Yamada T. Narcolepsy and disorders of excessive somnolence. *Prim Care*. 2005;32:389–413.

Hood BM, Harbord MG. Pediatric narcolepsy: complexities of diagnosis. *J Paediatr Child Health*. 2002;38(6):618–621.

Wise MS, Lynch J. Narcolepsy in children. *Semin Pediatr Neurol*. 2001;8(4):198–206.

A **10-year-old girl** with a 3-week history of persistent headaches presents to the neurology office for evaluation. Her headaches have never been present in a supine position. In an upright position, she experiences a severe headache associated with nausea and vomiting. Her headaches are described as a bifrontal pressure sensation. Occasionally they are associated with mild photophobia, but there is no history of visual aura or sonophobia. The headaches have been unresponsive to over-the-counter analgesics. She denies complaints of diplopia, blurry vision, loss of vision, tinnitus, hearing loss, numbness, paresthesia, or weakness. There is no recent history of fever, rash, abdominal pain, or diarrhea. There are no identifiable triggers for the headaches, but in retrospect, the family recalls that the patient had been on rides at a local fair around the time that the headaches began. Her headaches are now incapacitating and she has not attended school for 3 weeks. An initial work-up through the pediatrician's office included a normal head CT and unremarkable routine blood work.

Physical Examination General Examination: She has tall stature, arachnodactyly, joint hyperextensibility, and left lens dislocation. There is no nuchal rigidity, papilledema, or photophobia. Neurologic Examination: Mental Status: Alert. Language: Her speech is fluent without dysarthria. Cranial Nerves: Her pupils are equal, round, and reactive to light. Her visual fields are intact. Her face is symmetric. Her palate elevates symmetrically and her tongue is midline. Motor: She has normal bulk and tone with 5/5 strength throughout. Coordination: There is no dysmetria. Sensation: She has normal light touch, temperature, vibration, and proprioception. Gait: She is briefly able to stand and walk without ataxia. Reflexes: 1+ throughout with bilateral plantar flexor responses.

Guide to Case Discussion

- Briefly summarize this case.
- Localize the examination findings.
- Give the most likely diagnosis and provide a differential diagnosis.
- Discuss an appropriate diagnostic work-up.
- Discuss the management of this patient.

Diagnosis Spontaneous intracranial hypotension in a child with Marfan syndrome and dural ectasia.

Discussion Postural headache is a common complication of procedures interrupting the dura, such as lumbar puncture, spinal anesthesia, and myelography, but also may occur as a result of a spontaneous CSF leak. The majority of CSF leaks occur along the thoracic spine or at the cervicothoracic junction. Clinically, patients with spontaneous intracranial hypotension (SIH) present with a postural headache, the cardinal feature of this condition. A severe headache is experienced in an upright position and relieved in the recumbent position. It might occur in the frontal or occipital regions, or it might involve the whole head. Additional symptoms can include nausea, vomiting, dizziness, diplopia, blurred vision, photophobia, hearing abnormalities, visual field deficits, and neck pain, among others.

Two risk factors are associated with spontaneous CSF leaks: trivial trauma and meningeal weakness. Minor traumatic events that can cause CSF leaks include coughing, lifting, falls, or participation in sports. Weakness of the meningeal sac secondary to an underlying connective tissue disorder, such as Marfan syndrome, is increasingly recognized as an important cause of SIH. Dural ectasia are a common finding in Marfan patients and predispose individuals to SIH.

Marfan syndrome is a connective tissue disorder occurring in 1 in 5,000 individuals. The skeletal, cardiovascular, and ocular systems are primarily affected, but the skin, lungs, and dura might also be involved. Marfan syndrome is caused by a mutation in the fibrillin-1 (*FBN1*) gene on chromosome 15q15-q21.1 and is inherited in an autosomal dominant fashion. Fibrillins are extracellular matrix proteins found in elastic and nonelastic tissues. Hundreds of *FBN1* mutations have been identified in Marfan patients. There is great clinical variability among patients and no clear genotype–phenotype correlations have emerged.

Summary The patient is a 10-year-old girl with physical exam findings consistent with Marfan syndrome (tall stature, arachnodactyly, joint hyperextensibility, lens dislocation) who presents with a 3-week history of incapacitating postural headaches and a normal neurologic exam.

Localization Pain and neurologic symptoms in patients with SIH are usually caused by traction on or distortion of the pain-sensitive structures of the brain, including the dura, intracranial blood vessels, cervical roots, and cranial nerves. No localizing features were found on the neurologic exam in this case.

Differential Diagnosis The positional nature of this child's headache is strongly suggestive of SIH. However, other etiologies, such as a posterior fossa tumor, meningitis, and encephalitis, should be considered. A subdural hematoma is also in the differential diagnosis given that her symptoms began after a minor trauma. Tension headache or migraine are unlikely given the presentation.

Evaluation This patient should be referred for hospitalization for a work-up of her headaches. Her evaluation should begin with neuroimaging. A brain and spine MRI with and without gadolinium should be performed. They might reveal the classic finding of abnormal thickening and enhancement of the dura. A lumbar puncture should also be attempted but may show a low opening pressure or no CSF. Identifying the specific location of the dural tear may be challenging, but both radionuclide cisternography and CT myelography have been successful in individual cases.

Management   Initial management of SIH is usually conservative with bed rest and hydration in an attempt to allow closure of the leak. Caffeine and nonsteroidal anti-inflammatory medications might be helpful for the headache. Theophylline, corticosteroids, and abdominal binders have been tried but are of unproven benefit.

When more aggressive intervention is required, cervical, thoracic, and lumbar autologous epidural blood patches have been used with variable success. Continuous epidural saline infusion has been effective in some cases. Additional techniques may include epidural injection of fibrin glue, CSF shunting, and surgical repair of leaks. Despite these interventions, relapses with recurrent SIH are common.

If the diagnosis of Marfan syndrome had not previously been made, the patient should be referred to a geneticist for both confirmation of the diagnosis and for family genetic counseling. A cardiologist and ophthalmologist also need to be involved in her long-term management to monitor for complications associated with Marfan syndrome.

Additional Questions

1. How common is postural headache after a routine lumbar puncture?
2. How would your work-up and management change if this patient also had a fever?

References

Collod-Beroud G, Boileau C. Marfan syndrome in the third millennium. *Eur J Hum Genet.* 2002;10:673–681.

Mokri B. Spontaneous intracranial hypotension. *Curr Pain Headache Rep.* 2001;5(3):284–291.

Mokri B, Maher CO, Sencakova D. Spontaneous CSF leaks: underlying disorders of connective tissue. *Neurology.* 2002;58:814–816.

Rosser T, Finkel J, Vezina G, et al. Postural headache in a child with Marfan syndrome: case report and review of the literature. *J Child Neurol.* 2005;20(2):153–155.

A healthy 8-year-old girl is brought to the emergency room for complaints of facial asymmetry that has developed over 2 days. She has had symptoms of a viral illness over the last few days including low-grade fever, decreased appetite, and fatigue. Over the last week, she has also been intermittently clumsy with fine motor movements and has been bumping into things when she walks. She is on no medications. She has had no sick contacts or recent travel. The family history is unremarkable.

Physical Examination Vital Signs: Normal. General Examination: There is no nuchal rigidity, papilledema, or photophobia. Neurologic Examination: Mental Status: Awake and oriented. Language: She has normal comprehension, repetition, and naming. There is no dysarthria. Cranial Nerves: Her pupils are equal, round, and reactive to light. Her visual fields are full. She has difficulty fully abducting her right eye. There is weakness involving the upper and lower portions of her right face with difficulty closing her eye. Her palate elevates symmetrically but her gag seems weak and she has excessive oral secretions. Her tongue is midline without fasciculations. Motor: She has normal bulk and tone. Her strength is 5/5 throughout except there is a mild left pronator drift. Coordination: She has left more than right dysmetria on finger-to-nose and heel-to-shin testing. Some decrease in left rapid alternating movements is noted. Sensory: Intact to light touch, temperature, and vibration. Gait: Her gait is slightly wide-based and she is unable to perform tandem gait. Reflexes: 3+ in the left upper and lower extremities and 2+ in the right upper and lower extremities. She has a left plantar extensor and a right plantar flexor response.

Guide to Case Discussion

- Briefly summarize this case.
- Localize the examination findings.
- Give the most likely diagnosis and provide a differential diagnosis.
- Discuss an appropriate diagnostic work-up.
- Discuss the management of this patient.

Diagnosis　Brainstem glioma.

Discussion　Brainstem gliomas account for 10% to 20% of all pediatric central nervous system tumors. While brainstem gliomas can occur at any age, they generally develop in childhood with a mean age of diagnosis between 7 and 9 years.

Histologically, fibrillary astrocytomas of the brainstem are the most common intrinsic tumor of the brainstem. Other tumor types within the brainstem include lymphoma, ganglioglioma, oligodendroglioma, and primitive neuroectodermal tumor (PNET).

Several different classification systems have been devised for brainstem gliomas. Most simply, they are divided into focal or diffuse lesions. They may then be further subdivided into the following four subgroups depending on the tumor epicenter: focal, exophytic, cervicomedullary, and diffuse. Focal tumors are well-demarcated lesions of the midbrain, pons, and/or medulla. They may be solid or cystic. There is little evidence of edema or infiltration on neuroimaging. They are usually histologically benign (grade I or II) lesions. They may present over months to years and have a more benign course than diffuse brainstem gliomas.

Dorsally exophytic brainstem gliomas arise from the subependymal glial tissue, with the bulk of the tumor residing in the fourth ventricle. They do not typically infiltrate the brainstem. They are usually low-grade lesions and may present with the slow onset of symptoms. These lesions may be difficult to distinguish from ependymomas or choroid plexus papillomas on neuroimaging. Cervicomedullary tumors are also low-grade astrocytomas originating in the medulla or cervical spinal cord. They behave like intramedullary spinal cord gliomas and have limited infiltrative capacity.

Diffuse brainstem gliomas are the most common (58% to 75%) and deadliest tumor of the brainstem. Radiographically, they are characterized by diffuse infiltration and swelling of the brainstem. The epicenter usually lies within the pons but there may be rostral or caudal extension. On brain MRI, they have poorly distinguished margins. Histologically, these aggressive tumors are usually grade II or III malignant fibrillary astrocytomas. Patients typically present with a short history of multiple cranial nerve palsies (most notably sixth and seventh nerve palsies), pyramidal signs, and cerebellar deficits. Despite multimodality treatment, 90% of patients with diffuse intrinsic brainstem gliomas die within 18 months of diagnosis.

Summary　This patient is a previously healthy 8-year-old girl who presents with a 2-day history of right facial weakness associated with a 1-week history of clumsiness and ataxia, as well as a viral syndrome. Her neurologic exam demonstrates multiple cranial neuropathies (cranial nerves VI, VII, IX, X), cerebellar abnormalities (dysmetria, dysdiadochokinesis, ataxia), left-sided weakness (pronator drift), left-sided hyperreflexia, and a left plantar extensor response.

Localization　This child has difficulty fully abducting her right eye, which represents a right abducens nerve palsy. The abducens nucleus, fascicle, or nerve could be involved. This deficit may result from a variety of brainstem processes or from other causes, such as hydrocephalus in the case of nerve involvement. Difficulty moving the right upper and lower face (peripheral facial nerve palsy) can result from involvement of the right seventh cranial nerve nucleus, fascicle, or proximal peripheral nerve. However, combined involvement of the right abducens and right facial nerve suggests right-sided pontine involvement as a result of the proximity of these structures in the brainstem. There is also evidence of medullary involvement (cranial nerves IX and X), given the weak gag and excessive secretions, suggesting dysphagia. There is no evidence of impaired upgaze or pupillary abnormalities to suggest that the midbrain is affected.

The left-sided weakness (pronator drift), hyperreflexia, and plantar extensor response localize to the corticospinal tract. Given the right-sided abducens and facial nerve involvement, most likely the right corticospinal tracts in the pons have been affected before their decussation in the medullary pyramids, giving "crossed" motor weakness. Dysmetria, dysdiadochokinesis, and gait ataxia may localize to the spinocerebellar tracts that travel through the pons. This constellation of findings involving multiple cranial nerve palsies, crossed motor weakness, and cerebellar signs is consistent with a lesion in the right brainstem (pons and medulla).

Differential Diagnosis The differential diagnosis for a disorder causing multiple cranial neuropathies, motor weakness, and cerebellar signs includes many brainstem neoplastic and nonneoplastic processes. Brainstem tumors such as glioma, PNET, lymphoma, oligodendroglioma, and ganglioglioma, should be considered and are highly likely in this patient.

Given her history of low-grade fevers, decreased appetite, and fatigue, infectious and postinfectious causes are also high in the differential diagnosis. Brainstem encephalitis (Epstein-Barr virus, herpes simplex virus, Lyme disease) or basilar meningitis (tuberculosis, fungal infection) could potentially be causes. Demyelinating diseases such as multiple sclerosis and acute disseminated encephalomyelitis (ADEM) might also affect the brainstem, with symptoms developing over several days. Paraneoplastic phenomenon (limbic encephalitis), brainstem stroke, vascular malformations, and autoimmune conditions, such as sarcoidosis, also could be considered but are less likely given her presentation.

Evaluation In the emergency room, the evaluation of this child should begin with urgent neuroimaging. A head CT with and without contrast would be useful to rule out hydrocephalus or large structural lesions, although less useful for a detailed evaluation of the posterior fossa structures. A brain MRI with and without gadolinium will ultimately be needed to provide a more definitive diagnosis.

In brainstem gliomas, the MRI typically demonstrates hyperintensity on T_2-weighted images and hypointensity on T_1-weighted images. Gadolinium enhancement can often be variable and does not influence prognosis. Magnetic resonance (MR) spectroscopy can also be used as an adjuvant in the evaluation, revealing elevated choline/creatinine ratios, decreased N-acetylaspartate (NAA) and elevated lactate suggestive of necrosis. Even though leptomeningeal spread is rare at the onset, a complete MRI of the entire spinal axis with and without gadolinium, as well as a lumbar puncture for cytology, should be performed in the initial staging evaluation. Furthermore, patients with brainstem tumors should have a thorough skin examination to rule out stigmata of neurofibromatosis type 1 (NF1) as focal brainstem tumors in NF1 may have a more benign course.

Management This patient should be admitted to the hospital for further work-up and treatment. Her management should be coordinated by a multidisciplinary team and directed by an oncologist. Input from neurosurgery is usually obtained to help decide whether biopsy and/or excision of the lesion is necessary. However, the surgical management of brainstem gliomas is controversial given the possible resultant neurologic sequelae. The classification (diffuse versus focal) and location of the tumor help guide therapeutic options such as chemotherapy and/or radiation. Corticosteroids are used in most cases, but only temporarily improve neurologic symptoms. They do not affect long-term outcome.

Radiation therapy (RT) is the standard treatment for diffuse brainstem gliomas. RT produces neurologic improvement in 70% to 80% of patients. Adjuvant chemotherapeutic approaches and novel biologic agents have been used with limited success. There is no role for surgical excision or biopsy, except possibly in atypical cases, because of the high incidence of morbidity and mortality. The overall prognosis is very poor. Focal brainstem gliomas have a more favorable prognosis. Treatment can include surgery, chemotherapy, and/or focused irradiation, depending on the individual presentation.

Additional Questions

1. How are the clinical presentations of a mesencephalic glioma and a pontine/medullary glioma different?
2. What is the anatomic course of the facial nerve?
3. What are the most common pediatric supratentorial and infratentorial brain tumors?

References

Brazis PW, Masdeu JC, Biller J. *Localization in Clinical Neurology.* 3rd ed. Philadelphia, Pa: Lippincott Williams & Wilkins; 1996:271–291.

Broniscer A, Gajjar A. Supratentorial high-grade astrocytoma and diffuse brainstem glioma: two challenges for the pediatric oncologist. *Oncologist.* 2004;9(2):197–206.

Jallo GI, Biser-Rohrbaugh A, Freed D. Brainstem gliomas. *Childs Nerv Syst.* 2004;20(3):143–153.

Packer RJ. Brain tumors in children. *Arch Neurol.* 1999;56(4):421–425.

Patten J. *Neurological Differential Diagnosis.* 2nd ed. London, UK: Springer-Verlag; 1996:162–177.

You are contacted by the emergency room to see **a previously healthy 13-year-old girl** who presents with a 2-day history of worsening headaches and vision loss. She was well when her symptoms started, but now she also complains of nausea and fever. The resident in the emergency room notes that the patient seems drowsy and slow with mental processing but is cooperative for the exam. There is no past medical or family history for headaches, migraines, or other neurologic disorders.

Physical Examination Vital Signs: Temperature, 103°F. General Examination: There is no nuchal rigidity, papilledema, or photophobia. Neurologic Examination: Mental Status: The patient is awake but mildly drowsy. Language: Her speech is fluent. She has some difficulty naming objects and repeating phrases, as well as following complex commands. Cranial Nerves: Her pupils are equal, round, and reactive to light. Her extraocular muscles are intact. She has exaggerated lateral gaze nystagmus bilaterally. Finger counting is absent in the right nasal and left temporal visual fields. Facial sensation and strength are intact. Her gag is present and her tongue is midline. Motor: She has normal bulk and tone with 5/5 strength throughout. Coordination: She has pass pointing on finger-to-nose testing bilaterally. Sensory: Light touch, vibration, and temperature are intact. Gait: A wide-based, ataxic gait is noted. Reflexes: 2+ throughout with bilateral plantar extensor responses.

Guide to Case Discussion

▓ Briefly summarize this case.

▓ Localize the examination findings.

▓ Give the most likely diagnosis and provide a differential diagnosis.

▓ Discuss an appropriate diagnostic work-up.

▓ Discuss the management of this patient.

Diagnosis   Mitochondrial encephalomyopathy, lactic acidosis, and stroke-like episodes.

Discussion   Mitochondrial encephalomyopathy, lactic acidosis, and stroke-like episodes (MELAS) is a mitochondrial disorder involving progressive encephalopathy, seizures, and stroke-like events with onset usually in childhood. On MRI, however, the strokes result from a failure of mitochondrial energy metabolism and, thus, do not follow a vascular distribution. The occipital and temporal lobes are most frequently affected.

Children with MELAS typically present between 2 and 10 years of age. Most have had previously normal development and an unremarkable medical history. Common initial presentations include seizures, headaches/migraines, recurrent vomiting, and stroke-like episodes resulting in cortical blindness, hemianopia, and hemiparesis. Proximal muscle weakness, cortical blindness, gradual decline of mentation, and sensorineural hearing loss also occur. Less common features include myoclonus, ataxia, cardiomyopathy, ophthalmoplegia, diabetes mellitus, nephropathy, gastrointestinal dysmotility, and pigmentary retinopathy. Ragged red fibers are seen on muscle biopsy using the modified Gomori trichrome stain. Life expectancy is typically shortened with death reported as occurring between 10 and 35 years of age. Individuals, however, have been reported to live past 60 years of age.

The most common mutation in MELAS is an A-to-G nucleotide switch at position 3243 in the mitochondrial tRNA^{Leu} gene MTTL1 (80% frequency). Point mutations at locations 3271 (T-to-C) and 3252 (A-to-G) in the MTTL1 are each seen in approximately 7.5% of cases. Genotype–phenotype correlations are difficult to make because of heteroplasmy (relative abundance of mutant mitochondrial DNA), the tissue distribution of mutated mitochondrial DNA and individual tissue sensitivity to impaired oxidative metabolism.

Summary   The patient is a previously healthy 13-year-old girl who presents with a 2-day history of severe headache, vision loss, nausea, and fevers. On examination she is found to have fever, encephalopathy, aphasia, left homonymous hemianopia, lateral gaze nystagmus, bilateral dysmetria, gait ataxia, and bilateral plantar extensor responses.

Localization   The patient's headache localizes to the supratentorial pain-sensitive structures surrounding the brain, including the cerebral arteries, dural arteries, large veins, and venous sinuses. Pain sensation in these structures is mediated through the trigeminal nerve. Her encephalopathy is likely the result of a diffuse cortical process. A dense left homonymous hemianopia is caused by an abnormality in the right occipital lobe. She has fluent speech with difficulty naming, repeating, and comprehending. These deficits are consistent with a Wernicke aphasia and localize to the posterior part of the superior temporal gyrus in the dominant hemisphere. Nystagmus, bilateral dysmetria, and ataxic gait localize to the cerebellum and likely represent a pan-cerebellar process. Bilateral plantar extensor responses denote involvement of the corticospinal tracts. Overall, this pattern suggests a diffuse process affecting multiple parts of the central nervous system.

Differential Diagnosis   The patient in this vignette presents with a headache, nausea, and fever in addition to multifocal neurologic deficits. Common central nervous system disorders that may present with this constellation of symptoms include an acute infectious process (encephalitis, meningitis), acute disseminated encephalomyelitis (ADEM), and vasculitis. Although the presence of fever is suggestive of a systemic process, other diagnoses, such as a cerebrovascular ischemic event, intracranial hemorrhage, brain tumor, and complex migraines, should also be considered. Finally, given that her neurologic deficits do not fit a clear vascular distribution, the onset of MELAS is another possible diagnosis.

A detailed history and thorough physical examination may suggest certain diagnoses. For example, in this case, fever suggests that she may have an infectious or postinfectious process (like ADEM) affecting different parts of the brain, although nuchal rigidity and photophobia are not present. Systemic symptoms such as fever, malar rash, and joint pain would be suggestive of a central nervous system vasculitis associated with an autoimmune disease like lupus erythematosus, but she has no additional physical complaints. Fever could also trigger decompensation in a patient with an inborn error of metabolism such as MELAS. The acute onset of neurologic deficits could suggest an ischemic event. However, this patient's symptoms have developed subacutely over 2 days and her neurologic deficits do not follow the distribution of a single artery, making an acute stroke less likely.

Thus, screening laboratory tests, neuroimaging, and electrophysiologic monitoring typically are necessary to differentiate these diagnoses. Once a mitochondrial disorder is suspected, however, MELAS must be differentiated from other mitochondrial diseases that may have similar clinical features, such as Kearns-Sayre syndrome and chronic progressive external ophthalmoplegia.

Evaluation   The patient in this case has had the progressive onset of multiple neurologic deficits. She requires hospital admission as well as a prompt diagnostic work-up. Basic laboratory studies, including basic chemistry panel, CBC, liver function tests, blood culture, and urine toxicology screen, should be performed.

A head CT, possibly with contrast, should also be performed as soon as possible to evaluate for acute stroke, hemorrhage, and signs of infection. A lumbar puncture must then be done. CSF cell count, protein, glucose, and bacterial culture should be obtained. Extra CSF can be stored for additional studies if the work-up points to an infectious or demyelinating/postinfectious etiology. An ECG should also be performed in the emergency room to rule out arrhythmias, given that an acute stroke is also in the differential diagnosis.

As the patient is stabilized, performing a routine 18-channel EEG may be considered to rule out seizure activity, postictal state, or subclinical status epilepticus as possible contributors to her encephalopathy. An evaluation by an ophthalmologist is also warranted, given her ophthalmologic abnormalities. Formal visual fields should be performed when she is able to cooperate with testing.

A brain MRI with diffusion-weighted imaging and possible magnetic resonance (MR) angiography should also follow the initial head CT and will likely be the most useful test in a patient with this type of presentation. If clinical suspicion for an inheritable metabolic process is high, the addition of MR spectroscopy to evaluate for the presence of a lactate peak should be considered.

The diagnosis of MELAS can be made based on clinical symptoms in addition to the presence of elevated lactate in serum or CSF, mildly elevated CSF protein,

MRI changes suggestive of strokes but not following a vascular distribution, and MR spectroscopy with the presence of a lactate peak. The clinical features required are: (a) onset before 40 years of age; (b) stroke-like episodes; and (c) encephalopathy with seizures or dementia. The clinical suspicion can be confirmed with a muscle biopsy showing ragged red muscle fibers on a modified Gomori trichrome stain and/or with respiratory chain enzyme studies performed on the muscle tissue showing multiple partial defects.

Molecular genetics testing for mitochondrial DNA mutations for MELAS also is commercially available. Mutations can be detected in blood leukocytes. However, heteroplasmy in mitochondrial disorders leads to variable tissue distribution, and other tissues may need to be sampled. Prenatal diagnosis is not available because of heteroplasmy in mitochondrial disorders.

Management   As noted above, the patient's initial presentation is suggestive of several different serious diagnoses and she should be admitted to the hospital for a work-up and management. She should be placed on a cardiorespiratory monitor and a pulse oximeter. An intravenous line should be placed. After her work-up is initiated, empiric intravenous antibiotic and acyclovir coverage can be considered in the event that she has meningitis or herpes simplex virus encephalitis, respectively.

Currently, there are no specific treatments for MELAS or the associated exacerbations. Many patients are placed on coenzyme Q10 and levocarnitine as a daily mitochondrial cocktail. Some reports mention the use of idebenone, a form of coenzyme Q10, which may cross the blood–brain barrier more easily. Acute episodes may also be treated with an intravenous bolus of levocarnitine, dextrose, fluids, and possibly a benzodiazepine if seizures are also suspected.

Finally, this patient should receive physical and occupational therapy to help her recover from her neurologic deficits. She should also be evaluated by a geneticist who can provide genetic counseling and can assist in the evaluation of other family members who also may be affected. Ongoing monitoring by an ophthalmologist is also necessary given her visual disturbances.

Additional Questions

1. Name two other common mitochondrial disorders. Be able to distinguish them by clinical features.

2. Describe the difference between mitochondrial and nuclear inheritance patterns.

3. What is heteroplasmy?

References

Brazis PW, Masdeu JC, Biller J. *Localization in Clinical Neurology.* 3rd ed. Philadelphia, Pa: Lippincott Williams & Wilkins; 1996:449–534.

DiMauro S, Bonilla E. Mitochondrial encephalomyopathies. In: Rosenberg RN, Prusiner SB, DiMauro S, et al., eds. *The Molecular and Genetic Basis of Neurological Disease.* Boston, Mass: Butterworth-Heinemann; 1997:201–235.

Fenichel GM. *Clinical Pediatric Neurology: A Signs and Symptoms Approach.* 4th ed. Philadelphia, Pa: WB Saunders; 2001:77–89.

Hirano M, Pavlakis SG. Mitochondrial myopathy, encephalopathy, lactic acidosis, and stroke-like episodes: current concepts. *J Child Neurol.* 1994;9(1):4–13.

Schmiedel J, Jackson S, Schäfer J, et al. Mitochondrial cytopathies. *J Neurol.* 2003;250:267–277.

A healthy 5-year-old boy is referred to your office for evaluation after experiencing a new-onset unprovoked seizure. His parents report that several days ago he had a seizure while playing, described as whole-body rhythmic jerking with his eyes rolling back in his head and lasting 3 minutes. There was no fever or illness at the time. The parents also comment that their son was seen recently by a developmental pediatrician because over the last 2 months he has been speaking less and seems to be having increasing difficulty understanding things they tell him. His development had been normal up until that time. There is no family history of seizures or developmental delay.

Physical Examination General Examination: There are no dysmorphic facial features. Neurologic Examination: Mental Status: Alert and appropriate. Language: He says a two-word phrase with some difficulty in articulation. Cranial Nerves: The pupils are equal, round, and reactive to light. His extraocular muscles are intact. His face is symmetric. The tongue is midline. Motor: He has normal bulk with mild diffuse hypotonia. Formal strength cannot be assessed but he does not appear to be weak. Coordination: There is no dysmetria grabbing for toys. Gait: He has a normal flat gait and run. Reflexes: 2+ throughout with bilateral plantar flexor responses.

Guide to Case Discussion

- Briefly summarize this case.
- Localize the examination findings.
- Give the most likely diagnosis and provide a differential diagnosis.
- Discuss an appropriate diagnostic work-up.
- Discuss the management of this patient.

Diagnosis   Landau-Kleffner syndrome (acquired epileptic aphasia).

Discussion   Landau-Kleffner syndrome (LKS), or acquired epileptic aphasia, is a form of progressive epileptic encephalopathy. LKS is associated with self-limited seizures, acquired aphasia, and characteristic paroxysmal EEG abnormalities. LKS typically presents between the ages of 2 and 8 years, with a peak incidence between 5 and 7 years of age. Boys are affected more often than girls.

Approximately 60% of children present with seizures and 70% to 80% of affected children experience associated epilepsy. Generalized tonic-clonic, atypical absence, and simple partial seizures are seen, but complex partial and other seizure types are rare. Overall, seizures in LKS are infrequent and they are usually easily controlled with conventional anticonvulsants. Seizures typically remit in adolescence.

Aphasia occurs in previously healthy children who have already acquired normal speech. The onset is insidious and subacute. A verbal auditory agnosia (word deafness) with difficulty attaching semantic meaning to sounds is the classic finding, but likely a spectrum of aphasia is seen. Initial symptoms may include a paucity of speech, difficulty understanding spoken words, and inarticulation. Jargon speech, paraphrasias, and perseverations may subsequently occur. Further deterioration to mutism has also been reported. With time, the aphasia is characterized by exacerbations and remissions. Despite the decline in verbal abilities, affected children retain their nonverbal intelligence. Behavioral abnormalities, such as hyperactivity and aggression, are also common.

The EEG in LKS may demonstrate normal background activity in the awake state, but unilateral or multifocal epileptiform activity might be noted. Foci are most common in the temporal region, but are also observed in the parieto-occipital regions. Generalized discharges may also be seen. The EEG signature of LKS, however, is the finding of electrical status epilepticus in slow sleep (ESES). ESES is activated by the onset of sleep and demonstrates a pattern of continuous bilateral spike-and-wave discharges in more than 85% of nonrapid eye movement (non-REM) slow sleep. The term ESES is often used interchangeably with the term continuous spike and waves during slow sleep (CSWS). However, CSWS is a clinical syndrome that also can be considered as a distinct entity or, possibly, a variant of LKS, where the same EEG pattern is noted in sleep but patients experience a decline in cognition or behavior but not in language skills.

The duration of LKS is highly variable. Cases of spontaneous remission within months have been reported but complete recovery is less likely as symptoms persist. Aphasia usually stabilizes and improves before adulthood. This may correlate with improvements in the EEG.

Summary   The patient is a previously healthy, developmentally normal 5-year-old boy who presents with a new-onset, unprovoked, generalized tonic-clonic seizure in addition to the subacute regression of receptive and expressive language skills. His exam is significant for expressive difficulty and inarticulation.

Localization   The patient has experienced a generalized seizure that localizes to the cortex of both cerebral hemispheres. The progressive aphasia associated with LKS is thought to arise from functional interference from epileptiform discharges in the posterior temporal auditory association cortex. The neurologic exam does not have localizing features.

Differential Diagnosis   Although considerable overlap likely exists, LKS should first be differentiated from other age-related epileptic encephalopathy variants such as CSWS. Even though both conditions have similar EEG findings, acquired aphasia is the most prominent neuropsychological abnormality in LKS, whereas CSWS is more associated with behavioral and cognitive decline.

LKS should also be differentiated from Lennox-Gastaut syndrome (LGS). LGS can occur in a similar age group. It is associated with significant EEG abnormalities (generalized 2- to 2.5-Hz slow spike-and-wave discharges) and progressive deterioration of cognitive function, in addition to tonic, atonic, and atypical absence seizures. However, epilepsy is a prominent symptom in LGS and does not resolve with time.

Finally, acquired deafness from hereditary causes, infection, or an acoustic neuroma involving the eighth cranial nerve should be ruled out in a child presenting with aphasia. Elective mutism and autism also are in the differential diagnosis. However, although children with LKS show language regression, they do not have other features of autism, such as repetitive behaviors or restricted interests. Furthermore, language disturbance occurs earlier in autism than in LKS.

Evaluation   The patient in this vignette should first undergo an EEG containing sleep to evaluate for ESES as well as other epileptiform discharges. If a routine EEG does not reveal abnormalities, admission for a 24-hour video EEG containing a full night's sleep is warranted.

A brain MRI should be performed to rule out structural abnormalities. Although neuroimaging is typically normal in children with LKS, temporal lobe pathology has been reported.

This patient should also receive a thorough neuropsychological evaluation to document his language deficits and to assess other intellectual abilities. Hearing screening needs to be performed to exclude a hearing abnormality. Referral for speech therapy is also appropriate as the aphasia is likely to be ongoing.

Management   Seizures in LKS are usually easily controlled with conventional anticonvulsants. ESES, however, is suspected to be the underlying cause of language regression and the specific treatment of ESES with or without LKS is controversial. Conventional anticonvulsants, such as valproic acid and ethosuximide, reportedly have worked in some patients. Intravenous benzodiazepines may briefly suppress EEG abnormalities and improve language abilities but is a suboptimal long-term therapy. The use of steroids and intravenous immunoglobulin reportedly also stop ESES. Finally, surgical management with multiple transpial transections in the region of epileptiform discharges is an additional controversial intervention for ESES. Intracortical horizontal fibers are disrupted while vertical fibers are spared in an attempt to prevent synchronization of epileptiform activity and preserve normal cortical function.

As mentioned above, management of a patient with LKS necessitates neuropsychological, speech/language, and, often, behavioral evaluations. Academic and behavioral accommodations are usually required through the school system for affected children.

Additional Questions

1. What are the diagnostic features of autism?
2. Describe normal language development from infancy through early childhood.

References

Grote CL, Van Slyke P, Hoeppner JA. Language outcome following multiple subpial transection for Landau-Kleffner syndrome. *Brain*. 1999;122(pt 3):561–566.

Praline J, Hommet C, Barthez MA, et al. Outcome at adulthood of the continuous spike-waves during slow sleep and Landau-Kleffner syndromes. *Epilepsia*. 2003;44(11):1434–1440.

Sinclair DB, Snyder TJ. Corticosteroids for the treatment of Landau-Kleffner syndrome and continuous spike-wave discharge during sleep. *Pediatr Neurol*. 2005;32:300–306.

Tassinari CA, Rubboli G, Volpi L, et al. Electrical status epilepticus during slow sleep (ESES or CSWS) including acquired epileptic aphasia (Landau-Kleffner syndrome). In: Roger J, Bureau M, Dravet C, et al., eds. *Epileptic Syndromes in Infancy, Childhood and Adolescence*. 3rd ed. Eastleigh, UK: John Libbey; 2002:265–283.

Tatum W, Genton P, Bureau M, et al. Less common epilepsy syndromes. In: Wyllie E, ed. *The Treatment of Epilepsy: Principles and Practice*. 3rd ed. Philadelphia, Pa: Lippincott Williams & Wilkins; 2001:551–575.

The emergency room calls for an emergent neurology consult for **a previously healthy 15-year-old girl** with complaints of lower-extremity anesthesia and weakness. Her symptoms initially began 4 days prior when she sought emergency room treatment for new-onset back pain. At that visit, a work-up for a urinary tract infection with pyelonephritis was negative and the patient was discharged home. Since her first visit to the emergency room, the patient has become increasingly weak and now can no longer feel or move her legs. She has had difficulty with urination and defecation. There is no history of trauma, fevers, illness, or drug use.

Physical Examination   Vital Signs: Normal. General Examination: There is no lymphadenopathy, rash, nuchal rigidity, or Lhermitte sign. She has a palpable suprapubic mass. There is no focal back pain to palpation. Neurologic Examination: Mental Status: Alert. Language: She has fluent speech without dysarthria. Cranial Nerves: Her pupils are equal, round, and reactive to direct light and accommodation. There is no afferent pupillary defect. Her visual acuity is 20/20 bilaterally. Her extraocular movements are intact and her visual fields are full. Her face is symmetric. Her palate elevates symmetrically and her tongue is midline. Motor: She has normal bulk. Her upper extremity strength is 5/5 bilaterally. Her lower extremities are flaccid with 0/5 strength in all muscle groups. Coordination: There is no dysmetria in the upper extremities. Sensation: There is complete anesthesia to light touch, temperature, and pinprick to the level of the umbilicus. Vibratory sensation is also impaired in the lower extremities. There is poor rectal tone. The sensory exam in the remainder of the trunk and upper extremities is normal. Reflexes: 2+ in the upper extremities and absent in the lower extremities. The plantar responses are mute.

Guide to Case Discussion

▪ Briefly summarize this case.

▪ Localize the examination findings.

▪ Give the most likely diagnosis and provide a differential diagnosis.

▪ Discuss an appropriate diagnostic work-up.

▪ Discuss the management of this patient.

Diagnosis Acute transverse myelitis of the thoracic spine.

Discussion Acute transverse myelitis (ATM) is a focal inflammatory disorder of the spinal cord that affects motor, sensory, and autonomic fibers. It occurs in 1 to 4 million individuals each year and has no family or gender predisposition. There is a bimodal age of onset, with the highest incidence occurring between the ages of 10 and 19 years and 30 and 39 years. Patients experience acute or subacute onset of lower-extremity weakness, sensory loss, and autonomic symptoms (bowel/bladder incontinence, inability to void, constipation) over hours, days, or weeks. Dysesthesia, or pain, can be an important initial symptom. Fever or meningismus may also be present. The majority of cases (80%) occur in the thoracic region.

ATM can exist in isolation or as part of a demyelinating syndrome such as multiple sclerosis, Devic disease (neuromyelitis optica), or acute disseminated encephalomyelitis (ADEM). These disorders occur on a clinical continuum, making the classification of idiopathic ATM still controversial. It may also be seen in other immune-mediated or systemic inflammatory disorders. Recently proposed diagnostic criteria for ATM include: (a) the development of sensory, motor or autonomic dysfunction attributable to the spinal cord; (b) bilateral signs/symptoms; (c) a clearly defined rostral border of sensory dysfunction; and (d) inflammation of the spinal cord (demonstrated by CSF pleocytosis, elevated immunoglobulin IgG index or MRI abnormalities). In addition, there must be a progression to nadir from 4 hours to 21 days from the onset of symptoms.

The underlying pathogenesis of ATM is poorly understood but is thought to be caused by dysregulation of the immune system, as in other demyelinating diseases. Sixty percent of patients experience a preceding viral infection, a shared feature with ADEM.

The overall prognosis of ATM is variable. One third of affected individuals have no sequelae, one third have a moderate disability, and one third are left with a severe disability. Rapid progression, back pain, and symptoms of spinal shock carry a worse prognosis.

Summary The patient is a previously healthy 15-year-old girl who presents with a 4-day history of back pain, progressive lower-extremity weakness/anesthesia, and bowel/bladder dysfunction. Her exam is remarkable for symmetric, lower-extremity, flaccid paralysis, complete anesthesia to all sensory modalities to the umbilicus, absent lower-extremity reflexes, a palpable bladder, and poor rectal tone.

Localization This adolescent's constellation of findings (lower-extremity paralysis, anesthesia, areflexia, autonomic dysfunction) localize to the spinal cord. There is no apparent cortical involvement. The cranial nerves, cerebellar function, and upper extremities are unaffected.

Anesthesia to all sensory modalities (light touch, temperature, pain, vibration, and proprioception) is characteristic of a complete transverse myelitis. This patient has sensory loss to the level of the umbilicus, which localizes to one to three spinal segments above T10. The ventral spinothalamic tract (light touch) and lateral spinothalamic tract (pain and temperature) fibers enter the spinal cord ipsilaterally and ascend for several segments before decussating in the ventral white commissure to the contralateral side. The absence of vibratory sensation results from posterior column involvement. Her symmetric lower-extremity weakness can be explained by a lesion also involving the descending corticospinal tracts below the level of the lesion. Her bladder/bowel dysfunction is a result of involvement of the autonomic pathways that also pass through this portion of the spinal cord.

Absent reflexes could suggest a lower motor neuron process. However, given the relatively acute onset and associated symptoms, areflexia is more likely a result of an acute upper motor neuron (spinal shock) process. Back pain is a non-specific symptom but can accompany injury to the spinal cord. Thus, there appears to be complete thoracic cord transection with interruption of both ascending and descending tracts traveling through the lesion.

Differential Diagnosis   The diagnosis of idiopathic ATM is one of exclusion. When considering the differential diagnosis of acutely progressive lower-extremity weakness, anesthesia, and autonomic dysfunction, potentially reversible spinal cord processes must be considered first. Lesions of the spinal cord are divided into two groups by location. Extramedullary lesions lie outside the spinal cord and can be either extradural or intradural. They typically cause spinal cord compression. Intramedullary lesions lie within the spinal cord. Extramedullary tumors are more common in adults, whereas intramedullary tumors are more common in the pediatric population.

In children, extradural tumors can include neuroblastomas, ganglioneuromas, and sarcomas. An epidural abscess, hematoma, or metastasis may also occur in this region. Intradural lesions usually include meningiomas, neurofibromas, lipomas, and angiomas. Astrocytomas and ependymomas are the most common intramedullary tumors in childhood. Others include gangliocytomas, gangliogliomas, germinomas, primitive neuroectodermal tumors, and Langerhans cell histiocytosis. Congenital tumors (dermoids, epidermoids) or a syrinx may also be found in an intramedullary location.

Numerous other causes then need to be considered. Vascular abnormalities, such as a spinal arteriovenous malformation or spinal cord infarction, may produce an acute myelopathy. Symptoms usually evolve quickly (in less than 4 hours) in these cases, however. Systemic autoimmune conditions (systemic lupus erythematosus, sarcoidosis, Behçet disease, mixed connective tissue disease, Sjögren syndrome) deserve consideration. They may cause a vasculitis that results in a myelopathy. Parainfectious etiologies are also commonly responsible. A long list of pathogens that may be involved include *Borrelia burgdorferi* (Lyme disease), herpes simplex virus, HIV, West Nile virus, syphilis, Epstein-Barr virus, *Mycoplasma pneumoniae*, human T-cell lymphocytic virus-1 (HTLV-1), varicella virus, cytomegalovirus, and enterovirus, among others. Prior radiation to the spinal cord may also cause similar symptoms. Finally, in certain cases, adrenomyeloneuropathy, a leukodystrophy, may enter the differential diagnosis.

ATM must also be distinguished from other demyelinating syndromes seen in children and adolescents. Multiple sclerosis is uncommon in children. Children 12 years of age and older seem to be more predisposed to the development of multiple sclerosis whereas younger children experience ADEM. Multiple sclerosis is less likely than ATM and ADEM to have a preceding viral infection. Symptoms may fluctuate and usually begin with sensory (paresthesia) or visual disturbances (optic neuritis, diplopia). Although different specific diagnostic criteria for multiple sclerosis exist, in general, affected individuals experience two white matter lesions on brain MRI (separated by time) in addition to two discrete clinical attacks. Supportive lab data are also required for a more definitive diagnosis. In addition, ATM can be distinguished from multiple sclerosis by the symmetrical clinical motor/sensory findings, predominance of motor symptoms, MRI lesions extending greater than two spinal segments, and a normal brain MRI.

ADEM or postinfectious encephalomyelitis most often occurs in childhood (0.4 per 100,000 individuals) and accounts for 10% to 15% of acute pediatric encephalitis cases. It usually occurs in a previously healthy child following an infection or, rarely, vaccination. It is characterized by a monophasic, central nervous system demyelinating process involving both white and gray matter (thalami, basal ganglia). There is less predilection for the periventricular white matter as seen in multiple sclerosis. Neurologic symptoms may include seizures, altered consciousness, motor weakness, cranial neuropathy, sensory deficits, and/or ataxia. The pathogenesis is not completely understood, but likely involves autoreactive T-cell activation by viral/bacterial antigens.

Devic disease also tends to occur shortly after a viral infection or immunization. Optic neuritis and ATM might occur simultaneously or develop in succession. The optic neuritis is usually bilateral and ATM is usually severe. Many children who develop Devic disease after the age of 12 years will later develop multiple sclerosis.

Finally, other causes of an ascending paralysis, such as Guillain-Barré syndrome and tick paralysis, may initially enter the differential diagnosis. However, given that there is a clear sensory level, peripheral nervous system diseases such as these seem unlikely.

Evaluation This adolescent girl presents with an acute spinal cord process that is a neurologic emergency. She first requires an urgent MRI of the entire spine with and without gadolinium. Particular attention should be given to the mid to lower thoracic spinal cord, which appears to be affected on her neurologic exam. The MRI of the spine first helps to exclude extramedullary processes (discussed above) that might require immediate surgical intervention. Neurosurgery should be consulted immediately if a surgically amenable lesion is identified.

The spinal MRI is also helpful in demonstrating intramedullary lesions secondary to myelitis (demyelinating, infectious, postinfectious, autoimmune disorders) or spinal cord malignancies (primary, metastatic). Contrast enhancement may be seen with these lesions. Short-tau inversion recovery (STIR) and fast short-tau inversion recovery (FSE) are among the most sensitive means of detecting abnormalities of cord signal. However, the spinal MRI in transverse myelitis can initially be normal in approximately 5% of patients.

Once the diagnosis of transverse myelitis is confirmed, a brain MRI with and without gadolinium should be obtained to investigate possible involvement of the cerebral white matter that can occur with a demyelinating disease such as ADEM or multiple sclerosis. Also, the optic nerves should be carefully evaluated with contrast in the event that the patient has Devic disease. Depending on other clinical and lab findings, optic nerve involvement also may support a diagnosis of multiple sclerosis. In addition, leukodystrophies may demonstrate characteristic findings on brain MRI that might suggest a specific underlying diagnosis.

Once a structural cause has been ruled out by MRI and the diagnosis is more clear, a lumbar puncture should be performed to help distinguish inflammatory from noninflammatory processes. CSF should be sent for cell count, glucose, protein, myelin basic protein, oligoclonal bands, IgG synthesis, and cytology. CSF findings in ATM are abnormal in more than 60% of patients and often show a mild lymphocytic pleocytosis, elevated total protein, and myelin basic protein with occasional oligoclonal bands. If there is concern for an infectious or postinfectious process, extra CSF can be obtained to evaluate for infections such as Lyme disease, Epstein-Barr virus, or *Mycoplasma pneumoniae*, by using antibody titers or PCR testing for specific pathogens.

Serum studies are also typically done to exclude other possible diagnoses. Initial screening labs might include CBC, basic chemistry panel, liver function tests, erythrocyte sedimentation rate, ANA, vitamin B_{12} level, and thyroid function tests. If Devic disease is suspected, serum testing for the presence of the neuromyelitis optica (NMO) antibody can be clinically performed. It is positive in as many as 70% of cases and helps to distinguish Devic disease from multiple sclerosis. If an autoimmune vasculitis is suspected, testing with angiotensin-converting enzyme, anti–double-stranded DNA antibody, SS-A (Ro), SS-B (La), lupus anticoagulant, complement levels, and $beta_2$-glycoprotein 1 can be done. Under certain circumstances, additional testing might include HIV, HTLV-1, and very-long-chain fatty acids (adrenomyeloneuropathy). Serum antibody titers might also be done to evaluate for the infections mentioned above.

Electrodiagnostic studies (SSEPs, VERs, BAERs) may have value in determining the extent of neural injury and prognosis for recovery. In particular, VERs may detect subtle optic nerve involvement, consistent with several demyelinating diseases.

Management   This patient should be admitted to the hospital for further management. Given her distended bladder, a Foley catheter should be placed immediately. A bowel regimen should also be started.

There are no proven therapies for ATM. However, the majority of clinicians treat with corticosteroids, as ATM lies within the spectrum of demyelinating diseases seen in childhood and there is hope that some benefit may be gained. Although there are no clear guidelines on corticosteroid dosing, methylprednisolone at 20 mg/kg/day (maximum dose of 1 g) given intravenously for 3 to 5 days is commonly used. A taper of oral steroids for 3 to 6 weeks after the initial intravenous steroid therapy is also often prescribed. Gastric acid-reducing medications should be provided while a patient is on high-dose corticosteroids.

Once stabilized, this adolescent would benefit from physical and occupational therapy. Ongoing rehabilitation might also be required. Chronic immunomodulatory therapy is not typically prescribed in children or adolescents with ATM, although it has an important preventative role in the management of multiple sclerosis. In addition, intravenous immunoglobulin and plasmapheresis are occasionally used in the treatment of other demyelinating disorders (ADEM) but are not considered useful in ATM.

Additional Questions

1. How can one clinically distinguish conus medullaris from cauda equina syndrome?

2. What is the differential diagnosis for ascending and descending paralysis in childhood?

3. What are the side effects of corticosteroids?

References

Barkovich AJ. *Pediatric Neuroimaging*. 3rd ed. Philadelphia, Pa: Lippincott Williams & Wilkins; 2000:685–714.

Brazis PW, Masdeu JC, Biller J. *Localization in Clinical Neurology*. 3rd ed. Philadelphia, Pa: Lippincott Williams & Wilkins; 1996:79–108.

Krishnan C, Kaplin AI, Deshpande DM, et al. Transverse myelitis: pathogenesis, diagnosis and treatment. *Front Biosci*. 2004;9:1483–1499.

Leake JAD, Albani S, Kao AS, et al. Acute disseminated encephalomyelitis of childhood: epidemiologic, clinical and laboratory features. *Pediatr Infect Dis J*. 2004;23(8):756–764.

Lennon VA, Wingerchuk DM, Kryzer TJ, et al. A serum autoantibody marker of neuromyelitis optica: distinction from multiple sclerosis. *Lancet*. 2004;364:2106–2112.

Menge T, Hemmer B, Nessler S, et al. Acute disseminated encephalomyelitis. *Arch Neurol*. 2005;62:1673–1680.

Rust RS. Multiple sclerosis, acute disseminated encephalomyelitis, and related conditions. *Semin Pediatr Neurol*. 2000;7(2):66–90.

Scotti G, Gerevini S. Diagnosis and differential diagnosis of acute transverse myelopathy. The role of neuroradiological investigations and review of the literature. *Neurol Sci*. 2001;22(suppl 2):S69–73.

Transverse Myelitis Consortium Working Group. Proposed diagnostic criteria and nosology of acute transverse myelitis. *Neurology*. 2002;59(4):499–505.

A **16-year-old girl** is brought to the neurology office for complaints of muscle pain. She is having trouble with the school system because her gym teacher thinks she has a poor attitude. When participating in sports, she often stops playing because she says her muscles hurt. Her mother noted that even at a younger age she had less endurance and fatigued much more easily than her peers. After she tries to run, her mother sometimes has to rub her calves because she complains of stiffness and cramps that may last several hours. She is otherwise a healthy child. Her development has been normal.

Physical Examination General Examination: There are no dysmorphic features. Neurologic Examination: Mental Status: Alert. Cranial Nerves: Her pupils are equal, round, and reactive to light. Her extraocular muscles are intact. Her face is symmetric with normal strength. Her gag is strong. The tongue is midline without fasciculations. Motor: She has normal bulk and tone with 5/5 strength throughout. Sensory: No deficits are noted. Gait: She has a normal heel, toe, flat, and tandem gait. Reflexes: 2+ throughout with bilateral plantar flexor responses.

Guide to Case Discussion

- Briefly summarize this case.

- Localize the examination findings.

- Give the most likely diagnosis and provide a differential diagnosis.

- Discuss an appropriate diagnostic work-up.

- Discuss the management of this patient.

Diagnosis   Myophosphorylase deficiency (McArdle disease).

Discussion   McArdle disease is an autosomal recessive metabolic myopathy and glycogen storage disease caused by a mutation on chromosome 11q13. Myophosphorylase deficiency is also known as glycogen storage disease type V. This enzyme functions to break down glycogen in skeletal muscle. A deficiency of myophosphorylase results in symptoms such as myalgia, stiffness, cramps, fatigability, and myoglobinuria. Exercise intolerance is usually seen in younger children, whereas muscle cramps and myoglobinuria usually do not begin until adolescence or early adulthood. McArdle disease has a male predominance.

Symptoms are usually brought on by brief, intense exercise (heavy lifting), or by less-intense but sustained exercise (climbing stairs). Many affected individuals describe a "second wind" phenomenon. After a brief rest they may resume exercise without recurrent symptoms. Between attacks, patients may have mild proximal weakness (especially in adults at later stages of the disease) or may have normal muscle strength. Myoglobinuria occurs in approximately 50% of affected individuals and is associated with muscle necrosis. Myoglobinuria typically appears as "cola-colored" urine and may be mistaken for hematuria. Later in life, many patients develop secondary renal failure.

Summary   The patient is a healthy 16-year-old girl who presents with complaints of myalgia, muscle stiffness, cramps, and fatigability. Her neurologic exam is normal.

Localization   The patient in this vignette has a normal neurologic exam. However, symptoms of myalgia, muscle stiffness, cramps, and fatigability localize to the muscle.

Differential Diagnosis   The complaints of myalgia, cramps, and stiffness with exercise are strongly suggestive of a metabolic myopathy. Additional symptoms can include exercise intolerance, myoglobinuria, and proximal or distal weakness. Skeletal muscle has high energy demands. Enzymatic defects in glycogen, fatty acid oxidation, and mitochondrial (respiratory chain) pathways can cause very similar symptoms. A careful clinical history, family history, and physical exam, in addition to a thorough diagnostic work-up, are often necessary to arrive at a precise diagnosis.

Disorders of glycolysis and glycogenolysis, such as McArdle disease, are typically considered together. There are many of them and there is significant overlap in symptomatology. Enzyme deficiencies of phosphofructokinase, phosphorylase B kinase, phosphoglycerate kinase, phosphoglycerate mutase, and lactate dehydrogenase can closely clinically resemble McArdle disease, causing exercise intolerance, myalgias, cramps, and myoglobinuria (Table 31.1). Although myophosphorylase deficiency affects only muscle, other glycogenoses may have other organ involvement. Cardiomyopathy, hepatomegaly, and hepatic dysfunction are seen in many of the infantile forms. The clinical features of these disorders vary, depending on the level of enzyme deficiency and the age at presentation. In patients with myoglobinuria, common causes, such as trauma or infection, should be ruled out first.

Disorders of fatty acid oxidation (FAO) should also be considered in a child with a suspected metabolic myopathy. Fatty acids provide essential energy to muscle and brain tissue during fasting states, as liver glycogen stores are depleted after a few hours of starvation. This group of disorders presents with symptoms

TABLE 31.1

Glycogen Storage Diseases

Enzyme Defect	Type	Eponym	Onset	Exercise Intolerance, Myalgia, Cramps	Myoglobinuria	Cardiomyopathy	Hepatomegaly	Other
Alpha-glucosidase	II	Pompe	Infancy, childhood, adulthood			Yes (infancy)	Yes (infancy)	Profound weakness, hypotonia in infancy; proximal weakness in childhood and adulthood.
Debrancher	III	Cori-Forbes	Infancy, childhood, adulthood			Yes (infancy)	Yes (infancy)	Hypotonia, weakness, hypoglycemia in infancy; proximal weakness in childhood and adulthood.
Brancher	IV	Andersen	Infancy, childhood, adulthood			Yes (infancy)	Yes (infancy)	Hypotonia, weakness, hepatic failure in infancy; proximal weakness in childhood and adulthood.
Myophosphorylase	V	McArdle	Childhood, adulthood	Yes	Yes			

(Continued)

TABLE 31.1

Glycogen Storage Diseases (continued)

Enzyme Defect	Type	Eponym	Onset	Exercise Intolerance, Myalgia, Cramps	Myoglobinuria	Cardiomyopathy	Hepatomegaly	Other
Phosphofructokinase	VII	Tarui	Childhood, adulthood	Yes	Yes			Jaundice, hemolytic anemia, gout
Phosphorylase B kinase	VIII		Infancy, childhood, adulthood	Yes	Yes	Yes	Yes	
Phosphoglycerate kinase	IX		Infancy, childhood, adulthood	Yes	Yes			Seizures, retardation
Phosphoglycerate mutase	X		Adulthood	Yes	Yes			
Lactate dehydrogenase	XI		Adolescence, adulthood	Yes	Yes			Rash

such as recurrent myoglobinuria, progressive lipid storage myopathy, neuropathy, recurrent hypoglycemic hypoketotic encephalopathy (Reye-like syndrome), seizures, and mental retardation. FAO disorders are important to diagnose because many may be fatal if not promptly recognized and treated. Affected children are particularly vulnerable to metabolic decompensation with fasting, illness, exercise, or stress. There is also frequent chronic involvement of energy-dependent tissues such as the brain, muscle, and liver.

Examples of FAO disorders include carnitine palmityl transferase (CPT) I and II, short-chain acylcoenzyme-A dehydrogenase (SCAD), medium-chain acylcoenzyme-A dehydrogenase (MCAD), long-chain acylcoenzyme-A dehydrogenase (LCAD), and very-long-chain acylcoenzyme-A dehydrogenase (VLCAD) deficiencies. CPT II deficiency is an autosomal recessive disorder caused by a mutation on chromosome 1p32. In adolescents and adults, it can cause exercise intolerance and recurrent myoglobinuria. Symptoms of myalgia and muscle swelling occur after sustained aerobic exercise and sometimes after prolonged fasting. These patients are also at risk for malignant hyperthermia. VLCAD deficiency can occur during childhood and is associated with myalgia and myoglobinuria with prolonged exercise or fasting. Weakness during attacks can be profound. Frequent carbohydrate meals may prevent and alleviate symptoms in patients with both CPT II and VLCAD deficiency. The patient in this vignette is developmentally normal, has no other organ involvement, and has not become symptomatic with fasting. Consequently, an FAO disorder seems unlikely.

Mitochondrial diseases are a heterogeneous group of disorders. There is great variation in age of presentation, organ system involvement, and distribution of weakness. Defects in substrate transport, substrate oxidation, Krebs cycle, respiratory chain, and oxidative phosphorylation have been recognized. Although an isolated mitochondrial myopathy is possible, other organ system involvement is typical. Affected patients may have a history of developmental delay, hypotonia, peripheral neuropathy, seizures, ataxia, sensorineural hearing loss, retinopathy, ophthalmoplegia, and/or optic atrophy. Also, in contrast to McArdle disease, blood lactate levels are elevated during exercise in these patients. Again, the patient in this case does not fit the clinical picture of a mitochondrial disorder.

Myoadenylate deaminase deficiency (MAD) is also in the differential diagnosis of a patient with McArdle disease. MAD is an autosomal recessive disorder caused by a mutation in the *AMP1* gene on chromosome 1p. Onset is typically during late childhood. The characteristic clinical feature is myalgia on exertion. Muscle pain may be described as achy or cramping. Myoglobinuria occurs in a minority of patients. During attacks, the CK may be normal or elevated. The ischemic forearm test might be helpful in the diagnosis as ammonia levels fail to rise and lactate remains normal.

Finally, other muscle disorders such as inflammatory myopathies, infectious myopathies, toxic myopathies, endocrine myopathies, muscular dystrophies, congenital myopathies, myotonic dystrophy, and neuromuscular junction disorders seem unlikely given this adolescent's presentation and the fact that she is otherwise healthy and symptomatic only with exercise.

Evaluation Any patient presenting with a suspected myopathy should first have a serum CK level checked. In McArdle disease, it is typically mildly elevated at rest, which is in contrast to most other metabolic myopathies. A baseline electrolyte panel with BUN and creatine should also be checked to assess kidney function.

In the past, the diagnosis of McArdle disease required the ischemic forearm test. This test is useful in diagnosing defects in the glycogenolytic and glycolytic pathways. Baseline lactate and ammonia levels are drawn from the antecubital vein. A blood pressure cuff is then inflated around the patient's forearm to above the systolic blood pressure and the patient is asked to open and close the fist repeatedly. Repeat lactate and ammonia levels are drawn at regular intervals. Normally, the blood lactate level is increased to three to five times the baseline level and ammonia is elevated to five to ten times the baseline level 1 to 2 minutes after exercise. In McArdle disease, the absence of myophosphorylase prevents the breakdown of glycogen and the venous lactate response is flat with an exaggerated ammonia level. This test, however, is highly dependent on the patient's ability to cooperate and can be difficult to perform in children. Muscle cramping, myalgia, and myoglobinuria can occur during the test. A nonischemic forearm test has also been performed in these patients. It may be better tolerated and can also be useful in the diagnosis.

Currently, the diagnosis of McArdle disease can be made most easily by performing molecular genetic testing on leukocytes for common mutations in the myophosphorylase gene on chromosome 11q13. The availability of genetic testing has made the need for more invasive tests such as EMG and muscle biopsy unnecessary in many cases. However, if genetic testing is not available or the case is atypical, other studies might be required. The EMG may be normal or may show myopathic changes. Myophosphorylase activity is normal in erythrocytes, leukocytes, platelets, and fibroblasts, and only immunohistochemistry on muscle tissue can document abnormally low activity of the enzyme. The muscle biopsy in McArdle disease demonstrates subsarcolemmal and intermyofibrillar deposits of glycogen. Electron microscopy shows normal-appearing glycogen between myofibrils. Deficiency of myophosphorylase in muscle tissue is diagnostic.

In a patient who requires consideration of other metabolic myopathies, additional metabolic work-up may be warranted. Diagnostic testing for disorders of fatty acid oxidation include serum glucose measurement, liver function tests, serum ammonia, serum lactate, urine ketones, plasma total and free carnitine, serum acylcarnitines, urine acylcarnitines, and urine organic acids. Testing during an acute episode of metabolic decompensation is particularly important. Fasting studies are also occasionally performed, but must be done under controlled circumstances by experienced clinicians. Screening investigations for mitochondrial diseases might include a serum lactate/pyruvate and mitochondrial DNA testing. Muscle biopsy may be required, however, to arrive at a specific diagnosis.

Management There are no specific therapies available for McArdle disease. Management is usually symptomatic. Affected individuals should avoid strenuous or prolonged exercise. Patients who develop significant muscle necrosis with myoglobinuria should be closely monitored for renal failure. Muscle swelling caused by necrosis can also cause a compartment syndrome.

Several therapeutic interventions have been tried, unfortunately without clear benefit. Treatment strategies have been aimed at bypassing the metabolic block. Patients have been given additional glycolytic substrates of glucose, fructose, ribose, and amino acids. High-protein diets have also been tried, based on the hypothesis that branched-chain amino acids may serve as an alternative fuel source for glycogen. Vitamin B_6 has been given to patients because pyridoxal phosphate is depleted in McArdle disease. However, creatine supplementation in low doses was shown to improve muscle function in one study. In the future, gene therapy may hold promise for these patients.

Additional Questions

1. What is the typical clinical presentation of a child with MCAD deficiency?
2. What is Reye syndrome and what causes it?

References

Bruno C, Hays AP, DiMauro S. Glycogen storage diseases of muscle. In: Jones HR, De Vivo DC, Darras BT, eds. *Neuromuscular Disorders of Infancy, Childhood, and Adolescence: A Clinician's Approach.* Philadelphia, Pa: Butterworth-Heinemann; 2003:813–832.

Darras BT. Myoadenylate deaminase deficiency. In: Jones HR, De Vivo DC, Darras BT, eds. *Neuromuscular Disorders of Infancy, Childhood, and Adolescence: A Clinician's Approach.* Philadelphia, Pa: Butterworth-Heinemann; 2003:861–866.

Gordon N. Glycogenosis type V or McArdle's disease. *Dev Med Child Neurol.* 2003;45:640–644.

Kazemi-Esfarjani P, Skomorowska E, Jensen TD, et al. A nonischemic forearm exercise test for McArdle disease. *Ann Neurol.* 2002;52:153–159.

Tein I. Metabolic myopathies. In: Swaiman KS, Ashwal S, eds. *Pediatric Neurology: Principles and Practice.* 3rd ed. St. Louis, Mo: Mosby; 1999:1264–1289.

Victor M, Ropper AH. *Adams and Victor's Principles of Neurology.* 7th ed. New York: McGraw-Hill; 2001:1512–1528.

The patient is **a 12-year-old Hispanic girl** who presents for evaluation of a progressively abnormal gait. The patient began to have balance problems approximately 2 years prior to the clinic visit. She does not feel weak, but is often clumsy and falls. One year ago she was taken to the emergency room after a significant fall and her mother was told a head CT was normal. The patient also has slowly developed shakiness in her hands and will spill cups of fluid when drinking. Her birth history was unremarkable. She met all developmental milestones on time and is now an A and B student in regular classes. There is no family history of neurologic disease.

Physical Examination General Examination: Normal. Neurologic Examination: Mental Status: Alert. Language: She has fluent speech without dysarthria. Cranial Nerves: Her pupils are equal, round, and reactive to light. Her extraocular muscles are intact but she has dysmetric saccadic eye movements. Her facial movements are symmetric. Her palate elevates symmetrically and her tongue is midline. Motor: She has normal bulk and tone with 5/5 strength throughout. Coordination: There is significant dysmetria on finger-to-nose testing as well as dysdiadochokinesis bilaterally. Sensory: Vibration, pinprick, and cold sensation are intact. There is decreased proprioception in the toes. Gait: She has a wide-based and ataxic gait. Romberg testing is abnormal. Reflexes: Absent throughout. Bilateral plantar extensor responses are noted.

Guide to Case Discussion

- Briefly summarize this case.
- Localize the examination findings.
- Give the most likely diagnosis and provide a differential diagnosis.
- Discuss an appropriate diagnostic work-up.
- Discuss the management of this patient.

Diagnosis   Friedreich ataxia.

Discussion   Friedreich ataxia is the most common form of inherited ataxia. It usually presents in childhood or adolescence, but cases of onset in adulthood have been reported.

Friedreich ataxia is an autosomal recessive disorder caused by an expansion of the GAA triplet in the *FRDA* gene on chromosome 9q13. Normal individuals have fewer than 33 GAA repeats, whereas individuals affected with Friedreich ataxia have 67 to 1,000 repeats. This mutation results in a deficiency of the protein product frataxin. Even though the functions of frataxin are still under investigation, current research suggests that it has an important role in the biosynthesis of iron and sulfur cluster in mitochondrial proteins, including those involved in the respiratory chain such as complexes I, II, and III. The resultant decrease in iron/sulfur clusters causes a decrease in cellular energy production and an increase in free radicals. Iron storage builds up in the mitochondria as a secondary event. Understanding the biologic functions of frataxin in mitochondrial iron homeostasis and free radical toxicity is critical to developing therapies for this disorder.

Pathologically, degeneration of the cerebellum, pons, and medulla occurs. Spinal cord abnormalities are striking. There is early loss of the large sensory neurons in the dorsal root ganglia with subsequent involvement of the posterior columns, spinocerebellar tracts, and corticospinal tracts. The afferent visual pathways may be affected. Cardiomyocytes and beta-pancreatic islet cells also degenerate.

Clinically, affected individuals initially demonstrate truncal and gait ataxia, which is followed in time by dysarthria, dysphagia, upper-extremity ataxia, and lower-extremity weakness. Decreased vibratory and proprioceptive sensation, as well as areflexia (often most prominent in the lower extremities) with plantar extensor responses, may be noted on examination. Light touch, pain, and temperature sensation are usually initially preserved but can be affected in later stages of the disease. Gait ataxia primarily results from loss of proprioceptive sensation. Ocular findings may include optic atrophy, abnormal smooth pursuits, and saccades. Sensorineural hearing loss is also seen in a small number of patients.

Outside of the nervous system, hypertrophic cardiomyopathy occurs in the majority of affected individuals. Diabetes mellitus occurs in 10% and glucose intolerance is noted in up to 20% of patients. Scoliosis and pes cavus develop in later stages of the disease. It is also important to recognize that atypical cases of Friedreich ataxia occur with late presentation, slow progression, and retained deep tendon reflexes, and, very rarely, as spastic paraparesis without ataxia.

Friedreich ataxia is a neurodegenerative disease and most individuals lose the ability to perform activities of daily living independently 10 to 15 years after the diagnosis is made. Individuals die from complications of cardiac arrhythmias, diabetes, or aspiration pneumonia.

Summary   The patient is a previously healthy 12-year-old girl who presents for evaluation of a progressive ataxia. Her neurologic examination is remarkable for abnormal saccadic eye movements, dysmetria, dysdiadochokinesis, decreased proprioception, areflexia, gait ataxia, abnormal Romberg testing, and bilateral plantar extensor responses.

Localization   This disease process involves the central and the peripheral nervous systems. Bilateral dysmetria, dysdiadochokinesis, and gait ataxia localize to the cerebellum and spinocerebellar tracts. Control of saccadic eye movements is complex, and although frontal lobe, parietal lobe, or brainstem lesions may cause disruption of saccades, in the context of this patient, it is likely that a cerebellar process explains the abnormality. Abnormal proprioception localizes to the posterior columns of the spinal cord. An abnormal Romberg test may be a result of cerebellar and/or sensory ataxia in this case. Areflexia suggests involvement of the peripheral nerves. Bilateral plantar extensor responses demonstrate involvement of the corticospinal tracts.

Differential Diagnosis   The findings of abnormal eye movements, areflexia, posterior column involvement, and long tract signs in an adolescent with a progressive ataxia are fairly specific for Friedreich ataxia. However, Friedreich ataxia must then be differentiated from other clinically similar hereditary, neurodegenerative ataxia syndromes and metabolic diseases. These primarily include ataxia with vitamin E deficiency (AVED), autosomal dominant spinocerebellar ataxia syndromes, ataxia-telangiectasia, ataxia with oculomotor apraxia (types 1 and 2), Refsum disease, mitochondrial diseases, GM_2 gangliosidosis (Tay Sachs disease variants), and abetalipoproteinemia (Bassen-Kornzweig disease). Hereditary motor and sensory neuropathies (Charcot-Marie-Tooth disease) may also present with gait abnormalities, clumsiness, and peripheral neuropathy, which may be the only symptoms in early Friedreich ataxia.

AVED is caused by a mutation on chromosome 8 that results in an abnormality of the alpha-tocopherol transfer protein (TTPA). As a result, serum measurements of vitamin E are low. Although clinically very similar to Friedreich ataxia, the progression of AVED is slower and peripheral neuropathy is less prominent. Cardiac abnormalities rarely occur. Serum vitamin E levels are invariably low and are diagnostic. AVED is an especially important consideration in the differential as it is treatable with high doses of vitamin E.

Autosomal dominant spinocerebellar syndromes are a heterogeneous group of neurodegenerative disorders. Affected individuals present at different ages and display a variety of symptoms including progressive ataxia, dysarthria, extrapyramidal symptoms, ophthalmoplegia, retinal abnormalities, dorsal column dysfunction, deafness, and peripheral neuropathy. Ataxia-telangiectasia (AT) is an autosomal recessive disorder caused by a mutation of chromosome 11q22-23 (Table 32.1).[1] AT is also in the differential, but can be distinguished by the presence of visible telangiectasias, frequent sinopulmonary infections, and lymphoproliferative malignancies (leukemia, lymphoma). The serum alpha-fetoprotein is elevated and immunoglobulin levels are typically low.

Ataxia with oculomotor apraxia type 1 (AOA1) is an autosomal recessive disorder caused by a mutation on chromosome 9p13.3. It has been described in Japanese and Portuguese families. AOA1 presents with a progressive gait ataxia in early childhood. Oculomotor apraxia begins several years later and deteriorates to a progressive external ophthalmoplegia. A severe motor peripheral neuropathy also occurs, leading to areflexia and quadriplegia from neurogenic distal muscle atrophy. The onset of AOA2 is seen in later childhood through early adulthood. Ataxia, oculomotor apraxia, axonal sensorimotor peripheral neuropathy, dystonia, and choreoathetosis develop with time. AOA2 is also transmitted in an

TABLE 32.1

Inherited Ataxia Syndromes

	Ataxia-Telangiectasia	Friedreich Ataxia
Age of onset	3–6 yr	7–14 yr
Inheritance pattern	Autosomal recessive	Autosomal recessive
Chromosome	Chromosome 11q	Chromosome 9q
Gene	*ATM*	*FRDA*
Neurologic findings	Ataxia	Ataxia
	Dysarthria/dysphagia	Dysarthria/dysphagia
	Oculomotor apraxia	Oculomotor abnormalities
	Hyporeflexia/areflexia	Hyporeflexia/areflexia
		Dorsal column dysfunction
		Plantar extensor responses
Other clinical features	Telangiectasias	Cardiomyopathy
	Immunodeficiency	Pes cavus
	Leukemia/lymphoma	Scoliosis
		Diabetes mellitus
		Optic atrophy
		Sensorineural hearing loss

autosomal recessive manner and is caused by a mutation in the senataxin gene on chromosome 9q34.

Refsum disease is an autosomal recessive, peroxisomal disorder associated with retinal degeneration (causing night blindness), cerebellar degeneration, chronic sensorimotor polyneuropathy, sensorineural hearing loss, ichthyosis, and cardiac abnormalities. Corticospinal tracts are not involved though. Phytanic acid is elevated in the serum and symptoms of Refsum disease can be improved with dietary restriction of phytanic acid.

Mitochondrial diseases are also heterogeneous and frequently associated with central, as well as peripheral nervous system abnormalities. Because mitochondrial disorders can also be associated with ataxia, oculomotor abnormalities, retinitis pigmentosa, sensorineural hearing loss, and cardiac arrhythmias, they often enter the differential diagnosis of Friedreich ataxia. Leigh disease (subacute necrotizing encephalomyelopathy) and NARP syndrome (neuropathy, ataxia, retinitis pigmentosa) serve as examples.

A chronic form of GM_2 gangliosidosis has been reported to resemble atypical presentations of Friedreich ataxia with neurologic symptoms, sensory neuropathy, and oculomotor abnormalities. Finally, abetalipoproteinemia is another autosomal recessive condition in the differential diagnosis. It is a malabsorptive syndrome that usually presents earlier than Friedreich ataxia, in infancy or early childhood. Ataxia, posterior column abnormalities, and peripheral neuropathy probably result from vitamin E deficiency, pigmentary retinal degeneration, scoliosis, weakness, pes cavus, and failure to thrive can occur. Laboratory studies may demonstrate acanthocytosis, low levels of fat-soluble vitamins (vitamins A, E, K), low cholesterol, low triglycerides, and absent beta-lipoproteins (VLDL, low-density lipoproteins). Neurologic deterioration can be prevented by high-dose vitamin replacement.

Acquired disorders may also be considered in the differential diagnosis but are much less likely in this case. A slow growing posterior fossa tumor, like a pilocytic astrocytoma, may present with a chronic ataxia. In this vignette, a head CT performed after the onset of symptoms was normal, which makes a tumor less likely. Demyelinating diseases such as multiple sclerosis can be considered, but usually present as discrete attacks and would not be associated with a peripheral neuropathy. Subacute combined degeneration from vitamin B_{12} deficiency causes impairment of dorsal column function and sensory ataxia, but would be unusual in an otherwise healthy girl with a normal diet.

Evaluation Fortunately, clinical genetic testing for the abnormal expansion of the GAA tandem repeat in the *FRDA* gene on chromosome 9q13 is commercially available. This might be the first test performed in a patient with suspected Friedreich ataxia. Making this diagnosis genetically early in the work-up may spare the patient unnecessary timely or expensive diagnostic testing and is the most efficient way to confirm the presence of this disease. This methodology is almost 100% sensitive for Friedreich ataxia.

Patients with confirmed Friedreich ataxia should undergo a cardiac evaluation with ECHO and ECG. Glucose levels should be measured to rule out diabetes mellitus and referral to an endocrinologist should be made when appropriate. The family should also be referred for evaluation by a geneticist who can accurately document the family history, evaluate carrier status, and provide genetic counseling. Prenatal diagnosis is also available. Referral should also be made for physical therapy to help maximize an affected child's motor abilities as well as to provide any necessary orthotics or medical equipment. An orthopaedic evaluation is necessary in the later stages as scoliosis, spasticity, and contractures develop. A dilated ophthalmologic examination should also be performed to evaluate for optic atrophy and abnormal eye movements.

If the diagnosis is less clear or genetic testing is not available, a work-up for a progressive ataxia presenting in adolescence may begin with a brain and spinal MRI to evaluate for structural lesions. An ophthalmologic examination may be helpful in identifying possible findings such as optic atrophy, vision loss, retinitis pigmentosa, and eye movement abnormalities. EMG and NCS may delineate peripheral motor versus sensory nerve involvement. Screening laboratory testing might include a vitamin E level, vitamin A level, vitamin B_{12} level, CBC, basic chemistry panel, cholesterol, lipoproteins, triglyceride level, phytanic acid, lactate/pyruvate battery, mitochondrial DNA, alpha-fetoprotein, immunoglobulin levels, urine organic acids, and lysosomal enzymes.

Management Treatment of Friedreich ataxia is symptomatic at this time. Patients need to be monitored regularly by a multidisciplinary team that includes a neurologist, cardiologist, orthopedist, ophthalmologist, endocrinologist, and/or geneticist.

As the pathogenesis of Friedreich ataxia is increasingly understood, several therapeutic strategies are under investigation. Interventions have included antioxidants to detoxify excess free radicals that are generated in this disorder. Clinical trials using idebenone, vitamin E, coenzyme Q10, and mitoquidone have been performed. An excess of mitochondrial iron is suspected to contribute to the pathogenesis of Friedreich ataxia and iron chelators (desferoxamine, deferiprone, 2-pyridylcarboxyaldehyde isonicotinyl hydrazone [PCIH] analogues) have also been tried. Pharmacologic interventions or gene therapy to increase frataxin expression might also be possible in the future.

References

Bidichandani SI, Ashizawa T. Friedreich ataxia. 2004. Available at: www.genetests.org. Last accessed December 16, 2005.

Brazis PW, Masdeu JC, Biller J. *Localization in Clinical Neurology.* 3rd ed. Philadelphia, Pa: Lippincott Williams & Wilkins; 1996:155–250.

Federico A. Ataxia with isolated vitamin deficiency E, a treatable neurologic disorder resembling Friedreich's ataxia. *Neurol Sci.* 2004;25:119–121.

Ouvrier RA, McLeod JG, Pollard JD. *Peripheral Neuropathy in Childhood.* 2nd ed. London, UK: Mac Keith Press; 1999:136–156, 172–200.

Pandolfo M. Friedreich ataxia. *Semin Pediatr Neurol.* 2003;10(3):163–172.

Seznec H, Wilson RB, Puccio H. 2003 International Friedreich's ataxia research conference 14–16, February 2003, Bethesda, Md, USA. *Neuromuscul Disord.* 2004;14:70–82.

Swaiman KF, Zoghbi H. Cerebellar dysfunction and ataxia in childhood. In: Swaiman KS, Ashwal S, eds. *Pediatric Neurology: Principles and Practice.* 3rd ed. St. Louis, Mo: Mosby; 1999:787–800.

Voncken M, Ioannou P, Delatycki MB. Friedreich ataxia—update on pathogenesis and possible strategies. *Neurogenetics.* 2004;5:1–8.

You are contacted by the emergency room regarding the possible admission of **a 5-day-old female infant** presenting with episodes of right face and body twitching that began 2 days ago. She was born at full term without complications and was initially doing well at home without signs of fever or illness. Over the last 48 hours, however, she has had four stereotypic episodes of unresponsiveness with right-sided jerking lasting approximately 1 minute each. Before the emergency room resident hangs up the phone, he informs you that the infant also has a typical dry newborn rash involving her entire trunk and extremities.

Physical Examination Vital Signs: Afebrile. General Examination: Significant for a diffuse hyperpigmented, mildly erythematous rash with occasional vesicles. The rash is noted to be linear and appears to follow the lines of Blaschko on her trunk. Neurologic Examination: Mental Status: The newborn is easily arousable from sleep for the examination. She is alert and not irritable. Cranial Nerves: Her pupils are equal, round, and reactive to light. Her extraocular muscles are intact. Facial expression is symmetric. Her gag is present and her tongue is midline. Motor: She has normal bulk and tone. She moves all four extremities equally against gravity and has a symmetric Moro reflex. Reflexes: 2+ throughout with bilateral plantar flexor responses.

Guide to Case Discussion

- Briefly summarize this case.
- Localize the examination findings.
- Give the most likely diagnosis and provide a differential diagnosis.
- Discuss an appropriate diagnostic work-up.
- Discuss the management of this patient.

Diagnosis Incontinentia pigmenti with right focal seizures.

Discussion Incontinentia pigmenti (IP), also known as Bloch-Sulzberger syndrome, is an X-linked dominant neurocutaneous disorder that affects the skin, hair, teeth, nails, and eyes, as well as the central nervous system. IP occurs in 1 in 40,000 individuals and is usually lethal in males. The characteristic skin findings evolve over four defined stages that occur along the lines of embryonic and fetal skin development known as Blaschko lines. Blaschko lines are linear on the extremities and circumferential on the trunk.

The rash is usually present at birth or shortly afterwards. Stage 1 (bullous stage) is characterized by blister or vesicular-like eruptions that can be erythematous and appear infectious. Stage 2 (verrucous stage) is characterized by keratotic, warty papules and plaques that continue to follow the Blaschko lines. Stage 3 (hyperpigmentation stage) is noted for macular hyperpigmented whorls along the Blaschko lines ("marbled cake" appearance). The hyperpigmentation usually fades in the teens and early 20s, leading some individuals to proceed to stage 4. Stage 4 (atretic stage) is characterized by hairless hypopigmented streaks and patches with skin atrophy that may persist into adulthood.

Ocular manifestations are seen in almost 80% of affected individuals. They include mottled, hypopigmentation of the retina and abnormal peripheral vascularization of the retina, which can result in retinal detachment. Dental findings occur in 65% to 90%, with delayed tooth eruption, hypodontia, microdontia, and round, peg-shaped teeth. Dysplastic nails with ridging, pitting, onychogryposis, or subungual dyskeratomas occur in 40% to 60% of individuals. Woolly hair or alopecia may also be seen. Central nervous system manifestations occur in 10% to 40% of individuals with IP. They include microcephaly, mental retardation, spasticity, seizures, and strokes.

Summary The patient is a 5-day-old female infant born at full term without complications who presents with a 2-day history of right-sided seizure activity in the absence of encephalopathy, fever, or illness. She is found to have a prominent diffuse, erythematous, vesicular rash along Blaschko lines, and an otherwise normal neurologic exam.

Localization The presence of focal seizures in a newborn suggests an underlying cortical process and specifically in this case, in the left cerebral hemisphere. The presence of a diffuse erythematous, hyperpigmented rash along Blaschko lines suggests an underlying neurocutaneous disorder as an associated cause for seizures.

Differential Diagnosis The characteristic skin lesions of IP must be distinguished from other dermatologic possibilities. These include infections such as molluscum contagiosum, congenital HSV, varicella virus, bullous impetigo, and epidermolysis bullosa, as well as other neurocutaneous disorders such as hypomelanosis of Ito and Naegeli syndrome. In hypomelanosis of Ito, abnormal hypopigmentation is the primary skin manifestation. Naegeli syndrome is an extremely rare autosomal dominant skin disorder without the different stages of skin lesions.

Neonatal seizures have a broad differential diagnosis that can be primarily broken down into the following categories: infectious, metabolic, hypoxic-ischemic injury, intracranial hemorrhage, congenital stroke, structural abnormalities, and in-born errors of metabolism. In this case, the absence of fever, illness, and en-cephalopathy make infectious, metabolic, and inborn errors of metabolism less likely etiologies. However, strong consideration should be given to the possibility of HSV encephalitis in any infant presenting with focal seizures and a vesicular rash. HSV encephalitis is relatively common and is treatable with acyclovir.

The timing of the onset of seizures in newborns can also be helpful when the di-agnosis is less obvious. Hypoxic ischemic encephalopathy, bacterial meningitis, sep-sis, encephalitis, hemorrhage (subarachnoid, intraventricular), and pyridoxine de-pendency often present within the first 24 to 48 hours. Cerebral dysgenesis, drug withdrawal, urea cycle disorders, and neurocutaneous syndromes (tuberous sclerosis complex, IP) can present between 24 and 72 hours of life. Finally, inborn errors of metabolism such as aminoacidopathies (methylmalonic and propionic acidemia) frequently present after 72 hours of life as protein and glucose feeds are initiated.

Evaluation The patient in this case should be admitted to the hospital for appro-priate work-up and management. The prompt evaluation by a geneticist and/or der-matologist should help confirm the diagnosis of IP clinically. The decision can then be made regarding the need for more specific genetic testing.

The diagnosis of IP can be made based on clinical features or on molecular ge-netic testing. The clinical diagnosis of IP requires major and minor criteria. Major criteria are consistent skin lesions, which occur in stages. Minor criteria include the presence of a dental, hair, nail, or retinal finding as listed above. Histopathology on skin biopsy of dyskeratotic cells and deposition of melanin can help confirm the clinical diagnosis. Molecular genetic testing is commercially available for diagnos-tic confirmation, carrier testing, and prenatal diagnosis. Southern blot analysis is used to detect deletion of exons 4 through 10 of the *IKBKG* gene (NEMO protein) and identifies 80% of probands.

Dermatologic consultation is recommended for supportive skin care to mini-mize skin irritation, prevent infection, and perform skin biopsy confirmation. Ophthalmologic evaluation is recommended to identify ophthalmologic findings and monitor for retinal detachment.

The patient in this case also needs diagnostic testing for the etiology of her seizures. An EEG should be performed. In addition, neuroimaging, preferably with a brain MRI, should be done to evaluate for underlying structural abnormalities that might explain focal seizures. Magnetic resonance (MR) angiography of the head is also recommended as cerebrovascular abnormalities have been rarely reported with IP.

A thorough birth history, family history, physical examination, complete sepsis evaluation including CSF studies, basic chemistry testing, state newborn screen, and screening labs for inborn errors of metabolism (plasma amino acids, urine organic acids, lactate/pyruvate battery, ammonia level) also may be required to rule out other possible etiologies if there are questions regarding the diagnosis.

Management Surveillance evaluations by ophthalmology, dermatology, and den-tistry are recommended to monitor for retinal detachment, complications associ-ated with skin lesions, and dental care, respectively.

This patient will also require anticonvulsants for treatment of her seizure dis-order. In a neonate with frequent seizures, phenobarbital is the most appropriate medication choice. The patient can be loaded intravenously with up to 20 mg/kg/day and then placed on a maintenance dose of 3 to 4 mg/kg/day divided once or twice per day.

Genetic counseling is encouraged for parents and family as deletions of the *IKBKG* gene can be inherited or from a de novo gene mutation (commonly of paternal origin by germ line mosaicism). As the deletion is lethal in most males, a history of multiple miscarriages (males) is common in familial IP. Skewed X-chromosome inactivation in females can result in variable presentations.

Additional Questions

1. What patterns of inheritance occur with X-linked autosomal recessive disorders?

2. Name three other common neurocutaneous disorders that can present with seizures. Distinguish them by dermatologic characteristics, genetic pattern of inheritance, chromosome involved, and common neurologic manifestations.

References

Bourgeois BFD. Phenobarbital and primidone. In: Wyllie E, ed. *The Treatment of Epilepsy: Principles and Practice*. 3rd ed. Philadelphia, Pa: Lippincott Williams & Wilkins; 2001:869–879.

Fenichel GM. *Clinical Pediatric Neurology: A Signs and Symptoms Approach*. 4th ed. Philadelphia, Pa: WB Saunders; 2001:1–45.

Landy SJ, Donnai D. Incontinentia pigmenti (Bloch-Sulzberger syndrome). *J Med Genet*. 1993;30(1):53–59.

Parrish JE, Scheuerle AE, Lewis RA, et al. Selection against mutant alleles in blood leukocytes is a consistent feature in incontinentia pigmenti type 2. *Hum Mol Genet*. 1996;5(11):1777–1783.

Porksen G, Pfeiffer C, Hahn G, et al. Neonatal seizures in two sisters with incontinentia pigmenti. *Neuropediatrics*. 2004;35(2):139–142.

Smahi A, Courtois G, Vabres P, et al. Genomic rearrangement in NEMO impairs NF-kappaB activation and is a cause of incontinentia pigmenti. The International Incontinentia Pigmenti (IP) Consortium. *Nature*. 2000;405:466–472.

A pediatrician has referred **a 2-year-old girl** to your outpatient clinic emergently for evaluation of progressive loss of skills after a recent tonsillectomy. The patient was the product of a full term, uneventful gestation. Delivery was complicated by failure to progress and was assisted by vacuum extraction. In the neonatal period she was hospitalized in the NICU because of seizures that were easily controlled with phenobarbital. She initially had a poor suck, but it was transitory. The infant was weaned off of phenobarbital quickly and ultimately breast-fed well.

She was slow in attaining her initial milestones, but by 2 years of age she could hold a cup, sit, and stand with support. She did not have any words. At 2.5 years of age, however, she began to have a gradual loss of skills. Her mother coincides this with a tonsillectomy performed for obstructive sleep apnea. She has now lost the ability to sit and does not vocalize. Her mother is concerned that she neither hears nor sees well. When further questioned, the parents state that the child had always had difficulties with table food but now is fed pureed food exclusively and occasionally chokes when given a bottle.

Physical Examination General Examination: Facial dysmorphisms, including a prominent forehead, flat bridge of the nose, and micrognathia, are noted; otherwise her general exam is unremarkable and includes a normal head circumference. Neurologic Examination: Mental Status: She has minimal reaction to the examiner, although will smile to her mother's voice. Language: No words or vocalizations. Cranial Nerves: The pupils are equal, round, and reactive to light. There is no clear tracking, but she blinks to threat. There is an open-mouthed posture with drooling. Her gag is decreased. The tongue is midline without fasciculations. Motor: She has normal bulk and striking diffuse hypotonia with neck flexor weakness. There is spontaneous movement of the extremities in an antigravity fashion, but only in response to pain with localization. Coordination: No abnormal movements are noted. Reflexes: She is areflexic throughout with bilateral plantar extensor responses.

Guide to Case Discussion

- Briefly summarize this case.

- Localize the examination findings.

- Give the most likely diagnosis and provide a differential diagnosis.

- Discuss an appropriate diagnostic work-up.

- Discuss the management of this patient.

Diagnosis Peroxisomal disorder (D-bifunctional protein deficiency).

Discussion The peroxisomal disorders represent a clinically and genetically heterogeneous spectrum of heritable diseases. Peroxisomes are membrane-bound organelles that are found in most eukaryotic cells. They serve many critical functions, primarily involving the pathways of lipid metabolism. More specifically, they are involved in (a) ether phospholipid biosynthesis, (b) fatty acid beta-oxidation, and (c) fatty acid alpha-oxidation. Peroxisomal disorders are generally subdivided into two groups: (a) defects of peroxisomal biogenesis and (b) single peroxisomal enzyme disorders. Abnormal peroxisomal function may manifest with cerebral, peripheral nerve, hepatic, renal, bone, and cardiac involvement. A diverse number of peroxisomal diseases have been described.

Peroxisomal biogenesis disorders (PBDs) include Zellweger syndrome, neonatal adrenoleukodystrophy (NALD), infantile Refsum disease (IRD), and rhizomelic chondrodysplasia punctata (RCP). Zellweger syndrome, NALD, and IRD represent a spectrum of disorders with similar and overlapping clinical features. They are often referred to as the Zellweger spectrum disorders, with NALD and IRD being less severe. Children with Zellweger syndrome demonstrate facial dysmorphology with a prominent forehead, large anterior fontanelle, epicanthal folds, micrognathia, high-arched palate, and deformed ear lobes. The characteristic facies may resemble that of Down syndrome. Other features include profound hypotonia, hepatic dysfunction, hepatomegaly, retinal degeneration, sensorineural hearing loss, renal cysts, and calcific stippling of the epiphyses. Cortical migrational abnormalities and white matter dysmyelination that result in intractable seizures may be seen on brain MRI. Patients with NALD have hypotonia, intractable seizures, and progressive white matter disease on brain MRI. Children with IRD may demonstrate minor facial dysmorphisms, sensorineural hearing loss, cognitive dysfunction, failure to thrive, retinopathy, and hepatic dysfunction. The clinical features of RCP are in contrast to the other disorders of peroxisomal biogenesis. RCP is associated with characteristic facial features, dwarfism (shortened proximal extremities), spasticity, congenital contractures, profound mental retardation, and ocular abnormalities. The genetic abnormalities responsible for PBDs lie in the *PEX* genes (on many different chromosomes) and code for the peroxin proteins involved in the pathways of peroxisomal biogenesis.

X-linked adrenoleukodystrophy is the most common peroxisomal single-enzyme-defect disorder, resulting in abnormal peroxisomal beta-oxidation of very-long-chain fatty acids. Other peroxisomal single-enzyme defects include D-bifunctional protein deficiency (as seen in this patient), adult Refsum disease, and thiolase deficiency (pseudo-Zellweger syndrome), among many others.

D-bifunctional protein deficiency (DBP) is rare but is presented in this case to demonstrate the diverse clinical manifestations of peroxisomal disorders. DBP serves an important function in catalyzing a step of fatty acid beta-oxidation. Most patients present with neonatal hypotonia. Nystagmus, strabismus, and lack of fixation on objects may be noted early in the disease process. Progressive vision and hearing failure are also common. Other features have included developmental regression, peripheral neuropathy, failure to thrive, hepatomegaly, facial dysmorphism (resembling

Zellweger syndrome), macrocephaly, and neonatal seizures. The brain MRI commonly demonstrates cortical dysplasia, delayed white matter maturation, dilated ventricles, and cerebellar atrophy. Evolution is inexorable and death often occurs in infancy or early childhood.

Summary The patient is a 2-year-old dysmorphic girl with a history of neonatal seizures, poor feeding at birth, and global developmental delay who presents with subacute developmental regression after an elective surgery. Her history and physical exam are notable for depressed mental status, likely visual and auditory dysfunction, bulbar symptoms, severe hypotonia (with possible proximal weakness), areflexia, and bilateral plantar extensor responses.

Localization The child in this case presents with signs and symptoms of a disorder that affects both lower motor and upper motor neuron systems. The features of severe hypotonia and absent deep tendon reflexes make the possibility of a peripheral neuromuscular disorder a consideration. However, the child's severe hypotonia, depressed sensorium, antigravity movement of the extremities and bilateral plantar extensor responses suggest that central nervous system involvement is coexistent if not predominant. While her areflexia is likely caused by a peripheral neuropathy, it is clear that other features localize to the central nervous system. Altered mental status, developmental regression, bulbar dysfunction, and hypotonia suggest a disorder with diffuse involvement of central nervous system structures (both gray and white matter). Associated vision loss may localize to the retina, optic nerve, or visual cortex, depending on the disease process. Hearing loss is likely a result of involvement of the vestibulocochlear nerve or brainstem.

Differential Diagnosis The progressive deterioration of motor and cognitive skills after outpatient surgery seen in this dysmorphic child is most consistent with a neurodegenerative disorder. Other reversible disorders are less likely, particularly in light of her dysmorphic features and multiple neurologic abnormalities. However, subclinical seizures, sepsis, structural abnormalities (hydrocephalus, slow-growing brain tumors), central nervous system infections (meningitis, encephalitis), endocrine abnormalities (hypothyroidism), and electrolyte disturbances need to be excluded.

The differential diagnosis of inherited metabolic diseases that cause a chronic, progressive encephalopathy needs to be most seriously considered in this patient. Disorders in this category tend to affect global developmental skills. They tend to be progressive and may even occur after a period of normal or relatively normal development. Finally, they are usually associated with objective neurologic abnormalities, often involving different parts of the central and/or peripheral nervous system.

To initiate an appropriate work-up for a patient with a chronic encephalopathy, it must first be determined whether there is involvement outside of the central nervous system. Disorders that affect only the central nervous system are further broken down into diseases primarily affecting the gray matter (causing seizures, cognitive dysfunction, vision loss) and those primarily affecting the white matter (centrally and/or peripherally). Disorders with involvement outside of the central nervous system most commonly involve muscle, liver, spleen, bone, and/or skin.

Patterns of organ involvement then may suggest certain categories of diseases. The presence of facial dysmorphisms also helps point to certain diagnoses.

Disorders that can cause a chronic progressive encephalopathy in addition to facial dysmorphisms include peroxisomal disorders (Zellweger syndrome and its variants), lysosomal storage (mucopolysaccharidoses, Gaucher disease, GM_1 gangliosidosis, sialidosis), and mitochondrial disorders (electron transport disorders, pyruvate dehydrogenase deficiency, forms of glutaric aciduria). Diseases resulting from biosynthetic defects are also in the differential diagnosis (congenital disorders of glycosylation, mevalonic aciduria, Smith-Lemli-Opitz syndrome, Menkes disease, homocystinuria). However, the facial characteristics and neurologic findings in this case are most suggestive of a peroxisomal disorder.

Evaluation At initial presentation, basic laboratory tests including a CBC, basic chemistry panel, blood gas, liver function tests, thyroid function tests, urinalysis, and creatine kinase should be done. An initial investigation for inborn errors of metabolism should be performed, including an ammonia level (urea cycle defects), plasma lactate/pyruvate battery (mitochondrial disorders), lysosomal enzymes, urine organic acids (organic acidurias), plasma amino acids (amino acidopathies), plasma acylcarnitine profile (fatty acid oxidation defects), urine mucopolysaccharides/oligosaccharides (mucopolysaccharidoses), and very-long-chain fatty acids (peroxisomal disorders). Given the presence of dysmorphic features, it would also be reasonable to send a high-resolution karyotype.

As diseases are ruled in or out, more refined genetic testing may be necessary. More specifically, although very-long-chain fatty acids may screen for peroxisomal disorders, additional specialized, biochemical testing is required to delineate individual syndromes and to make an accurate diagnosis. For example, single-enzyme defects such as D-bifunctional protein deficiency may have a clinical presentation and very-long-chain fatty acid profile indistinguishable from the PBDs. Plasma pipecolic acid deserves mention, however, as it may be elevated in peroxisomal single-enzyme defects but normal in the PBDs.

Neuroimaging should also be performed promptly. A brain MRI with magnetic resonance (MR) spectroscopy would be most helpful in the assessment of intracranial findings consistent with certain inborn errors of metabolism. A dilated ophthalmologic examination might also be helpful in determining whether optic nerve or retinal involvement is present. These may be important factors when considering possible metabolic and genetic diagnoses. Electrodiagnostic testing with an electroretinogram (ERG), VERs, and BAERs can aid in the assessment of vision and hearing impairments, respectively. Finally, EMG and NCS may help to evaluate the patient's apparent peripheral neuropathy.

Management Given that the patient appears to have more subacute symptoms superimposed on chronic but progressive neurologic symptoms, she should be admitted to the hospital for a thorough diagnostic work-up. An intravenous line should be placed and she should be placed on a cardiorespiratory monitor and a pulse oximeter until her diagnosis is more clear. She should not be given anything by mouth until her swallowing is evaluated as she is at risk for aspiration by history.

There are no accepted therapies for disorders of peroxisomal fatty acid oxidation and treatment is directed at the management of complications. Severe hypotonia and bulbar dysfunction result in feeding difficulties and frequent respiratory complications. There is a significant risk of respiratory failure. Input from a pulmonologist, gastroenterologist, and nutritionist is often required. As symptoms progress, swallowing studies and evaluation by appropriate therapists are necessary to assess the safety of oral intake.

Seizures may occur and are often intractable. EEG and video EEG are often required in the diagnosis and management of an associated seizure disorder. Treatment with multiple anticonvulsants may be needed.

Genetic counseling is also an important aspect of the management of this disorder. There is an autosomal recessive inheritance pattern and each pregnancy results in a 25% risk of an affected child. Once a genetic defect is identified, prenatal testing is available.

Additional Questions

1. Describe the typical presentation and clinical features of adrenoleukodystrophy.

2. What is the presentation of other causes of encephalopathy caused by the following heritable disorders of metabolism: urea cycle disorders, organic acidopathies, and disorders with lactic acidosis?

3. How would you address a parent's wish to have the patient's siblings screened for carrier status for this disorder?

References

Clarke JTR. *A Clinical Guide to Inherited Metabolic Disorders*. 2nd ed. Cambridge, UK: Cambridge University Press; 2002:18–64, 134–168.

Ferdinandusse S, Denis S, Mooyer PA, et al. Clinical and biochemical spectrum of D-bifunctional protein deficiency. *Ann Neurol*. 2006;59:92–104.

Raymond GV. Peroxisomal disorders. *Curr Opin Neurol*. 2001;14:783–787.

Wanders RJA. Peroxisomes, lipid metabolism, and peroxisomal disorders. *Mol Genet Metab*. 2004;83:16–27.

Wanders RJA, Waterham HR. Peroxisomal disorders: biochemistry and genetics of peroxisome biogenesis disorders. *Clin Genet*. 2004;67:107–133.

A 6-year-old girl with no significant past medical history presents to the emergency department for concerns of new-onset right-sided weakness that was first noted when she tried to get out of bed that morning. Her speech was also slurred. Her symptoms seemed to improve throughout the morning but did not completely resolve. There was no history of trauma, fever, flu-like symptoms, nausea, vomiting, or headache. There were no witnessed convulsions or associated loss of consciousness. The patient's birth history was uncomplicated and her development has been age appropriate. The family history is negative for stroke in young individuals.

Physical Examination   Vital Signs: Normal. General Examination: There are no birthmarks. Her heart has a regular rate and rhythm without murmurs, rubs, or gallops. Neurologic Examination: Mental Status: Awake and alert. Language: She has dysarthric speech in short phrases. She seems to have difficulty understanding basic commands. Cranial Nerves: Her pupils are equal, round, and reactive to light. Her visual fields are full. There is flattening of the right nasolabial fold. Her tongue is midline. Motor: She has normal bulk with a slight decrease in right-sided tone. Right-sided upper- and lower-extremity strength is 4/5 with 5/5 strength on the left side. Coordination: There is no dysmetria on the left but coordination is difficult to assess on the right because of weakness. Sensation: No deficits are noted. Gait: Not assessed. Reflexes: 2+ on the left and 1+ on the right. Right plantar extensor and left plantar flexor response.

Guide to Case Discussion

▓ Briefly summarize this case.

▓ Localize the examination findings.

▓ Give the most likely diagnosis and provide a differential diagnosis.

▓ Discuss an appropriate diagnostic work-up.

▓ Discuss the management of this patient.

Diagnosis Moyamoya vasculopathy presenting as an acute left-middle cerebral artery infarction.

Discussion Idiopathic moyamoya vasculopathy is a noninflammatory, progressive cerebrovascular occlusive disease that slowly causes stenosis or occlusion of the cerebral arteries, especially those surrounding the circle of Willis or the arteries that feed it. There is a predilection for the internal carotid arteries. The cause of idiopathic moyamoya disease is unknown. Moyamoya is Japanese for "puff of smoke" and it describes the characteristic angiographic appearance of abnormal collateral arterial networks that develop around occluded vessels. Moyamoya disease is usually bilateral, but unilateral involvement does not rule the condition out. Its peak incidence is in the first decade of life. In children, the mortality is around 4%. There is a slight female preponderance. Although Asian populations seem to be particularly affected, it can occur in any race.

Pathologically, intimal thickening of vessel walls can be seen. In addition to vessel stenosis, autopsy usually shows evidence of stroke or hemorrhage. Aneurysms are also associated with it. A family occurrence of 10% and clustering of the disease in Japan and other Asian countries suggest a genetic etiology. Some cases of familial moyamoya have been linked to chromosome 17q25.

Moyamoya vasculopathy can be divided into primary and secondary syndromes. Secondary causes are associated with a variety of medical conditions (Table 35.1). Clinically, moyamoya syndrome results in repeated ischemic events. Hemiparesis, speech difficulties, visual field defects, and sensory impairment frequently occur. More than half of patients have progressive cognitive decline, presumably from repeated ischemia. Intracerebral hemorrhage usually presents with headache and impaired consciousness. Symptoms and signs depend on the location and severity of the insults. Seizures are a frequent complication. Both seizures and ischemic events are more prevalent in children, whereas hemorrhage is more common in adults. Moyamoya is a progressive disease with increasing neurologic decline. In children, the progression is more rapid and the prognosis poorer.

Summary The patient is a previously healthy 6-year-old girl who presents with the acute onset of aphasia (receptive and expressive), dysarthria, right hemiparesis (involving the face, arm, and leg), depressed right-sided reflexes, and a right plantar extensor response.

TABLE 35.1

Disease States Associated with Moyamoya Vasculopathy

Neurofibromatosis type 1	Infectious or postinfectious vasculopathy
Fibromuscular dysplasia	Congenital heart disease
Marfan syndrome	Sickle cell disease
Down syndrome	Fanconi anemia
Radiation vasculitis	Atherosclerosis
Vasculitis	Head trauma

TABLE 35.2

Differential Diagnosis of Acute Hemiparesis

Ischemic infarction	Focal seizure with Todd paralysis
Intracranial hemorrhage	Complicated migraine
Encephalitis/meningitis	Alternating hemiplegia of childhood
Cerebral abscess	Demyelinating disease
Brain tumor	Malingering/conversion disorder

Localization   The patient's findings of aphasia and dysarthria in addition to a right hemiparesis with depressed reflexes and a right plantar extensor response localize to the left cerebral hemisphere. These deficits can be explained by a lesion in the distribution of the left middle cerebral artery. Cortical language areas, as well as the motor cortex, are affected. A discrete subcortical lesion in the internal capsule could explain a hemiparesis and plantar extensor response, but would not present with cortical signs such as an aphasia.

Differential Diagnosis   The potential causes of acute hemiparesis in childhood are numerous and are summarized in Table 35.2. The patient in this case has no history of trauma, fever, illness, or headache, which helps narrow the differential. There has been no witnessed seizure activity and there is no indication that she has a conversion reaction. Thus, it is most likely that she has had an acute stroke.

Childhood stroke has a broad differential diagnosis (Table 35.3). Congenital heart disease is a common cause of pediatric stroke. It can cause ischemia via emboli or a hyperviscous state. Central nervous system infections such as meningitis or encephalitis can cause vessel wall inflammation and lead to ischemia. Various hematologic disorders can cause pediatric stroke. A hypercoagulable state can cause thromboembolic phenomena, and hemoglobinopathies, such as sickle cell disease, frequently cause ischemic infarcts. Hyperviscosity syndromes such as polycythemia can result in arterial occlusion. Vasculitis from a variety of causes and vasculopathy can also cause pediatric stroke.

TABLE 35.3

Differential Diagnosis of Childhood Ischemic Stroke

Idiopathic	Trauma
Congenital heart disease	Vasculitis
Inborn errors of metabolism	Vasculopathy
Drugs	Vasospastic disorders
Hematologic disorders	
Coagulopathies	
Hemoglobinopathies	

Several inborn errors of metabolism are associated with cerebral infarction. Homocystinuria can present as a thrombotic syndrome. Mitochondrial disorders such as mitochondrial encephalomyopathy with lactic acidosis and stroke-like episodes (MELAS) mimic stroke symptomatology, but neurologic deficits do not follow a clear vascular distribution. Autoimmune disorders lead to cerebrovascular disease by causing either vasculitis or a hypercoagulable state. An autoimmune hypercoagulable state is usually associated with antiphospholipid antibodies such as lupus anticoagulant or anticardiolipin antibody. Trauma to the neck can predispose to carotid thrombosis or dissection. Various drugs (cocaine, phencyclidine, and amphetamines) can cause vasospasm, vasculitis, or platelet adhesion. One-third of childhood strokes have no recognizable cause.

Evaluation   At presentation, the patient is presumed to have had a stroke and a thorough work-up for an underlying etiology is warranted. A head CT should be performed immediately to document the presence or absence of ischemic change and to rule out cerebral hemorrhage. This should be followed up with a brain MRI with diffusion-weighted imaging and a brain and neck MRA to evaluate for vascular abnormalities.

The diagnosis of moyamoya disease is suspected when multiple acute and/or chronic cortical and subcortical strokes are seen. The patient should also have an ECG performed in the emergency room to rule out arrhythmias. An ECHO may be indicated at a later time if there is suspicion of a cardioembolic event.

Laboratory studies for a pediatric stroke of unclear etiology should include an infectious, hypercoagulable, and vasculitic evaluation. Hematologic labs might include a homocysteine level, PT/PTT, hemoglobin electrophoresis, protein C studies, protein S studies, factor V Leiden gene mutation, prothrombin G20210A mutation, antithrombin III, and lipid profile. Erythrocyte sedimentation rate, complement levels, ANA, and antiphospholipid antibodies should be measured to rule out vasculitis. In some clinical circumstances, a lumbar puncture with cerebrospinal fluid analysis might be required to rule out inflammatory and/or infectious etiologies.

Once the diagnosis of moyamoya disease is strongly suspected, cerebral angiography is the gold standard for diagnosis and may be required to delineate both the degree of vessel involvement and the presence of collateral blood supply. It might also be necessary if surgical intervention is planned. Finally, an investigation for the presence of the various disease states associated with moyamoya disease should be done.

Management   The child in this case presents with an acute stroke. She should be stabilized in the emergency room, initially by evaluation of her airway, breathing, and circulation. An intravenous line needs to be placed and she should be put on cardiorespiratory and pulse oximeter monitoring. She should be provided nothing by mouth until her ability to swallow safely is evaluated. She should be given intravenous isotonic fluids without dextrose to maintain normovolemia. Hypo- and hyperglycemia should be avoided. Further monitoring in the intensive care unit should be considered.

In the acute phase of pediatric ischemic stroke, medical treatment is primarily symptomatic. Antiplatelet therapy and anticoagulation can be considered to prevent further ischemic events in children with moyamoya disease, but they are not approved by the FDA specifically for this use. Aspirin, low-molecular-weight heparin, and heparin have all been used in individual cases. However, specific treatment guidelines have not yet been developed for the management of pediatric stroke.

Surgical procedures to bypass focal areas affected by the underlying vasculopathy might also be considered, but they are controversial. The goal is to restore circulation so as to prevent further ischemia. More specifically, this is done with either direct or indirect anastomoses. Direct interventions include superficial temporal artery (STA) to middle cerebral artery (MCA) bypass and middle meningeal artery to MCA bypass. Indirect techniques include encephaloduroarteriosynangiosis (EDAS), encephalomyosynangiosis (EMO), and encephaloarteriosynangiosis (EAS). Surgery is more effective in children with ischemic lesions than in adults. Rehabilitation with physical, occupational, and speech therapy should also be initiated when the patient is stable.

References

Biller J, Love BB. Ischemic cerebrovascular disease. In: Bradley WG, Daroff RB, Fenichel GM, et al., eds. *Neurology in Clinical Practice*. 4th ed. Philadelphia, Pa: Butterworth-Heinemann; 2004:1197–1249.

Fenichel GM. *Clinical Pediatric Neurology: A Signs and Symptoms Approach*. 4th ed. Philadelphia, Pa: WB Saunders; 2001:243–256.

Fukui M. Guidelines for the diagnosis and treatment of spontaneous occlusion of the circle of Willis ("moyamoya" disease). Research Committee on Spontaneous Occlusion of the Circle of Willis (Moyamoya Disease) of the Ministry of Health and Welfare, Japan. *Clin Neurol Neurosurg*. 1997;99(suppl 2):S238–S240.

Fung LW, Thompson D, Ganesan V. Revascularization surgery for pediatric moyamoya: a review of the literature. *Childs Nerv Syst*. 2005;21(5):358–364.

Golby AJ, Marks MP, Thompson RC, et al. Direct and combined revascularization in pediatric moyamoya disease. *Neurosurgery*. 1999;45(1):50–58.

Heros RC, Heros DO, Schumacher JM. Principles of neurosurgery. In: Bradley WG, Daroff RB, Fenichel GM, et al., eds. *Neurology in Clinical Practice*. 4th ed. Philadelphia, Pa: Butterworth-Heinemann; 2004:963–993.

Hoffman HJ. Moyamoya disease and syndrome. *Clin Neurol Neurosurg*. 1997;99(suppl 2): S239–S244.

Hutchison JS, Ichord R, Guerguerian AM, et al. Cerebrovascular disorders. *Semin Pediatr Neurol*. 2004;11(2):139–146.

Kim SK, Seol HJ, Cho BK, et al. Moyamoya disease among young patients: its aggressive clinical course and the role of active surgical treatment. *Neurosurgery*. 2004;54(4): 840–844.

A 9-month-old male infant is brought to your office for evaluation of developmental delay. The patient was born at full term by normal, spontaneous vaginal delivery. There were no pregnancy complications and fetal movement was reported to be normal. There were no feeding or breathing difficulties after birth. He appeared to be developing normally until age 5 months when he seemed to get weaker. His parents noted that he was having difficulty holding his head up and stopped reaching up with his arms to grab toys. At age 7 months he still could not roll over or sit up. He recently started to have some difficulty swallowing and may cough with meals. The pediatrician has done an initial work-up, including electrolytes, CBC, creatine kinase, thyroid function tests, TORCH titers, and a head CT, all of which are normal.

Physical Examination Vital Signs: Normal. Weight in the fifth percentile. General Examination: The patient is a thin, small, 9-month-old boy with a bell-shaped chest, paradoxical respirations, and frog-leg positioning. There are no dysmorphic facial features. No hepatosplenomegaly is noted. Neurologic Examination: Mental Status: Alert and visually attentive. Language: No babbling is heard. Cranial Nerves: The pupils are equal, round, and reactive to light. He tracks well in all directions. His face moves symmetrically. A gag is present. The tongue is midline with fasciculations. Motor: He has slightly decreased bulk with marked hypotonia. There is diffuse weakness and the patient is unable to lift his arms or legs against gravity; however, he does have some movement of his hands and feet. There is very poor head control. Sensory: He has some withdrawal and grimacing to pain. Reflexes: Absent throughout with bilateral plantar flexor responses.

Guide to Case Discussion

- Briefly summarize this case.
- Localize the examination findings.
- Give the most likely diagnosis and provide a differential diagnosis.
- Discuss an appropriate diagnostic work-up.
- Discuss the management of this patient.

Diagnosis Spinal muscular atrophy.

Discussion Spinal muscular atrophy (SMA) describes a spectrum of clinical syndromes caused by a mutation in the survival motor neuron (*SMN*) gene mapped to chromosome 5q13. SMA is inherited in an autosomal recessive fashion and occurs in approximately 1 in 6,000 to 10,000 individuals. SMA causes degeneration of the anterior horn cells and cranial nerve nuclei, resulting in progressive weakness as a consequence of widespread denervation.

Three primary clinical SMA syndromes are generally described, although the use of these names is increasingly controversial as the spectrum of this disease becomes better understood. SMA type 1 (Werdnig-Hoffmann disease) occurs in infants younger than 6 months of age who never attain the ability to sit up. SMA type 1 carries a very poor prognosis and the majority of patients die from respiratory failure by the age of 2 years. SMA type 2 (intermediate form) manifests later, typically between 6 and 18 months of age. These children are usually able to achieve an upright sitting posture independently. Many patients with SMA type 2 survive into their 20s but may experience complications such as kyphoscoliosis and contractures. Individuals with SMA type 3 (Kugelberg-Welander disease) present after 18 months of age and are able to ambulate, although typically with assistance and bracing. Life expectancy in these individuals is almost normal.

Summary The patient is a small 9-month-old boy with significant gross motor delay, progressive weakness, and dysphagia who is found to have a bell-shaped chest, paradoxical respirations, tongue fasciculations, severe hypotonia (frog-leg position), proximal weakness, and areflexia on exam.

Localization Both central and peripheral nervous system etiologies must be considered in the differential diagnosis of a hypotonic infant. The fact that the patient is alert and visually attentive helps to rule out cerebral causes. Given the history and cranial nerve findings, a spinal cord process is unlikely. The presence of tongue fasciculations, progressive proximal weakness, and absent deep tendon reflexes further points to a lower motor neuron problem. Disorders of the anterior horn cell, peripheral nerve, neuromuscular junction, and muscle must be considered. However, tongue fasciculations indicate involvement of the twelfth cranial nerve motor unit and are usually indicative of anterior horn cell disease.

Differential Diagnosis This patient's presentation is pathognomonic for a diagnosis of SMA, a degenerative disorder of the anterior horn cell and cranial nerve motor nuclei. He appears cognitively bright. His extraocular muscles are intact. There is quivering of the tongue, generally referred to as fasciculations, which is caused by tonic contraction of surviving motor units. Profound hypotonia with frog-leg positioning in addition to weakness (proximal more than distal) and respiratory muscles (diaphragmatic breathing) are present. There is also absence of the deep tendon reflexes, which can be very helpful in making the diagnosis.

Although a spinal cord injury could be considered in the case of a hypotonic infant, there is no history of birth or other trauma in this patient. There is no apparent sensory level and no sphincter abnormalities.

Peripheral neuropathies are rare in infancy but are the primary alternative diagnostic consideration in a patient with this presentation. Polyneuropathies can be distinguished from anterior horn cell disease because they tend to primarily affect distal musculature and involve both sensory and motor nerves. The most common primary congenital neuropathies in the differential diagnosis include congenital hypomyelinating neuropathy, a disease of myelin formation, and Déjérine-Sottas disease (hereditary motor and sensory neuropathy type III), a disorder with overlapping clinical features. Peripheral neuropathies in infancy might also be associated with metabolic disease (lysosomal storage diseases, peroxisomal defects, mitochondrial diseases), but these disorders typically also affect the central nervous system as well as other organs. Acquired peripheral neuropathies such as Guillain-Barré syndrome have been reported to cause hypotonia, ascending paralysis, and areflexia in infants, but are exceptionally rare.

Disorders of the neuromuscular junction might also be considered. Transient neonatal myasthenia gravis, congenital myasthenia gravis, and infantile botulism are the primary considerations. Transient neonatal myasthenia is an autoimmune disorder occurring in 10% of infants of mothers with myasthenia gravis. It may present with respiratory distress, feeding difficulty, and ptosis but resolves within the first 6 to 8 weeks of life. Congenital myasthenia gravis results in a similar syndrome of hypotonia, feeding abnormalities, poor suck, respiratory distress, and ptosis. Infants with botulism typically present with constipation followed by a descending paralysis. A poor suck, ophthalmoplegia, ptosis, pupillary dilatation, hyporeflexia, and weakness subsequently develop.

Finally, myopathic disorders such as congenital myopathies (nemaline, central core, centronuclear myopathy), muscular dystrophies, and myotonic dystrophy are in the differential diagnosis and all have similar clinical characteristics. They all may present in infancy with hypotonia, proximal weakness, feeding difficulty, and respiratory distress. Metabolic myopathies, such as acid maltase deficiency, can also present with hypotonia and progressive weakness, but are also associated with organomegaly (hepatomegaly, macroglossia, cardiomegaly). However, these neuromuscular and myopathic diseases do not cause tongue fasciculations and these clinical patterns do not fit that of the patient in the vignette.

Evaluation This child presents with very typical findings of SMA. A screening work-up was already done by the pediatrician. The availability of specific genetic testing for the *SMN* gene greatly simplifies the evaluation for SMA. Serum DNA testing is the first recommended step in the evaluation of a child with suspected SMA. Polymerase chain amplification of exons 7 and 8 of the *SMA* genes (*SMN1* and *SMN2*) will detect a mutation in approximately 95% of patients. Although the genetics of SMA are complex, the *SMN1* gene is responsible for the pathogenesis, but the *SMN2* gene is a contributing pathogenic factor.

For patients who do not have genetically proven SMA, more conventional testing is warranted. Serum muscle enzymes, EMG, NCS, and muscle biopsy can help to confirm the diagnosis. Serum creatine kinase may be mildly elevated but is usually normal. EMG in severely affected infants demonstrates fibrillations and positive sharp waves consistent with acute denervation. In less severely affected children, abnormal spontaneous activity is rare, but the duration and amplitude of motor unit potentials are increased, indicating fiber type grouping with reinnervation. Denervation atrophy causes decreased amplitude of compound muscle action potentials (CMAPs) on motor nerve conduction testing. Sensory nerve action potentials (SNAPs) are normal in SMA and help to distinguish this condition from infantile polyneuropathies.

The muscle biopsy in SMA reveals denervation (neurogenic atrophy). Small fibers are found adjacent to normal and hypertrophied fibers with type grouping that is seen in reinnervation.

Management The treatment for spinal muscular atrophy is symptomatic and supportive at this time. Joint contractures and spinal deformities may be helped with physical and occupational therapy or bracing devices. SMA patients are at risk for failure to thrive because of a progressive fatigability and weak suck. Nutritional support is often required. It is also important to observe patients' respiratory status as neurologic deterioration occurs. Involvement of a pulmonologist can be helpful in addressing long-term respiratory issues. Children with SMA should also be evaluated by a geneticist to assist in family counseling and assessment of carrier status.

References

Crawford TO. Spinal muscular atrophies. In: Jones HR, De Vivo DC, Darras BT, eds. *Neuromuscular Disorders of Infancy, Childhood, and Adolescence: A Clinician's Approach*. Philadelphia, Pa: Butterworth-Heinemann; 2003:145–166.

Fenichel GM. *Clinical Pediatric Neurology: A Signs and Symptoms Approach*. 4th ed. Philadelphia, Pa: WB Saunders; 2001:149–169.

Hirtz D, Iannaccone S, Heemskerk J, et al. Challenges and opportunities in clinical trials for spinal muscular atrophy. *Neurology*. 2005;65:1352–1357.

A healthy 7-year-old boy has been referred for an evaluation several months after starting the second grade because his teacher has noted that he frequently day-dreams. His reading and math skills were average but now are slightly below grade level. On questioning, his mother reports that there are times when he stops talking, stares, and blinks his eyes for several seconds. These spells do not seem to bother him, however, and he is fine afterwards.

Physical Examination General Examination: Normal. Neurologic Examination: Mental Status: Alert. Language: His speech is fluent without dysarthria. Cranial Nerves: II through XII intact. Motor: He has normal bulk and tone with 5/5 strength throughout. Coordination: He has normal finger-to-nose testing bilaterally. Sensory: There are no sensory deficits. Gait: He has a normal heel, toe, flat, and tandem gait. Reflexes: 2+ throughout with bilateral plantar flexor responses.

Guide to Case Discussion

- Briefly summarize this case.
- Localize the examination findings.
- Give the most likely diagnosis and provide a differential diagnosis.
- Discuss an appropriate diagnostic work-up.
- Discuss the management of this patient.

Diagnosis　Childhood absence epilepsy.

Discussion　Childhood absence epilepsy (petit mal epilepsy) is an idiopathic, primary, generalized epilepsy that occurs in otherwise healthy children. Seizure onset is between 4 and 10 years of age with a peak at 5 to 7 years of age. Girls are more commonly affected than boys. A strong genetic predisposition for absence epilepsy exists, although specific causative genes have not yet been identified.

Typical absence seizures last approximately 10 seconds but are almost always less than 30 seconds in duration. Multiple seizures usually occur in a day. The onset and termination of absence seizures are abrupt. The ictal state impairs consciousness and causes a cessation of voluntary activities. Clonic movements, such as eye fluttering or mouth movement, may be noted during seizures. Automatisms, such as chewing, perseverative hand movements, and changes in postural tone, can also occur. Patients are usually unaware of the event and recommence activities after a seizure is over. If postictal confusion occurs, it is brief, lasting only 2 to 3 seconds. There is also a risk of experiencing generalized tonic-clonic seizures.

The EEG background is normal in children with childhood absence epilepsy. An ictal event is characterized by bilaterally synchronous, symmetric, rhythmic 3-Hz spike-and-wave complexes. Similar interictal discharges also may be seen. Hyperventilation activates absence seizures in the majority of untreated individuals. Photic stimulation precipitates epileptiform activity on the EEG in approximately 15% of patients. Intermittent rhythmic delta activity may also be seen in the occipitoparietal regions.

Typical absence seizures in the setting of childhood absence epilepsy have a generally favorable prognosis, with approximately 80% of affected children outgrowing their seizures by adolescence. Some patients, however, may go on to experience juvenile absence epilepsy or juvenile myoclonic epilepsy.

Summary　The patient is a healthy 7-year-old boy who presents with a decline in academic performance and staring spells.

Localization　The patient is having generalized seizures that localize to the neurons of the cerebral cortex. Research suggests that the thalamocortical networks have a role in the generation of absence seizures. There are no localizing features on his neurologic exam.

Differential Diagnosis　The differential diagnosis of a child with difficulties in school and daydreaming includes various types of absence, as well as complex, partial seizures. In certain cases, typical absence seizures may need to be differentiated from eyelid myoclonia with absence seizures when parents report associated rhythmic eye blinking or fluttering. In this seizure type, children experience rhythmic eyelid myoclonia with a minor impairment of consciousness during seizures. These patients are highly photosensitive. Absence seizures with perioral myoclonia, as well as myoclonic absence, are additional generalized epilepsies that may need to be considered. The EEG in these cases usually demonstrates generalized discharges with polyspikes.

Atypical absences are another distinct seizure type. However, they occur most often in patients with mental retardation or other neurologic impairments and complex epilepsies, such as Lennox-Gastaut syndrome. Atypical absence seizures tend to last 5 to 10 seconds. The EEG typically demonstrates less-well-organized slow spike-and-wave discharges of 1.5 to 2.5 Hz. Atypical absence seizures are not precipitated by hyperventilation or photic stimulation.

In contrast to typical absence seizures, complex partial seizures may begin with an aura. They tend to last more than 1 minute and have more prominent automatisms, such as lip smacking and semipurposeful hand movements. Complex partial seizures are also more often associated with a postictal state. The EEG in complex partial seizures demonstrates focal rather than generalized epileptiform discharges.

Nonepileptic conditions such as learning disabilities, attention deficit disorder, daydreaming, depression, and other behavioral disorders must be considered. In these cases, a detailed history of the spells may help differentiate them from seizures. Children can usually be brought out of nonepileptic spells by having their name called or shoulder touched. They also do not interrupt ongoing activities, such as talking, chewing, or walking, as seizures do. Simple motor tics should also be considered in a child with brief episodes of eye blinking or fluttering. Tics are not associated with impaired consciousness.

Evaluation   A child with suspected absence seizures may be hyperventilated in the office, which will often provide the diagnosis. However, an EEG with hyperventilation and photic stimulation should be performed to confirm the diagnosis. Video EEG might be indicated in some patients to further clarify the diagnosis. Neuroimaging is not warranted in an otherwise healthy child with absence seizures unless the EEG or neurologic examination shows focal or atypical features. The child in this vignette also has poor school performance. Although untreated absence seizures may account for this, psychological and educational testing should be performed through the school system to rule out an underlying learning disability.

Management   Treatment with anticonvulsants is indicated in childhood absence epilepsy because seizures are frequent and ongoing seizure activity can adversely affect cognitive function. Accidents may also occur during seizures. Treatment options include ethosuximide, valproic acid, and lamotrigine.

Ethosuximide is usually reserved as first-line monotherapy for cases of simple absence seizures without other seizure types, such as generalized tonic-clonic. Initial doses of 10 to 15 mg/kg/day divided one to three times per day are typically used. Doses may be increased to 30 to 40 mg/kg/day if necessary. Common dose-related side effects of ethosuximide include gastrointestinal upset (nausea, vomiting, abdominal pain), anorexia, headaches, and sedation. Idiosyncratic reactions include blood dyscrasias (aplastic anemia, thrombocytopenia), systemic lupus erythematosus, lupus-like syndrome, autoimmune thyroiditis, allergic dermatitis, and Stevens-Johnson syndrome.

Valproic acid is a broader spectrum anticonvulsant and is used when other generalized seizure types occur. It can be used alone or in combination with ethosuximide when seizures are refractory to one medication. Doses of 15 to 60 mg/kg/day divided two or three times per day are used. Dose-related valproic acid side effects include gastrointestinal distress, increased appetite, weight gain, thrombocytopenia, hepatic dysfunction, menstrual irregularities, polycystic ovary disease, tremor, and hair loss. Idiosyncratic reactions include fatal hepatotoxicity and pancreatitis. Young age and polytherapy are risk factors for severe hepatotoxicity.

Finally, lamotrigine has also shown efficacy as monotherapy in the management of absence seizures. The metabolism of lamotrigine is significantly affected by the use of concomitant anticonvulsants. When used as monotherapy in children, an initial dose of 0.5 mg/kg/day is typically given with escalation to a maintenance dose of 2 to 12 mg/kg/day (divided twice per day). When used in conjunction with an enzyme-inducing anticonvulsant (phenytoin, phenobarbital, carbamazepine), an initial dose of 0.6 mg/kg/day is recommended, with a goal dose of 5 to 15 mg/kg/day. Valproic acid prolongs the elimination half-life of lamotrigine so when using a combination of these two drugs, patients should be started at 0.15 mg/kg/day with a maintenance goal of 1 to 5 mg/kg/day. Because of the risk of rash, the initial dose is usually maintained for 2 weeks, with subsequent dose increases made once per week.

Alergic rash is the most serious side effect associated with lamotrigine and is seen in approximately 10% of patients. It usually occurs in the first 8 weeks of administration. Rash leading to hospitalization, including erythema multiforme and Stevens-Johnson syndrome, has been reported in 1% of children and 0.03% of adults. Rapid titration and use in conjunction with valproic acid increases the risk of experiencing a rash. The neurotoxic effects of lamotrigine appear to be fewer than those of other anticonvulsants. However, headache, dizziness, sedation, nausea, and vomiting have been reported. The long titration period required to achieve a therapeutic level of lamotrigine may be a disadvantage for patients who are having frequent seizures.

Additional Questions

1. What is a serious teratogenic side effect of valproic acid?
2. Are the anticonvulsant treatment options limited for a child with absence seizures who cannot swallow a pill?

References

Berkovic SF, Benbadis S. Absence seizures. In: Wyllie E, ed. *The Treatment of Epilepsy: Principles and Practice.* 3rd ed. Philadelphia, Pa: Lippincott Williams & Wilkins; 2001: 357–367.

Coppola G, Auricchio G, Federico R, et al. Lamotrigine versus valproic acid as first-line monotherapy in newly diagnosed typical absence seizures: an open-label, randomized, parallel-group study. *Epilepsia.* 2005;45(9):1049–1053.

Coppola G, Liccardi F, Sciscio N, et al. Lamotrigine as first-line drug in childhood absence epilepsy: a clinical and neurophysiological study. *Brain Dev.* 2004;26(1):26–29.

Guberman AH, Besag FM, Brodie MJ, et al. Lamotrigine-associated rash: risk/benefit consideration in adults and children. *Epilepsia.* 1999;40(7):985–991.

Loiseau P, Panayiotopoulos P, Hirsch E. Childhood absence epilepsy and related syndromes. In: Roger J, Bureau M, Dravet C, et al., eds. *Epileptic Syndromes in Infancy, Childhood and Adolescence.* 3rd ed. Eastleigh, UK: John Libbey; 2002:285–303.

Pearl PL, Holmes GL. Absence seizures. In: Pellock JM, Dodson WE, Bourgeois BFD, eds. *Pediatric Epilepsy: Diagnosis and Therapy.* 2nd ed. New York: Demos Medical; 2001: 219–231.

A healthy 5-year-old girl presents to the neurology clinic because her mother has noted that over the last several weeks she has started bumping into things on her right side. The child articulates that she is having difficulty seeing out of her right eye. There is no history of headaches, nausea, or vomiting. She is currently in kindergarten, doing well, but she did require physical and speech therapy when she was a toddler. There is no family history of neurologic disease.

Physical Examination General Examination: Multiple brown macules are noted on her trunk. Freckles are seen in the axillary regions bilaterally. Neurologic Examination: Mental Status: Alert and cooperative. Language: Her speech is fluent without dysarthria. Cranial Nerves: Her visual acuity is 20/20 on the left and 20/200 on the right. Her pupils are equal, round, and reactive to light when light is placed in the left eye. When the light is quickly moved to the right eye, the right pupil dilates slowly. Her extraocular muscles are intact. She has difficulty cooperating with visual field testing but there does appear to be some degree of vision loss in the right eye. Facial sensation and movement are intact. A gag is present. The tongue is midline. Motor: She has normal bulk and tone with 5/5 strength throughout. Coordination: There is no dysmetria. Sensory: No deficits are noted. Gait: She has a normal heel, toe, and flat gait. Reflexes: 1+ throughout with bilateral plantar flexor responses.

Guide to Case Discussion

- Briefly summarize this case.
- Localize the examination findings.
- Give the most likely diagnosis and provide a differential diagnosis.
- Discuss an appropriate diagnostic work-up.
- Discuss the management of this patient.

TABLE 38.1

National Institutes of Health Diagnostic Criteria for Neurofibromatosis Type 1

Two or more of the following features must be present for the diagnosis of neuro-fibromatosis type 1 (NF1).

1. Six or more café-au-lait spots with a diameter greater than 0.5 cm before puberty and 1.5 cm after puberty
2. Axillary or inguinal freckling
3. Two or more neurofibromas or a single plexiform neurofibroma
4. Two or more Lisch nodules (iris hamartomas)
5. Optic pathway glioma
6. A distinctive osseous lesion such as a sphenoid wing dysplasia or thinning of long bone cortex
7. A first-degree relative with NF1 by the above criteria

Diagnosis Right optic nerve glioma in a child with neurofibromatosis type 1.

Discussion Neurofibromatosis type 1 (NF1) is a common autosomal dominant multisystem genetic disorder caused by a mutation on chromosome 17. NF1 occurs in approximately 1 in 3,000 individuals. Fifty percent of cases occur sporadically; the other 50% of cases are familial in origin. NF1 most commonly affects the skin (café-au-lait spots, axillary/inguinal freckling, neurofibromas), the eyes (optic gliomas, Lisch nodules), and the musculoskeletal system (pseudoarthrosis, scoliosis). Learning disabilities and developmental delays are also common in children with NF1. The diagnosis of NF1 is made clinically according to the National Institutes of Health (NIH) NF1 Diagnostic Criteria (Table 38.1). Two of seven features must be present to have the diagnosis.

Optic pathway gliomas (OPGs) are the most common intracranial tumor in the pediatric NF1 population, occurring in approximately 15% of children with NF1. However, only half of patients with OPGs experience symptoms such as decreased visual acuity, optic atrophy, pupillary dysfunction, nystagmus, proptosis, and/or decreased color vision. Precocious puberty can be seen when there is extension of an OPG into the chiasm and hypothalamus. Involvement of the chiasm occurs in two-thirds of patients with OPGs. Pathologically, OPGs are typically benign pilocytic astrocytomas by the World Health Organization (WHO) classification system. Children with NF1 who are younger than age 6 years are at the greatest risk for development of OPGs, although OPGs can occur in older children. For reasons that are poorly understood, OPGs in NF1 also tend to have a much more benign course than in patients without NF1.

Summary The patient is a 5-year-old girl with a history of mild gross motor and speech delays who presents with subacute right-sided vision loss. Her exam is remarkable for decreased right visual acuity and a right afferent pupillary defect in addition to café-au-lait spots and axillary freckling, which suggest a diagnosis of NF1.

Localization Gross motor and speech delays suggest a generalized encephalopathy that localizes diffusely to the cortex. Her right-sided vision loss and afferent pupillary defect localize to the right anterior visual pathway. Afferent pupillary defects are most common with lesions of the retina, optic nerve, and optic chiasm, but can also be seen with lesions involving the optic tract, brachium of the superior colliculus, and pretectal nucleus. Given this patient's probable diagnosis of NF1, it is most likely that her vision loss is a result of a lesion in the right optic nerve. Chiasmatic involvement cannot be ruled out, but vision appears to be normal in the left eye. There are no other cranial neuropathies to suggest brainstem involvement.

Differential Diagnosis The child in this vignette can be diagnosed with NF1 because of the presence of multiple café-au-lait spots, axillary freckling, and an OPG. Knowing that the patient has NF1 significantly narrows the differential diagnosis, making an OPG the most likely etiology of her symptoms.

However, demyelinating disease (Devic disease), immune-mediated disorders (lupus erythematosus), and infectious etiologies causing an inflammatory optic neuritis should also be considered. Suprasellar masses, such as pituitary adenomas or craniopharyngiomas, can compress the optic nerves and/or chiasm, causing progressive unilateral or bilateral vision loss, as well as endocrine abnormalities. Hereditary optic neuropathies seen in mitochondrial disorders (Leber hereditary optic neuropathy, Wolfram disease) can cause progressive vision loss but also may be associated with other neurologic abnormalities. Multiple inborn errors of metabolism (Refsum disease, abetalipoproteinemia, neuronal ceroid lipofuscinosis) are associated with retinal degeneration that results in progressive vision loss and deserve consideration. Finally, toxins, drugs (chemotherapy, antibiotics), and nutritional deficiencies (vitamins B_1, B_2, B_6, B_{12}) also enter the differential diagnosis. Drug toxicity is more likely to cause central vision loss though.

Evaluation A brain MRI with and without contrast should be performed immediately to evaluate for a lesion affecting the right afferent visual pathway. The patient also should be seen by an ophthalmologist to document a complete eye exam. If there is extension of the lesion into the optic chiasm and/or hypothalamus, an endocrinologist should be consulted for an appropriate screening evaluation.

Management Evidence-based medicine has not shown a benefit to routine screening brain MRIs for the detection of OPGs in asymptomatic children with NF1. In asymptomatic children younger than age 6 years, a complete ophthalmologic exam should be performed annually. Older asymptomatic children may have less frequent, abbreviated eye exams. Children found to have an OPG but who are without symptoms are typically managed conservatively with clinical observation, frequent ophthalmologic exams, and regular brain MRI scans. However, when OPGs become symptomatic, intervention is often required. Treatment options include chemotherapy (usually vincristine and carboplatin), radiation, and, rarely, globe-sparing tumor resection, but the type of therapy depends on the location and extent of the tumor. In addition, children with NF1 should be followed in a clinical setting by physicians familiar with their disease to monitor for complications. This patient should also be referred to a geneticist to discuss the implications of her NF1 diagnosis and to provide genetic counseling to the family.

Additional Questions

1. Describe the visual field defects associated with lesions of the optic chiasm.
2. Discuss the differential diagnosis of acute vision loss.

References

Brazis PW, Masdeu JC, Biller J. *Localization in Clinical Neurology.* 3rd ed. Philadelphia, Pa: Lippincott Williams & Wilkins; 1996:115–154.

Fenichel GM. *Clinical Pediatric Neurology: A Signs and Symptoms Approach.* 4th ed. Philadelphia, Pa: WB Saunders; 2001:317–330.

Habiby R, Silverman B, Listernick R, et al. Precocious puberty in children with neurofibromatosis type 1. *J Pediatr.* 1995;126(3):364–367.

Listernick R, Charrow J, Gutmann DH. Intracranial gliomas in neurofibromatosis type 1. *Semin Med Genet.* 1999;89:38–44.

Listernick R, Ferner RE, Piersall L, et al. Late-onset optic pathway tumors in children with neurofibromatosis 1. *Neurology.* 2004;63:1944–1946.

Listernick R, Louis DN, Packer RJ, et al. Optic pathway gliomas in children with neurofibromatosis 1: consensus statement from the NF1 optic pathway glioma task force. *Ann Neurol.* 1997;41(2):143–149.

National Institutes of Health Consensus Development Conference. Neurofibromatosis: conference statement. *Arch Neurol.* 1988;45(5):575–578.

North KN. Neurofibromatosis 1 in childhood. *Semin Pediatr Neurol.* 1998;5:231–242.

A **15-year-old boy** is brought to the office by concerned parents for complaints of unusual behavior. The patient had been sleeping almost continuously over the last 3 weeks. If his family tries to wake him up, he becomes very angry and quickly goes back to sleep. At times, he awakens to go to the bathroom or to eat voraciously. While awake, he seems confused and irritable. His parents had a very difficult time getting him out of the house to make the appointment. There is no history of head trauma, fever, or illness. There is no family history of neurologic disease.

Physical Examination General Examination: A 15-year-old boy sleeping on the exam table with a normal general exam. Neurologic Examination: Mental Status: He is arousable and able to perform the exam but very irritable. Language: He speaks in full sentences without dysarthria. Cranial Nerves: His pupils are equal, round, and reactive to light. His extraocular muscles are intact and there are no visual field deficits. His face is symmetric. The tongue is midline. Motor: He has normal bulk and tone with 5/5 strength throughout. Coordination: There is no dysmetria or tremor. Sensory: Light touch, temperature, and vibration are intact. Reflexes: 2+ throughout with bilateral plantar flexor responses.

Guide to Case Discussion

- Briefly summarize this case.
- Localize the examination findings.
- Give the most likely diagnosis and provide a differential diagnosis.
- Discuss an appropriate diagnostic work-up.
- Discuss the management of this patient.

Diagnosis Kleine-Levin syndrome.

Discussion Kleine-Levin syndrome is a rare disorder that is characterized by a classic triad of hypersomnia, compulsive hyperphagia, and hypersexuality. Other symptoms, such as compulsions, behavioral disturbance, derealization, hallucinations, delusions, and depression, commonly occur. Associated cognitive abnormalities have included confusion, as well as deficits in memory, attention, and concentration.

Hypersomnia is present in all cases, with most patients sleeping 18 to 24 hours per day. Affected individuals may briefly awaken to eat or void but they are extremely agitated if woken from sleep. Depressed mood and irritability typically occur during the episodes. Most affected individuals have increased food intake with intense food cravings. A desire for eating sweets is very common. Hypersexual behaviors have included overt masturbation, exposing oneself, making unwanted sexual advances, and genitalia fondling.

Symptoms typically last 2 to 4 weeks and then resolve spontaneously. Episodes commonly recur weeks to months later. There is a 2:1 male predominance, but females may be more severely affected. The average age of onset is 15 years. The disorder usually lasts between 4 and 8 years. It typically resolves by early adulthood and overall has a good prognosis.

The underlying pathophysiology of this unique disorder is poorly understood. Most cases are primary, but secondary causes, like stroke, multiple sclerosis, hydrocephalus, posttraumatic intracranial hematoma, and encephalitis, have been reported. Secondary cases have a later age of onset as well as a worse prognosis. Precipitating factors for Kleine-Levin syndrome have included head trauma, viral infection (flu-like illness, gastroenteritis, upper respiratory tract infection), alcohol or marijuana use, and menses. However, during episodes, cerebrospinal fluid studies, hormone tests, and neuroimaging are all typically normal. EEGs performed during the episodes are also normal or diffusely slow. It has been hypothesized that Kleine-Levin syndrome may represent an infectious or postinfectious autoimmune process that targets the hypothalamus. The human leukocyte antigen (HLA) subtype DQB1*02 is associated with the disorder and supports this theory.

Summary The patient is a healthy 15-year-old boy who presents during a 3-week-long episode of hypersomnia and hyperphagia. He is sleepy and irritable, but has a normal neurologic exam.

Localization There are no focal features to the patient's neurologic exam. However, symptoms of hypersomnolence and hyperphagia suggest an abnormality of the hypothalamus.

Differential Diagnosis The symptoms of episodic and extreme hypersomnia, hyperphagia, and hypersexuality are relatively specific for Kleine-Levin syndrome. However, the differential diagnosis of Kleine-Levin syndrome includes other intrinsic sleep disorders, as well as many secondary organic etiologies. Narcolepsy presents with excessive daytime sleepiness, but prolonged periods of sleep are not characteristic of it. It also manifests with sleep attacks, cataplexy, sleep paralysis, and hypnagogic hallucinations. Obstructive sleep apnea, periodic limb movement disorder, and restless leg syndrome are not associated with the extreme sleepiness or behavioral changes seen in this case.

Hypersomnia can occur posttraumatically and may be part of a postconcussive syndrome. However, the patient in this case has no history of head trauma. Psychiatric disorders, such as major depression or bipolar disorder, may be characterized by excessive sleepiness, irritability, and appetite change and should be ruled out. Drug dependency or addiction can cause similar symptoms and are common during adolescence. Endocrinopathies such as hypothyroidism or adrenal abnormalities should also be considered. Complex partial seizures may be associated with episodic alteration of consciousness and behavior change, but are unlikely to explain this teenager's symptoms.

Several intracranial processes may be associated with the symptoms of Kleine-Levin syndrome. Lesions affecting the diencephalon and mesencephalon should be considered. Brain tumors, meningoencephalitis, vasculitis, vascular lesions, demyelinating disease, stroke, hypoxic-ischemic/metabolic/toxic encephalopathy, and hypothalamic sarcoidosis enter the differential diagnosis. Finally, Prader-Willi syndrome is associated with a deletion on chromosome 15. It is characterized by extreme hyperphagia and obesity. Given that the patient in this vignette has otherwise been normal and healthy, this is an unlikely cause of his symptoms.

Evaluation The diagnosis of Kleine-Levin syndrome is one of exclusion and organic etiologies must first be ruled out. Baseline laboratory studies, including a CBC, basic chemistries, liver function tests, kidney function tests, and urine toxicology screen, may be performed. Abnormalities of the hypothalamic-pituitary axis can be excluded with assessment of thyroid function tests, cortisol levels, adrenocorticotropic hormone analysis, and growth hormone analysis. Neuroimaging with a brain MRI with and without gadolinium is mandatory to rule out structural abnormalities that involve the diencephalon and/or mesencephalon such as tumor, infection, demyelinating disease, vascular lesions, and trauma. A lumbar puncture might also be considered to rule out meningoencephalitis or other inflammatory processes. An EEG helps exclude seizure activity. A polysomnogram can also be helpful in assessing overall sleep patterns and ruling out other intrinsic sleep disorders, such as narcolepsy, restless leg syndrome, period limb movement disorder, and obstructive sleep apnea. A psychiatric assessment is also important to exclude an underlying depression or other psychiatric disorder.

Management Kleine-Levin syndrome is particularly refractory to pharmacologic management. Stimulant medications are successfully used to combat excessive sleepiness but may exacerbate other symptoms, such as hypersexuality. Neuroleptics, antidepressants, anticonvulsants, and lithium have been tried in the management of a variety of the associated symptoms, but rarely are of clear benefit. Antidepressants and phototherapy have been used to prevent relapses, but are not usually helpful. Lithium, however, may have some role in preventing relapses.

The psychosocial impact of Kleine-Levin syndrome on affected adolescents and their families is profound. Discussion of the diagnosis must occur with the school system and specific accommodations need to be made. Involvement of a neurologist and/or psychiatrist is also necessary to help manage symptoms during attacks.

References

Arnulf I, Zeitzer JM, File J, et al. Kleine-Levin syndrome: a systematic review of 186 cases in the literature. *Brain*. 2005;128(pt 12):2763–2776.

Capp PK, Pearl PL, Lewin D. Pediatric sleep disorders. *Prim Care*. 2005;32:549–562.

Dauvilliers Y, Mayer G, Lecendreux M, et al. Kleine-Levin syndrome: an autoimmune hypothesis based on clinical and genetic analyses. *Neurology*. 2002;59:1739–1745.

Wise MS, Lynch J. Narcolepsy in children. *Semin Pediatr Neurol*. 2001;8(4):198–206.

A 10-year-old boy is referred to the neurology office for evaluation because he is having difficulty keeping up with his friends on the soccer team. When practice begins, he feels like his muscles are stiff and he has a hard time starting to exercise. This improves after he exercises for a few minutes and practice continues. There is no muscle pain or cramping. He is otherwise healthy and his development has been normal. His father has similar symptoms but they do not interfere with his activities of daily living and he has never discussed them with his doctor.

Physical Examination General Examination: There are no dysmorphic facial features. Neurologic Examination: Mental Status: Alert and cooperative. Language: His speech is fluent without dysarthria. Cranial Nerves: His pupils are equal, round, and reactive to light. His extraocular muscles are intact. His face is symmetric with normal strength. It takes several seconds for him to open his eyes after closing them. The tongue is midline without fasciculations. Motor: There is mild hypertrophy of the calves bilaterally. He has normal tone with 5/5 strength throughout. Coordination: There is no dysmetria or tremor. Sensory: Light touch, temperature, and vibration are intact throughout. Gait: Before getting up to walk, he hesitates and complains of muscle stiffness. He then has a normal flat, heel, toe, and tandem gait. Reflexes: 2+ throughout with bilateral plantar flexor responses.

Guide to Case Discussion

- Briefly summarize this case.
- Localize the examination findings.
- Give the most likely diagnosis and provide a differential diagnosis.
- Discuss an appropriate diagnostic work-up.
- Discuss the management of this patient.

Diagnosis   Myotonia congenita.

Discussion   Myotonia congenita is a hereditary intrinsic disorder of the muscle characterized by myotonia. Myotonia causes impairment of relaxation of skeletal muscle after a contraction. Myotonia congenita is caused by a mutation in the skeletal muscle chloride channel gene *CLCN1* on chromosome 7. It results in an abnormality of a subunit of the skeletal muscle voltage-gated chloride channel CLC-1. Chloride conductance is essential to maintaining the resting membrane potential in skeletal muscle. An imbalance in the delicate system of sodium, potassium, and chloride conductance in muscle cells can result in myotonia, as well as weakness.

Myotonia congenita has two similar clinical presentations, Thomsen disease and Becker disease (Table 40.1). Although both are caused by mutations in the *CLC1* gene, Thomsen disease follows an autosomal dominant inheritance pattern whereas Becker disease is transmitted in an autosomal recessive manner. Becker disease is much more common. Onset is highly variable but usually occurs in childhood. Males may be more severely affected than females. Individuals with myotonia congenita usually experience complaints of painless muscle stiffness at rest, which improves with repeated muscle contraction or exercise. This "warm-up" phenomenon is difficult to explain on a physiologic basis. All striated muscle groups may be affected, so myotonia may be seen in the face, tongue, or extremity musculature. Other organ systems are not involved.

Thomsen disease typically has an earlier onset and milder symptoms than Becker disease. Myotonia is usually mild to moderate. Heterozygotes are usually symptomatic. Becker disease generally has a later onset and more severe symptoms. Myotonia is moderate to severe and some individuals experience a mild, but persistent distal weakness. Brief attacks of weakness may also occur after complete relaxation in Becker disease. Muscle hypertrophy is more prominent than in Thomsen disease. Heterozygotes are typically asymptomatic.

Symptoms of myotonia congenita are usually stable and lifelong. Some women report worsening of myotonia during pregnancy. Many affected individuals also report some worsening with cold. There also appears to be a clinical spectrum of the severity with myotonia congenita. There is a high degree of intrafamilial variation that occurs in individuals who carry the same mutation. In addition, several

TABLE 40.1

Forms of Myotonia Congenita

	Thomsen Disease	Becker Disease
Inheritance	Autosomal dominant	Autosomal recessive
Chromosome	Chromosome 7q35	Chromosome 7q35
Gene	*CLCN1*	*CLCN1*
Age of onset	Earlier onset	Later onset
Myotonia	Mild-moderate	Moderate-severe
Calf hypertrophy	Mild	Moderate
Strength	Normal	Distal weakness

autosomal dominant mutations are associated with unusual phenotypes, including fluctuating symptoms, a paramyotonia-like syndrome, and a form with proximal weakness and dysphagia, as well as a form with distal myopathy.

Summary The patient is a healthy, developmentally normal, 10-year-old boy who presents with complaints of painless muscle stiffness when initiating movement, symptoms that are also reported by his father. His exam is remarkable for eyelid myotonia and mild calf hypertrophy but is otherwise normal.

Localization This child's complaints of stiffness and eyelid myotonia localize to the muscle. Calf hypertrophy also supports localization to the muscle.

Differential Diagnosis Myotonia congenita must be differentiated from other conditions that cause myotonia (Table 40.2). This may prove challenging in many cases, as there is significant clinical overlap with other chloride and sodium channelopathies. Several of the myotonic disorders are associated with periodic paralysis, which is not present in this patient. However, distinguishing clinical features may be determined by factors that precipitate or alleviate myotonia, presence of other organ system involvement, and findings on electrodiagnostic studies.

Myotonia congenita should first be differentiated from the more common myotonic dystrophy. Myotonic dystrophy is an autosomal dominant disorder caused by an expansion of the CTG trinucleotide repeat on chromosome 19 that codes for a serine/threonine protein kinase. The age of onset of myotonic dystrophy varies widely. It may present as a severe congenital form with respiratory distress, poor feeding, and hypotonia. Onset in childhood is usually associated with nonmuscular symptoms such as cognitive delay, clumsiness, cardiac arrhythmias, and gastrointestinal dysmotility. Patients may have a characteristic facies with myopathy of the face and eyes that also affects the arms, hands, and legs, but calf hypertrophy does not occur. Myotonia worsens with rest and cold. A "warm-up" phenomenon may be described by some patients. The child presented in this case does not have a myopathy or other extramuscular symptoms, making it an unlikely etiology of his symptoms.

Proximal myotonic myopathy (PROMM) is an another autosomal dominant myotonic condition, but its genetic defect is unknown. It is only rarely seen in childhood, typically presenting in adolescence or adulthood. Affected children usually

TABLE 40.2
Differential Diagnosis of Myotonia Congenita
Myotonic dystrophy Proximal myotonic myopathy Myotonia fluctuans Myotonia permanens Acetazolamide-responsive sodium channel myotonia Paramyotonia congenita

complain of myotonia and pain in the hands and legs. Calf hypertrophy may occasionally be seen. Later in life, affected individuals demonstrate weakness of the proximal thighs, hips, and neck flexors in addition to muscle pain, cataracts, and arrhythmias. Consequently, because of the age of onset, PROMM is unlikely in the patient in this vignette.

Three autosomal dominant myotonic conditions are associated with a mutation in the skeletal muscle sodium channel gene on chromosome 17: myotonia fluctuans, myotonia permanens, and acetazolamide-responsive sodium channel myotonia. They do not cause periodic paralysis. All three disorders present during the first decade of life and have clinical features similar to myotonia congenita. Only myotonia fluctuans, however, is associated with calf hypertrophy. Symptoms fluctuate in severity, particularly after exercise, which is not described by the patient in this case. Myotonia permanens causes severe myotonia of the face, extremities, and respiratory muscles, and can result in hypoxia. Acetazolamide-responsive sodium channel myotonia affects the eyelids, face, extremities, and paraspinous muscles. Symptoms are precipitated by fasting, cold, potassium, and infections.

Finally, paramyotonia congenita is an autosomal dominant condition also caused by a mutation in the skeletal muscle sodium channel gene on chromosome 17. Like myotonia congenita, it can present with generalized stiffness and muscle cramps in early to mid-childhood. Myopathy and muscle hypertrophy, however, are not seen. Also, in contrast to myotonia congenita, children with paramyotonia congenita are extremely sensitive to cold. Stiffness, myotonia, and weakness occur on cold exposure. Although children with myotonia congenita experience an improvement in symptoms with exercise, children affected with paramyotonia have worsening of their stiffness with repeated muscle contraction.

Calf hypertrophy is also a classic physical exam finding in Duchenne muscular dystrophy. However, affected children present at a much younger age with progressive proximal weakness and motor delays. Myotonia is not seen in muscular dystrophies. The child in this case has a very different clinical presentation, making Duchenne muscular dystrophy unlikely.

Evaluation   Making the diagnosis of a myotonic disorder can be challenging. A thorough history of alleviating measures and provocative stimuli must be taken. It must also be determined whether the patient has associated symptoms of periodic paralysis as there is significant overlap between these channelopathies. A family history is essential as many of these disorders are hereditary. Other organ involvement also may help to suggest a specific disease. The evaluation should start by obtaining a CK level. The CK level in myotonia congenita may be normal or slightly elevated to three to four times the upper limit of normal. EMG usually confirms the presence of myotonia.

Fortunately, now that the underlying genetic abnormality has been identified, specific DNA testing can be performed for myotonia congenita. Sequence analysis detects a causative mutation in more than 95% of affected individuals with both autosomal dominant and recessive forms of the disease, and currently is the most efficient, least-invasive means of arriving at a definitive diagnosis.

A muscle biopsy can be very helpful in determining the etiology of a myopathy. However, in myotonia congenita the muscle biopsy is typically normal and a biopsy is usually not indicated because genetic testing is available.

Management   A variety of pharmacologic treatments has been used to control myotonia. The antiarrhythmic drug mexiletine is probably most effective. Tocainide, procainamide, quinine, and phenytoin also have been found to be beneficial in some patients, as have carbamazepine, dantrolene, and acetazolamide. Depolarizing muscle relaxants, beta-adrenergic agonists, beta-antagonists (propranolol), and colchicines may worsen myotonia. In addition, many individuals with myotonia congenita need to adapt their lifestyle and exercise to avoid factors that precipitate symptoms. Stretching exercises should be encouraged to avoid the development of heel cord and elbow contractures.

Finally, any child found to have a myotonic disorder should be referred to a geneticist. Other family members should undergo an appropriate work-up and genetic counseling should be provided.

Additional Questions

1. What are the characteristics of myotonia on EMG?
2. What are the clinical features of myotonic dystrophy in adulthood?

References

Colding-Jørgensen E. Phenotypic variability in myotonia congenita. *Muscle Nerve.* 2005;32: 19–34.

Dunø M, Colding-Jørgensen E. Myotonia congenita. 2005. Available at: http://www. genetests.org. Last accessed April 28, 2006.

Moxley RT, Tawil R, Thornton CA. Channelopathies: myotonic disorders and periodic paralysis. In: Swaiman KS, Ashwal S, eds. *Pediatric Neurology: Principles and Practice.* 3rd ed. St. Louis, Mo: Mosby; 1999:1299–1310.

Moxley RT. Channelopathies affecting skeletal muscle: myotonic disorders including myotonic dystrophy and periodic paralysis. In: Jones HR, De Vivo DC, Darras BT, eds. *Neuromuscular Disorders of Infancy, Childhood, and Adolescence: A Clinician's Approach.* Philadelphia, Pa: Butterworth-Heinemann; 2003:783–812.

Zhang J, Bendahhou S, Sanguinetti MC, et al. Functional consequences of chloride channel gene (*CLCN1*) mutations causing myotonia congenita. *Neurology.* 2000;54:937–942.

A 12-year-old girl from South America presents to the office for evaluation of frequent falls. Over the past 2 years, she has had increasing difficulty walking and she often trips. She recently stopped playing on the school soccer team because of difficulties with running and kicking the ball. Her schoolwork is also suffering because she has trouble holding the pencil and writing as quickly as her classmates. Her father, as well as several relatives who reside in her home country, has similar neurologic problems but no definitive diagnosis has ever been made.

Physical Examination General Examination: Normal except mild pes cavus bilaterally. Neurologic Examination: Mental Status: She is pleasant and cooperative. Cranial Nerves: Her pupils are equal, round, and reactive to light. Her extraocular muscles are intact. There are no visual field deficits. Her face is symmetric with normal strength. The tongue is midline without fasciculations. Motor: There is mild atrophy of the thenar eminences and foot intrinsic muscles. Her strength is 5/5 in the proximal muscle groups. The strength in the hands is 4+/5, her ankle dorsiflexion is 3/5, and her plantar flexion is 4/5. Coordination: No dysmetria or tremor is noted. Sensory: There is slightly decreased vibratory sensation and proprioception in her toes more than her fingers. Gait: She has a mild steppage gait with some evidence of bilateral footdrop. She is able to ambulate on her toes but not her heels. Reflexes: Cannot be obtained even with reinforcement. She has bilateral plantar flexor responses.

Guide to Case Discussion

▦ Briefly summarize this case.

▦ Localize the examination findings.

▦ Give the most likely diagnosis and provide a differential diagnosis.

▦ Discuss an appropriate diagnostic work-up.

▦ Discuss the management of this patient.

Diagnosis Hereditary motor and sensory neuropathy type 1A (Charcot-Marie-Tooth disease type 1A).

Discussion The hereditary motor and sensory neuropathies (HMSN) are a heterogeneous group of hereditary polyneuropathies. Classification of these disorders has proven challenging because of their diverse clinical manifestations and complex inheritance patterns. Currently, the HMSN are categorized according to histologic and neurophysiologic findings. Both demyelinating and axonal forms of the disease exist. Demyelinating variants include HMSN1, HMSN3, and HMSN4. HMSN2 describes axonal neuropathies. The incidence of these disorders is approximately 1 in 2,500 individuals.

HMSN1A, 1B, 1C, and 1D follow an autosomal dominant inheritance pattern. HMSN1A is most common and is caused by a duplication in the peripheral myelin protein 22 (*PMP22*) gene on chromosome 17p11.2-12. Rarely, it is caused by a point mutation in the *PMP22* gene. The precise function of the *PMP22* gene is not yet understood. HMSN1B maps to chromosome 1q and is the result of a mutation in the myelin protein zero (*Po*) gene.

HMSN2 is much less common than HMSN1. HMSN2 is the axonal form of the disease and, again, there are various subtypes (HMSN2A, 2B, 2C, 2D). Several of the associated genes have been identified. HMSN2C has a distinct presentation with vocal cord paralysis and respiratory muscle weakness.

HMSN1 and HMSN2 share very similar clinical features. They both cause an insidious and progressive, distal polyneuropathy that begins in the intrinsic muscles of the feet and then progresses to cause proximal weakness as well as involvement of hand muscles. Onset is usually during the first two decades of life. Initial complaints may include ankle instability, tripping, and gait abnormalities (steppage gait, toe walking). Early in the course there may be difficulty with heel walking, mild pes cavus, calf atrophy, and depressed or absent reflexes. With time, pes cavus, peroneal atrophy, and hammer toes become more prominent. Progressive impairment of vibration and proprioception may also be noted and contribute to difficulties with balance and walking. Touch, pain, and temperature sensation are less commonly involved. Pain, paresthesias, and cranial neuropathies are not characteristic of the disorder. As the hands become involved, fine motor tasks, such as writing and doing buttons, become more difficult. Clawing of fingers may eventually occur. In general, HMSN2 has a later onset (during the 20s) with less involvement of hand intrinsic musculature. Also, HMSN1 may be associated with palpable peripheral nerves, which are not seen in individuals with HMSN2.

The classification of HMSN3 is controversial but it is also known as Déjérine-Sottas disease (DSD). Autosomal dominant and autosomal recessive forms exist. Several variants have been described. HMSN4 is a diverse group of neuropathies also with autosomal dominant and autosomal recessive inheritance patterns. HMSN4 is also known as congenital hypomyelination neuropathy (CHN). DSD and CHN have significant clinical overlap and present in infancy with a severe demyelinating polyneuropathy, hypotonia, areflexia, generalized weakness, and developmental motor delay.

Summary The patient is a 12-year-old girl who presents with progressive distal weakness involving the lower extremities more than the upper extremities and a positive family history of a similar neurologic disease. Her exam is remarkable for pes cavus, atrophy of hand and foot intrinsic musculature, distal weakness, and areflexia, in addition to mild impairment of distal vibration and proprioceptive sensation.

Localization   The adolescent in this case presents with many signs and symptoms of a lower motor neuron disease process. Pes cavus, muscle atrophy, distal weakness, sensory loss, and areflexia all point to a disorder of the peripheral nerve. The patient has both weakness and sensory loss, which suggests a motor and sensory neuropathy. Loss of vibratory and proprioceptive sensation localize to the nerve fibers subserved by the posterior columns.

Differential Diagnosis   The differential diagnosis of polyneuropathy in childhood and adolescence is broad. Both hereditary and acquired conditions must be considered. It is helpful to determine the distribution of the neuropathy (symmetric versus asymmetric), the destructive process (demyelinating versus axonal), the nerves involved (motor versus sensory), the location (distal versus proximal) and the time course of development of the neuropathy (acute versus chronic). However, as in this case, a positive family history can help narrow the differential diagnosis significantly.

Although HMSN1 is most common, other forms of hereditary neuropathy should also be considered. HMSN1A must be differentiated from other subtypes of HMSN1, HMSN2, and hereditary neuropathy with susceptibility to pressure palsy (HNPP). HNPP often develops in adolescence. Affected individuals experience recurrent mononeuropathies with focal motor and/or sensory deficits. The patient in this vignette has a more generalized neuropathy, however. Hereditary motor neuropathies represent a subgroup of the HMSN but patients experience a pure motor neuropathy on clinical exam as well as on electrophysiologic studies. These patients may have atypical features such as vocal cord or diaphragmatic paralysis. Hereditary sensory and autonomic neuropathies, such as Riley-Day syndrome, are another heterogeneous group of disorders characterized by autonomic and sensory findings. Pain fibers are typically affected. Four forms of the disease are recognized. The patient in this case reports no autonomic symptoms or pain, however.

Acquired disorders also need to be ruled out, particularly when the family history is negative. Special attention should be given to any treatable conditions that may be responsible for an affected patient's symptoms. First, chronic inflammatory demyelinating polyneuropathy (CIDP) must be considered in any child presenting with a subacute polyneuropathy. CIPD is an immune-mediated demyelinating polyneuropathy and is distinguished from Guillain-Barré syndrome by its clinical course. Weakness of the lower extremities is the predominant symptom although cranial neuropathies can also occur. These children may demonstrate one of three clinical syndromes: (a) a monophasic illness with symptoms lasting more than 2 months, (b) a slow progressive course, or (c) a relapsing/remitting course. NCS demonstrate demyelination with slowing of motor nerve conduction velocity, prolonged distal latencies, absent or prolonged F-wave latencies, and dispersion of the compound muscle action potential or conduction block. The CSF protein is usually elevated.

Second, systemic conditions (diabetes, uremia, porphyria), endocrinopathies (hypothyroidism), vitamin deficiencies (vitamin B_{12}, vitamin E), and chronic exposure to toxins such as heavy metals (arsenic, lead, thallium) should be considered.

Mononeuritis multiplex is a vasculitis that affects peripheral nerves asymmetrically and can be seen in autoimmune disorders like lupus erythematosus, rheumatoid arthritis, and polyarteritis nodosa. Infections such as Lyme disease can also cause a peripheral neuropathy.

Finally, a wide variety of metabolic diseases can present with peripheral nerve involvement, but this is rarely the primary manifestation. For example, leukodystrophies (metachromatic leukodystrophy, Krabbe disease, Pelizaeus-Merzbacher disease), lipid storage diseases (Tay-Sachs, Fabry disease, Gaucher disease), peroxisomal disorders (Refsum disease, adrenoleukodystrophy), and mitochondrial disorders can manifest with peripheral neuropathy. Inborn errors of metabolism would be unusual in the patient presented in this case, however. She has not had any other symptoms of an inborn error of metabolism such as developmental regression, facial dysmorphisms, seizures, cognitive decline, myopathy, ophthalmologic abnormalities, or hepatosplenomegaly.

Evaluation Any child who presents with signs and symptoms of a polyneuropathy requires a thorough birth, medical, developmental, and family history, in addition to a general and neurologic exam. A history of exposure to toxins, medications or infections is relevant. Features suggestive of systemic illness or metabolic disease should be noted. A positive family history may also help point to a specific etiology.

For the patient in this vignette, the presentation and family history are highly suggestive of an HMSN. Electrodiagnostic studies are the next step in the work-up and will help to determine whether a demyelinating or axonal process is involved. An NCS in a patient with HMSN1 typically shows moderate to severely slowed motor and sensory nerve conduction velocities. The compound muscle action potentials are usually normal with normal morphology. EMG may demonstrate normal- or high-amplitude, rapidly firing motor unit potentials, reduced recruitment, and little spontaneous activity. Molecular genetic testing is commercially available for many of the HMSNs and can significantly aid in the diagnosis. It should be done for the patient in this vignette in an attempt to identify a specific causative mutation.

In the absence of a family history of neuropathy, ruling out other causes of polyneuropathy is warranted. An initial screening evaluation might include a CBC, basic chemistry panel, glucose, urinalysis, erythrocyte sedimentation rate, ANA, liver function tests, thyroid function tests, vitamin B_{12} level, vitamin E level, and urine toxicology/heavy metal screen. A lumbar puncture might also be considered to rule out CIDP, Guillain-Barré syndrome, and an infectious process.

Management Management of HMSN is aimed at maintaining mobility, comfort, and stability. Early in the disease course, orthotic devices such as splints, shoe insoles, and ankle-foot orthoses, can be very helpful. Stretching and limited exercise might also be beneficial. Because a variety of surgical procedures are available for joint stability and management of deformities, physical therapists, occupational therapists, and an orthopaedics team should follow an affected patient. Patients should also be monitored closely for the development of scoliosis as orthopaedic surgeries may be required for spine stabilization.

Any child presenting with an HMSN should also be evaluated by a geneticist. A geneticist is helpful in interpreting any genetic tests used to establish the diagnosis. The geneticist can also help to evaluate and counsel other family members.

Additional Questions

1. What are the treatment options for a child with CIDP?
2. What are the clinical features of giant axonal neuropathy?
3. Which peripheral neuropathies predominantly affect motor nerves? Sensory nerves?

References

Bennett CL, Chance PF. Molecular pathogenesis of hereditary motor, sensory and autonomic neuropathies. *Curr Opin Neurol.* 2001;14:621–627.

Chance PF, Escolar DM, Redmond A, et al. Hereditary neuropathies in late childhood and adolescence. In: Jones HR, De Vivo DC, Darras BT, eds. *Neuromuscular Disorders of Infancy, Childhood, and Adolescence: A Clinician's Approach.* Philadelphia, Pa: Butterworth-Heinemann; 2003:389–406.

Ouvrier RA, McLeod JG, Pollard JD. *Peripheral Neuropathy in Childhood.* 2nd ed. London, UK: Mac Keith Press; 1999:29–41, 67–135, 172–200.

Reilly MM. Classification of the hereditary motor and sensory neuropathies. *Curr Opin Neurol.* 2000;13:561–564.

Ryan MM, Ouvrier R. Hereditary peripheral neuropathies of childhood. *Curr Opin Neurol.* 2005;18:105–110.

A healthy 7-year-old girl is brought to the emergency department by her parents for complaints of right-sided weakness and an abnormal, limping gait that has developed over 3 days. She was well until 2 weeks prior when she began to have low-grade fevers, headaches, and emesis. During this time, she also experienced some rhinorrhea and cough, which the pediatrician diagnosed as a viral infection. While in the emergency room, she is witnessed having four episodes of right-gaze deviation with jerking of the right face and tonic-clonic movements of the right upper and lower extremities lasting 1 minute each. The patient is developmentally normal with no significant past medical history.

Physical Examination   Vital Signs: Temperature = 100.5°F. General Examination: Her fundi are difficult to visualize but there appears to be blurring of the right disc margin. Otherwise she has a normal general exam. Neurologic Examination: Mental Status: Alert but irritable. Language: She is able to follow commands well and speaks in full sentences without dysarthria. Cranial Nerves: Her pupils are equal, round, and reactive to light. Her extraocular muscles are intact, except she is unable to completely abduct her right eye. Her visual fields are intact. There is mild flattening of the right nasolabial fold. The tongue is midline. Motor: She has normal bulk but the right upper and lower extremities are slightly hypotonic. Her strength is 3 to 4/5 in the right upper and lower extremities. She has normal tone, with 5/5 strength on the left. Coordination: There is no dysmetria on finger-to-nose testing on the left but it is difficult to assess on the right because of weakness. Sensory: Light touch, temperature, and vibration are intact. Gait: She ambulates with some assistance and circumduction of the right leg. Reflexes: 3+ on the right and 2+ on the left. Right plantar extensor and left plantar flexor responses.

Guide to Case Discussion

▧ Briefly summarize this case.

▧ Localize the examination findings.

▧ Give the most likely diagnosis and provide a differential diagnosis.

▧ Discuss an appropriate diagnostic work-up.

▧ Discuss the management of this patient.

Diagnosis Cerebral sinus venous thrombosis and mastoiditis resulting in subacute left frontal lobe venous infarction.

Discussion Cerebral sinus venous thrombosis (CSVT) likely accounts for 25% of ischemic cerebrovascular disease in children. The incidence is estimated to be 0.67 per 100,000 children. Children of all ages can be affected, but neonates and younger children appear to be particularly at risk. Neonates typically present with fever, irritability, lethargy, and respiratory distress, whereas older children may have fever and lethargy in addition to signs of elevated intracranial pressure such as headache, vomiting, papilledema, and abducens nerve palsy. Focal seizures are also common at presentation in all age groups. In some cases, small intraparenchymal hemorrhages may occur.

Several mechanisms can cause thrombosis in the cerebral venous system, including venous stasis, hypercoagulable conditions, and endothelial damage. Impaired venous drainage leads to ischemia as a consequence of congestion of the underlying white matter. Superior sagittal sinus thrombosis can cause bilateral cortical infarcts whereas thrombosis involving the deep venous system can cause cerebellar or basal ganglia infarcts. Neurologic deficits caused by venous infarction may less clearly localize than those caused by arterial stroke.

A wide variety of local and systemic conditions predispose to the development of CSVT in childhood (Table 42.1). Cerebral hypoperfusion as a result of dehydration, shock, or congestive heart failure may result in CSVT. Infectious processes, such as mastoiditis, otitis media, and bacterial meningitis, predispose children to developing CSVT, and sepsis in neonates can also be a risk factor. A hypercoagulable state is found in many children with CSVT and may be related to a broad range of conditions. Autoimmune diseases (systemic lupus erythematosus, rheumatoid arthritis), malignancy, hereditary thrombophilia (protein C deficiency, protein S deficiency, antithrombin III deficiency, factor V Leiden gene mutation, prothrombin G20210A gene mutation), and medications (oral contraceptive pills) should be considered. Antiphospholipid

---

TABLE 42.1

Risk Factors for Pediatric Cerebral Sinus Venous Thrombosis

Infection
  Mastoiditis
  Otitis media
  Bacterial meningitis
  Sepsis (neonates)

Hematologic Thrombophilia
  Protein C deficiency
  Protein S deficiency
  Antithrombin III deficiency
  Factor V Leiden gene mutation
  Prothrombin G20210A gene mutation
  Antiphospholipid syndrome

Autoimmune Disorders
  Systemic lupus erythematosus
  Rheumatoid arthritis
  Behçet disease

Cerebral Hypoperfusion
  Dehydration
  Congestive heart failure

Other
  Malignancy
  Head trauma
  Medications (oral contraceptive pills)
  Nephrotic syndrome
  Liver disease

syndrome occurs in childhood, predisposing to both arterial and venous infarction. Classically, affected children experience headaches, livedo reticularis, pulmonary hypertension, and recurrent deep vein thromboses in addition to strokes. A variety of other conditions deserves mention as potential causes of CSVT in childhood, including head trauma, nephrotic syndrome, and liver disease. Nevertheless, the underlying cause of CSVT remains idiopathic in as many as 25% of cases.

Although treatment of CSVT is controversial, patients with partial or complete resolution of their thrombosis may have a normal neurologic outcome. However, residual neurology deficits are very common.

Summary The patient is a previously healthy 7-year-old girl who presents with a 2-week history of low-grade fever, upper respiratory tract infection, headaches, and emesis in addition to the subacute development of right-sided weakness and now with right focal seizures. Her exam is remarkable for a low-grade fever, papilledema, a right abducens nerve palsy, right hemiparesis, and hyperreflexia with a right plantar extensor response.

Localization Papilledema is caused by elevated intracranial pressure. Given that there are no additional cranial nerve abnormalities, the right abducens nerve palsy is likely a nonspecific sign associated with increased intracranial pressure.

Increased ICP leads to downward displacement of the brainstem, which stretches the sixth cranial nerve as it passes out of the brainstem and through the subarachnoid space. This, in turn, produces weakness of the ipsilateral lateral rectus muscle. It is likely that her headaches and emesis are also related to increased intracranial pressure.

Her right-sided weakness could localize to the precentral gyrus in the left frontal lobe or to the left internal capsule. However, right focal seizures are more consistent with involvement of the left cortex. This upper motor neuron involvement of the corticospinal tracts likely also explains her brisk right-sided reflexes and right plantar extensor response.

Differential Diagnosis The patient in this case presents with symptoms of a nonspecific systemic illness and elevated intracranial pressure with focal neurologic deficits and focal seizures. Thus, there is obvious involvement of the central nervous system, but in the emergency room her underlying diagnosis is unclear. A variety of different disorders can be considered. Low-grade fever may be seen in many conditions, including infection, malignancy, and autoimmune disease. This patient's presentation is suggestive of an infectious cause with recent cold symptoms. She has not had rash or joint pain/swelling/erythema that might indicate an autoimmune or rheumatologic condition. There is no history of weight loss, anorexia, or malaise that would suggest an underlying malignancy.

Infections could place this child at risk for venous, and possibly arterial, stroke. CSVT with venous infarction could explain her signs of elevated intracranial pressure, abducens nerve palsy, and right hemiparesis with focal seizures, and should be considered high in the differential diagnosis. In general, it is important that the clinician maintain a high degree of suspicion for the variety of presentations of CSVT in the correct clinical setting. In any patient presenting with a viral syndrome, fever, headache, and focal seizures, HSV encephalitis needs to be excluded.

Causes of arterial stroke should also be considered as they are the primary type of stroke in infants and children. A high degree of suspicion for arterial strokes should be maintained, especially in children with hemoglobinopathies, such as sickle cell disease, or complex congenital heart disease. In general, cyanotic heart lesions produce secondary polycythemia and anemia, consequently increasing the risk of thromboembolism. Moreover, intracardiac right-to-left shunts enable paradoxical emboli from the venous circulation. Other causes of childhood arterial strokes include vasculitis related to meningitis/encephalitis, postradiation vasculopathy, and inflammatory vasculitis secondary to autoimmune disease. Arterial dissection of the carotid or vertebral arteries may occur following intraoral trauma or manipulation of the neck. More infrequent etiologies of pediatric stroke include moyamoya syndrome, familial hyperlipidemia, migraine, and metabolic diseases such as homocystinuria, Fabry disease, and mitochondrial encephalomyopathy with lactic acidosis and stroke-like episodes (MELAS).

Once a CSVT is diagnosed, risk factors for CSVT in childhood should be assessed (Table 42.1). In many cases, the cause is obvious. For example, an otitis media might be seen on examination; mastoiditis might be noted on neuroimaging (as in this case); the patient already might have a diagnosis of an autoimmune disease, malignancy, or kidney disease; gastroenteritis with vomiting and diarrhea might be responsible for dehydration. In other cases, the underlying cause is less clear and these patients deserve a thorough evaluation for potential etiologies.

Evaluation   In the emergency room, an initial evaluation should begin with neuroimaging with a head CT with and without contrast. This will help guide further work-up as it may clarify whether or not there has been an arterial or venous infarction. It may also help to determine if there is an underlying infection, such as mastoiditis and/or meningitis. She should also have baseline labs done, including a CBC, basic chemistry panel, liver function tests, and erythrocyte sedimentation rate. A chest radiograph might also be considered given that she has had cold symptoms.

Several findings on head CT may confirm the diagnosis of CSVT. Opacification of the torcula as a consequence of freshly thrombosed blood (dense triangle sign) may be seen on a noncontrast study. A contrast study may demonstrate an empty delta sign with an area of hypodensity in the torcula correlating with the contrast-enhanced thrombus in the sinus. A cord sign may also be seen as a linear hyperdense thrombus in the sinus on a noncontrast study, but this is rare. A follow-up brain MRI (with and without gadolinium) with magnetic resonance venography (MRV) is always indicated. Head CT may miss a CSVT in 10% to 40% of cases and may also underestimate its extent. MRV demonstrates low venous flow. Venous clot appears as a hyperintensity on T_1- and T_2-weighted images. Cerebral angiography is rarely required but may demonstrate partial or complete lack of filling of cerebral veins/sinuses or slow venous drainage.

Once this patient is stabilized and her work-up is initiated, she will require a formal ophthalmologic examination to document the extent of her papilledema. A lumbar puncture is also indicated after the head CT is performed to rule out signs of central nervous system infection. An opening pressure should be obtained and CSF should include cell count, protein, glucose, bacterial culture, and possibly HSV PCR testing. Additional CSF may be held if further studies are required. Given that she experienced several seizures, an EEG is also indicated once she is stabilized.

In cases where the etiology cannot quickly be identified, a thorough evaluation for an underlying cause of CSVT must be undertaken. A family history of any hypercoagulable conditions must be elicited. Consideration must be given to the possibility of an underlying malignancy or autoimmune condition, looking for appropriate history and physical exam symptoms and signs. Additional labs for prothrombotic conditions can include protein C antigen/activity, activated protein C resistance, protein S clottable/total antigen, PT/PTT, antithrombin III function/antigen, factor V Leiden gene mutation, prothrombin G20210A mutation, homocysteine level, lipid profile, methylenetetrahydrofolate reductase (MTHFR) polymorphism, lipoprotein a, antiphospholipid antibody panel, lupus anticoagulant assay, fibrinogen activity/antigen, factor VIII assay, and ANA.

Management   This patient should be admitted to the hospital for further work-up and management. Her current medical problems include mastoiditis, headache, CSVT, increased intracranial pressure, right hemiparesis, and focal seizures.

Aggressive antibiotic treatment is required for mastoiditis and may best be provided under the guidance of infectious disease specialists. Otolaryngology should also be consulted as surgical debridement of mastoiditis is generally recommended. Her headache may be treated with acetaminophen or ibuprofen. Stronger analgesics such as ketorolac or narcotics are sometimes required.

There is little data regarding the safety and efficacy of anticoagulation in children with CSVT but the primary aim of management is limitation or elimination of the thrombus. Anticoagulation improves outcome in patients with this condition in some studies. The overriding concern is the risk for intracranial hemorrhage.

Traditionally, anticoagulation with intravenous heparin has been the mainstay of treatment. Even if some intracranial hemorrhage is present, the risks of not treating with heparin may outweigh the risk of clot progression. More recently, the use of subcutaneous low-molecular-weight heparin has been evaluated but its efficacy compared to intravenous heparin is still unclear, particularly in the pediatric population. Recombinant tissue-type plasminogen activator (rtPA) has also been used in individual cases in adults. After a period of stabilization and improvement, most patients are transitioned to oral therapy with warfarin for 3 to 6 months. The need for long-term anticoagulation may arise in patients who are proven or presumed to have an underlying hypercoagulable state. Repeat neuroimaging with brain MRI and MRV is also required periodically through the recovery process to monitor for recanalization.

Elevated intracranial pressure does not require specific intervention in most patients with CSVT. Often a lumbar puncture with removal of adequate amounts of CSF can reduce intracranial pressure sufficiently. Extreme measures to control elevated intracranial pressure, such as elevation of the head of the bed to 30 degrees, hyperventilation, and osmotic diuretics, are rarely required.

Regarding her right hemiparesis, occupational and physical therapy should be consulted for the direction of appropriate rehabilitative activities. Seizure management is also required. In the short-term, she may be loaded and maintained on phenytoin. However, transition to alternative anticonvulsants may be needed, depending on the anticipated course of treatment, which is determined on an individual basis.

Additional Questions

1. Discuss the adjustment and monitoring of intravenous heparin therapy.
2. What are the clinical manifestations of superior sagittal sinus venous infarction?

References

Barnes C, Newall F, Furmedge J, et al. Cerebral sinus venous thrombosis in children. *J Pediatr Child Health.* 2004;40:53–55.

Carvalho KS, Garg BP. Cerebral venous thrombosis and venous malformations in children. *Neurol Clin.* 2002;20:1061–1077.

Hutchinson JS, Ichord R, Guerguerian A, et al. Cerebrovascular disorders. *Semin Pediatr Neurol.* 2004;1(2):139–146.

Kline LB, Bajandas FJ. *Neuro-Ophthalmology.* 5th ed. Thorofare, NJ: Slack; 2001:93–102.

Masuhr F, Mehraein S, Einhaupl K. Cerebral venous and sinus thrombosis. *J Neurol.* 2004;251:11–23.

A 6-month-old boy is brought to the emergency room by his parents for complaints of worsening respiratory distress. They are from out of town and do not have the child's medical records with them. He has been diagnosed with a genetic disease, but the parents do not know the name of it. He has not had a fever, cough, rhinorrhea, diarrhea, vomiting, or irritability. He was born at full term by vaginal delivery and there were no pregnancy complications. At birth he was noted to have a heart murmur and now he sees a cardiologist regularly for his "large heart." He has had poor weight gain and has difficulty feeding. He has never rolled over, crawled, or sat without support. He smiles but does not babble.

Physical Examination Vital Signs: Afebrile with tachypnea. General Examination: Ill-appearing 6-month-old boy. There are no dysmorphic facial features but his tongue is large and protrudes from his mouth. A heart murmur is present. There is mild hepatomegaly but no splenomegaly. Neurologic Examination: Mental Status: Alert. Cranial Nerves: His pupils are equal, round, and reactive to light. He is able to track in all directions. His face is symmetric. A gag is present and the tongue is midline without fasciculations. Motor: He has normal bulk with severe axial hypotonia and little head control. He is lying with frog-leg positioning with little spontaneous movement. He is able to move his extremities against gravity but appears weak. Sensory: There is some withdrawal to tickle. Reflexes: 1+ throughout with bilateral plantar flexor responses.

Guide to Case Discussion

■ Briefly summarize this case.

■ Localize the examination findings.

■ Give the most likely diagnosis and provide a differential diagnosis.

■ Discuss an appropriate diagnostic work-up.

■ Discuss the management of this patient.

Diagnosis   Pompe disease (glycogen storage disease type II).

Discussion   Pompe disease (glycogen storage disease type II) is a rare autosomal recessive disorder caused by a deficiency of alpha-glucosidase (also called acid maltase), a critical enzyme in the degradative pathway of lysosomal glycogen. Pompe disease is also known by the names glycogen storage disease II and acid maltase deficiency. It can be considered a metabolic myopathy, glycogen storage disease, and lysosomal storage disease. The enzyme deficiency results in the accumulation of glycogen in many tissues but primarily affects skeletal muscle. The responsible gene lies on chromosome 17q. The incidence is estimated to be 1 in 40,000 individuals.

The three distinct forms of the disease vary by the age at onset (infancy, childhood, adulthood), severity of symptoms, and the rate of progression. Classic infantile Pompe disease usually presents within the first few months of life with hypotonia, developmental delay, and progressive weakness, in addition to feeding and breathing problems. Massive macroglossia, hypertrophic cardiomegaly, and hepatomegaly result from deposition of glycogen in these tissues. Hypertrophic cardiomyopathy is usually diagnosed before 6 months of age. ECG abnormalities may be unique, showing a shortened PR interval and large, broad QRS complexes. These infants usually die of respiratory or cardiac failure by the end of the first year of life.

The juvenile form presents in childhood or adolescence with mild gross motor delays and slowly progressive proximal weakness. There is no cardiomegaly or hepatomegaly. Death usually occurs in the second or third decade from respiratory failure. The adult form of the disease is characterized by onset in the 20s or 30s with complaints of impaired motor function. This is followed by progressive proximal weakness and respiratory difficulties caused by diaphragmatic involvement. This form may resemble a limb-girdle muscular dystrophy.

Summary   The patient is a 6-month-old boy with a history of global developmental delay, failure to thrive, and cardiomyopathy who presents for evaluation of respiratory distress. His examination is remarkable for macroglossia, cardiac murmur, hepatomegaly, severe hypotonia, generalized weakness, and hyporeflexia.

Localization   The infant presented in this case has multiorgan system involvement, which suggests an inborn error of metabolism. Although hypotonia can be caused by both central and peripheral causes, a primary peripheral process seems most likely given the presence of generalized muscle weakness and other organ involvement. In consideration of peripheral causes of hypotonia, disorders of the anterior horn cell, peripheral nerve, neuromuscular junction, and muscle could be possible. The fact that the cardiac muscle is involved points to a myopathic process that also involves skeletal muscle.

Anterior horn cell diseases, such as spinal muscular atrophy (SMA), can cause hypotonia, and proximal more than distal weakness but not organomegaly. Although it is hard to exclude peripheral nerve involvement given the patient's hyporeflexia, a peripheral nerve disorder alone would not explain the patient's constellation of symptoms. Neuromuscular junction disorders such as myasthenia gravis cause ptosis, bulbar dysfunction, and generalized weakness but no organomegaly. Thus, a myopathic process is likely responsible for this patient's symptoms of hypotonia and generalized weakness.

Differential Diagnosis The differential diagnosis for an infant presenting with hypotonia and weakness is broad. However, the fact that this patient presents with organomegaly involving the tongue, heart, and liver helps narrow the differential diagnosis significantly and is highly suggestive of an inborn error of metabolism and more specifically, a metabolic storage disease. As discussed above, there also appears to be significant involvement of skeletal muscle.

Pompe disease can sometimes be mistaken for SMA type I (Werdnig-Hoffmann disease), an anterior horn cell disorder. Although SMA may result in infantile hypotonia and proximal weakness, it does not cause organomegaly. SMA may also cause tongue fasciculations, which can be a distinguishing feature. In addition, other myopathies such as congenital muscular dystrophies, congenital myopathies, congenital myotonic dystrophy, and inflammatory myopathies do not cause organomegaly and would be unlikely to explain this patient's constellation of symptoms.

The differential diagnosis is then mostly limited to other metabolic diseases that produce cardiac, hepatic, and skeletal muscle involvement. There is also significant clinical overlap in many of these syndromes, further complicating the diagnosis in many children. Other disorders of glycogen metabolism and glycolysis should first be considered as they most closely resemble Pompe disease. Debrancher enzyme deficiency (glycogen storage disease III), as well as brancher enzyme deficiency (glycogen storage disease IV), can cause hypotonia, muscle weakness, cardiomyopathy, and hepatomegaly in addition to an elevated CK in infancy. Phosphorylase b kinase deficiency (glycogen storage disease VIII) is associated with four clinical phenotypes, which variably cause exercise intolerance, myalgias, myoglobinuria, weakness, hepatic dysfunction, and cardiomyopathy. Even though liver and cardiac abnormalities may arise in infancy, myopathic symptoms typically occur in childhood or adolescence, in contrast to infantile-onset Pompe disease.

Mitochondrial cytopathies are a heterogeneous group of disorders with multisystem organ involvement and can also be considered in the differential diagnosis of this patient. Because of the nonuniform distribution of mitochondria in various tissues and the critical role of mitochondria in oxidative metabolism, a wide range of symptoms may be seen. Abnormalities of the respiratory chain, in particular cytochrome c oxidase (COX) deficiency can frequently be demonstrated in affected patients.

Mitochondrial cytopathies variably involve muscle, heart, the CNS, the peripheral nervous system, and endocrine tissues. Muscle disease may present as hypotonia, exercise intolerance, weakness, ptosis, and external ophthalmoplegia. Hypertrophic cardiomyopathy and arrhythmias may occur. Seizures, cognitive delay, optic atrophy, pigmentary retinopathy, ataxia, stroke, and sensorineural hearing loss demonstrate CNS involvement. A peripheral axonal neuropathy is reported in many mitochondrial diseases. Finally, endocrine manifestations such as diabetes mellitus and short stature may be noted. A mitochondrial cytopathy would need to be excluded if testing for Pompe disease and other glycogen storage diseases was negative.

Certainly other storage diseases such as the mucopolysaccharidoses, peroxisomal disorders, and the gangliosidoses could also be considered in the differential diagnosis. However, cardiomyopathy and/or hepatomegaly are less frequently the primary symptoms in these disorders. They also often present with dysmorphisms that are not characteristic of Pompe disease.

Evaluation The patient in this case presents with acute respiratory distress that is likely related to his underlying genetic disease. In the emergency room, his initial management should focus on stabilization of his respiratory status. He should be placed on a pulse oximeter and cardiorespiratory monitor. Basic laboratory tests (CBC, arterial blood gas, liver function tests, basic chemistry panel) should be done to screen for signs of infection and metabolic abnormalities. A CK level can be sent to screen for neuromuscular involvement. A chest radiograph should be performed to rule out pneumonia and to evaluate for cardiac abnormalities. He will also need an ECG and ECHO to be performed under the supervision of a cardiologist to establish his cardiac status. As this patient has an established diagnosis, attempts should be made to contact his regular team of physicians to help further coordinate his care.

For an undiagnosed patient, a CK level is useful as a screening test and is usually moderately elevated (may be as high as 2,000 UI/L) in Pompe disease. However, it may be normal in adult forms. Liver function tests may also be elevated because of hepatic involvement. EMG typically shows a myopathic pattern. Pseudomyotonic discharges, positive sharp waves, and fibrillation potentials may be seen. Motor and sensory nerve conduction studies are typically normal. As discussed above, a chest radiograph, ECG, and ECHO demonstrate cardiac involvement and can be useful in ruling out other conditions.

Once Pompe disease is strongly suspected, the diagnosis can be definitively established by demonstrating an absence or decrease in alpha-glucosidase activity in muscle tissue or skin fibroblasts obtained from a skin biopsy. Lysosomal vacuoles are filled with glycogen. Electron microscopy also demonstrates the presence of glycogen in lysosomes and in the cytoplasm.

For patients presenting with a storage syndrome and/or dysmorphic features in whom the diagnosis is less clear, a screening work-up includes urine mucopolysaccharides and oligosaccharides (mucopolysaccharidoses), urine organic acids, plasma amino acids, lactate/pyruvate (mitochondrial disease), phytanic acid (Refsum disease), and plasma very-long-chain fatty acids (peroxisomal disorders).

Management   Treatment of Pompe disease is supportive. Patients need to be followed by a multidisciplinary team of pulmonologists, cardiologists, and neurologists. A geneticist should also be involved early on to aid in the diagnosis, assess carrier status of family members, and to provide counseling, particularly if the parents wish to have other children. In patients with infantile-onset, respiratory and cardiac supportive care can prolong life, but do not resuscitate orders eventually need to be discussed with parents.

Enzyme replacement therapy is currently under investigation for Pompe disease. The administration of recombinant alpha-glucosidase from rabbit milk benefits patients with infantile as well as adult-onset forms of the disease.

Additional Questions

1. What are the clinical features of the mucopolysaccharidoses?
2. What is Zellweger syndrome?

References

Bruno C, Hays AP, DiMauro S. Glycogen storage diseases of muscle. In: Jones HR, De Vivo DC, Darras BT, eds. *Neuromuscular Disorders of Infancy, Childhood, and Adolescence: A Clinician's Approach.* Philadelphia, Pa: Butterworth-Heinemann; 2003:813-832.

Clarke JTR. *A Clinical Guide to Inherited Metabolic Diseases.* 2nd ed. Cambridge, UK: Cambridge University Press; 2002:134-168.

Hagemans MLC, Winkel LPF, Van Doorn PA, et al. Clinical manifestation and natural course of late-onset Pompe's disease in 54 Dutch patients. *Brain*. 2005;128:671–677.

Kishnani PS, Howell RR. Pompe disease in infants and children. *J Pediatr*. 2004;144(suppl 5): S35–S43.

Schiedel J, Jackson S, Schafer J, et al. Mitochondrial cytopathies. *J Neurol*. 2003;250:267–277.

Van den Hout HMP, Hop W, Van Diggelens OP, et al. The natural course of infantile Pompe's disease: 20 original cases compared with 133 cases from the literature. *Pediatrics*. 2003;112(2):332–340.

A 17-month-old boy is seen in the neurology office for evaluation of spells. The patient has experienced two stereotypic episodes in which he abruptly stopped breathing, lost consciousness, and had shaking of all four extremities. Both episodes occurred after his older brother took away a favorite toy. After a few cries, he stopped breathing, turned blue, and went limp. As his mother went to pick him up during the spells, he became stiff and had jerking of his extremities for a few seconds. The child then quickly responded to his mother's voice and his color returned to normal. Both spells lasted less than 1 minute. The boy was the product of a normal pregnancy and delivery. He has no significant past medical history and his development is age appropriate. The family history is noncontributory.

Physical Examination General Examination: Unremarkable. Neurologic Examination: Awake, alert, and playful. Language: He babbles and says several words. Cranial Nerves: II through XII are intact. Motor: He has normal bulk and tone. He moves all four extremities equally against gravity. Coordination: There is no dysmetria grabbing for toys. Gait: He has a normal toddler gait. Reflexes: 2+ throughout with bilateral plantar flexor responses.

Guide to Case Discussion

- Briefly summarize this case.

- Localize the examination findings.

- Give the most likely diagnosis and provide a differential diagnosis.

- Discuss an appropriate diagnostic work-up.

- Discuss the management of this patient.

Diagnosis   Cyanotic breath-holding spells.

Discussion   Breath-holding spells (BHS) are a benign, nonvolitional, paroxysmal event of childhood. They are typically classified as cyanotic or pallid, depending on the color change during the spell. Some children may experience both types. BHS are most common in children between the ages of 6 and 18 months. They are seen in approximately 5% of children and may occur with variable frequency. BHS typically resolve by 3 to 4 years of age and are rare in children older than 6 years of age. There is support for a genetic basis of BHS and a family history is reported in as many as 20% to 35% of cases.

Cyanotic BHS are more common. They are usually precipitated by crying in response to pain, anger, frustration, or minor trauma. The crying is brief (less than 15 seconds) and followed by cessation of respiration, usually after exhalation. Apnea with cyanosis occurs and the child goes limp. In some cases, short, anoxic-clonic seizures may follow. The pathophysiologies of cyanotic and pallid BHS are believed to be different. Cyanotic spells involve complex factors such as intrapulmonary shunting and autonomic dysregulation.

Pallid BHS are more associated with sudden pain or fright, such as an unexpected minor fall or bump on the head. The child lets out a brief gasp or cry and then becomes pale during a short loss of consciousness. The body stiffens and brief clonic jerks of the eyes and extremities may be seen. The child becomes limp but quickly becomes alert again, with the whole spell lasting less than 1 minute. Children are more likely to be fatigued or sleep after these episodes. Pallid BHS are caused by excessive vagally mediated cardiac inhibition that leads to cerebral hypoperfusion. Experiments using ocular compression show that a pallid BHS can be associated with bradycardia and asystole. Prolonged asystole can subsequently result in reflex anoxic seizures.

Summary   The patient is a healthy, developmentally normal 17-month-old boy who presents after two provoked episodes of crying, apnea with cyanosis, loss of consciousness, and brief jerking of the extremities. His neurologic exam is normal.

Localization   There are no focal findings on the child's neurologic exam. A generalized anoxic seizure may have occurred as a result of hypoperfusion and localizes to the bilateral cerebral cortex.

Differential Diagnosis   The description of this child's spells is most consistent with a diagnosis of cyanotic BHS. Both spells were provoked by anger and were associated with a brief cry followed by apnea and cyanosis. The stiffness and generalized jerking of the extremities likely represent a brief anoxic reflex seizure. Immediately thereafter he returned to his usual state of good health.

BHS primarily need to be differentiated from epileptic seizures and cardiac phenomena such as syncope or arrhythmias. A thorough history usually helps distinguish BHS from epileptic seizures. Epileptic seizures are not provoked. They are typically longer than a BHS and are associated with a postictal state. Moreover, in a BHS, the color change occurs before the loss of consciousness and the seizure, whereas in epileptic seizures, color change, when present, occurs after the loss of consciousness as the convulsion evolves.

Syncope results from a sudden loss of cerebral perfusion and causes a loss of postural tone as well as a loss of consciousness. Cardiac vasovagal (neurocardiogenic dysregulation) can be precipitated by fear, emotion, or pain. This usually affects older children and adolescents. Other cardiac conditions, such as shunts, impaired inflowing/filling, bradyarrhythmias, and tachyarrhythmias, must also be considered. In addition, congenital long QT syndrome can cause syncope and anoxic seizures precipitated by exercise, fright, injury, or emotion.

Other disorders that can be considered in the differential diagnosis of BHS include benign paroxysmal vertigo, brainstem lesions, and central or obstructive apneas. BHS have been described in children with congenital structural abnormalities such as Arnold-Chiari malformations. Developmental disorders, such as Rett syndrome, can include breath holding and abnormal respiratory patterns. Patients with Riley-Day syndrome, a familial dysautonomia, also can have similar episodes. Finally, BHS are associated with hematologic abnormalities, such as transient erythroblastopenia of childhood and iron-deficient states.

Evaluation BHS usually can be diagnosed with a careful history. A thorough cardiac exam should be performed. Laboratory and ancillary tests are usually not needed but in cases where the diagnosis is less clear, a work-up might be required. A CBC to evaluate for anemia might be performed. A 12-lead ECG can exclude arrhythmias such as long QT syndrome. Holter monitoring and/or a cardiology referral may be necessary if a cardiac abnormality is suspected. If the history is suspicious for epileptic seizures, a routine EEG might be considered. If spells are frequent, video EEG monitoring might also help to arrive at a diagnosis.

Management The mainstay of management is parental education and support. BHS are frightening to observe. Parents need to be informed that the attacks are benign and involuntary. The fact that the long-term outcome is excellent should be reinforced. Although BHS are provoked, it is unreasonable for parents to alter discipline practices or to avoid situations where the child may become upset or frustrated. It is impossible to prevent every conflict or mishap in childhood. When a BHS begins, parents should be instructed to place the child in a lateral decubitus position to maximize cerebral blood flow. Cardiopulmonary resuscitation should be avoided.

Pharmacologic intervention is usually not required in the management of BHS. Anticonvulsants are not indicated in patients with reflex anoxic seizures. Supplemental iron therapy reduces the frequency of breath-holding spells, especially with concomitant iron-deficiency anemia. The length of treatment has varied from 3 to 16 weeks and consisted of 5 to 6 mg/kg/day of ferrous sulfate. Rarely, atropine is indicated for the management of severe pallid BHS.

References

Boon R. Does iron have a place in the management of breath-holding spells? *Arch Dis Child.* 2002;87(1):77–78.

Breningstall GN. Breath-holding spells. *Pediatr Neurol.* 1996;14(2):91–97.

DiMario FJ. Prospective study of children with cyanotic and pallid breath-holding spells. *Pediatrics.* 2001;107:265–269.

Fejerman N. Nonepileptic disorders imitating generalized idiopathic epilepsies. *Epilepsia.*
2005;46(suppl 9):80–83.

Mocan H, Yildiran A, Orhan F, et al. Breath-holding spells in 91 children and response to treatment with iron. *Arch Dis Child.* 1999;81:261–262.

Roddy SM. Breath-holding spells and reflex anoxic seizures. In: Swaiman KS, Ashwal S, eds.
Pediatric Neurology: Principles and Practice. 3rd ed. St. Louis, Mo: Mosby; 1999:759–762.

A **6-year-old girl** is brought to the emergency room because of complaints of worsening headache and vomiting. Her headache began about 2 months ago. It is now described as constant, pounding, severe, and all over her head. The pain has woken her up from sleep the last three nights. She vomited a few times earlier in the week but was brought to the hospital after five episodes of vomiting today. She has had no fever, diarrhea, or ill contacts. She had seizures described as staring, drooling, and right-sided jerking in early childhood while in her home country of Mexico, but none recently. Her mother recalls that she was briefly treated with phenobarbital but the patient never underwent an EEG or neuroimaging. Her birth history is unremarkable. She walked at 16 months and did not speak in phrases until she was almost 3 years old. She is now in first grade. Difficulties in math and reading have been attributed to the fact that Spanish is her native language. The family history is noncontributory.

Physical Examination Vital Signs: Afebrile. General Examination: There is no nuchal rigidity. Her fundi are difficult to visualize but the margins of the optic discs are blurred. Several small white macules are noted on the trunk and right leg. Small, raised, erythematous papules are seen on the nose and cheeks. Neurologic Examination: Mental Status: Alert but irritable. Language: She has fluent speech. Cranial Nerves: Her pupils are equal, round, and reactive to light. She tracks objects in all directions. Her facial movements are symmetric. She has a normal gag. The tongue is midline without fasciculations. Motor: She has normal bulk and tone. Her strength is 5/5 throughout. Coordination: There is no dysmetria. Sensory: Light touch, vibration, and temperature are intact. Reflexes: 3+ symmetrically throughout with bilateral plantar extensor responses.

Guide to Case Discussion

▨ Briefly summarize this case.

▨ Localize the examination findings.

▨ Give the most likely diagnosis and provide a differential diagnosis.

▨ Discuss an appropriate diagnostic work-up.

▨ Discuss the management of this patient.

Diagnosis   Tuberous sclerosis complex with subacute hydrocephalus caused by a subependymal giant cell astrocytoma.

Discussion   Tuberous sclerosis complex (TSC) is a multisystem genetic disorder that occurs in approximately 1 in 6,000 to 10,000 individuals. TSC causes hamartomatous lesions of all organs, but primarily affects tissues of the skin, central nervous system, kidney, eye, heart, and lung. The current clinical diagnosis of definite, possible, or probable TSC is based on the presence of major and/or minor features of the disease (Table 45.1).

TSC occurs by a spontaneous mutation in approximately 70% of affected individuals. Mutations in the *TSC1* gene, on chromosome 9q34, and the *TSC2* gene, on chromosome 16p13.3, result in a similar phenotypic presentation. *TSC1* is more common in familial cases and results in less-severe disease. The pathogenesis of TSC lies in the expression and function of the associated gene products, hamartin in *TSC1* and tuberin in *TSC2*, in tissue. The tuberin-hamartin complex is critical to multiple intracellular signaling pathways, especially those in control of cell growth.

TABLE 45.1

Diagnostic Criteria for Tuberous Sclerosis Complex

Major Features
  Facial angiofibroma or forehead plaque
  Nontraumatic ungual or periungual fibroma
  Hypomelanotic macules (more than 3)
  Shagreen patch (connective tissue nevus)
  Cortical tuber
  Subependymal nodule
  Subependymal giant cell astrocytoma
  Multiple retinal nodular hamartomas
  Cardiac rhabdomyoma, single or multiple
  Lymphangiomyomatosis
  Renal angiomyolipoma

Minor Features
  Multiple, randomly distributed pits in dental enamel
  Hamartomatous rectal polyps
  Bone cysts
  Cerebral white matter radial migration lines
  Gingival fibromas
  Nonrenal hamartoma
  Retinal achromic patch
  "Confetti" skin lesions
  Multiple renal cysts

Definite TSC = Either 2 major features or 1 major feature plus 2 minor features
Probable TSC = One major plus 1 minor feature
Suspect TSC = Either 1 major feature or 2 or more minor features

The neurologic complications of TSC are the most common, and often the most impairing, aspect of this disease. The classic TSC central nervous system findings of cortical tubers, subependymal nodules (SENs), subependymal giant cell astrocytomas (SEGAs), and white matter abnormalities are seen on neuroimaging studies.

Tubers occur in up to 95% of patients. They involve the surface cortical and subcortical areas of the brain. SENs are also seen in the majority of TSC patients. Radiographically, SENs appear as small protrusions into the walls of the lateral ventricles. SEGAs are benign tumors that occur in approximately 10% of patients with TSC. They are thought to arise from SENs at the origin of the foramen of Monro. SEGAs are clinically significant because enlargement of these lesions may obstruct the flow of CSF at the foramen of Monro, causing obstructive hydrocephalus, as in this case.

Seizures occur in most patients with TSC. The onset usually occurs during infancy or early childhood, but can happen at any age. Partial motor and complex partial seizures, with or without generalization, are most common, likely as a consequence of focal cerebral pathology. Infantile spasms develop in approximately one-third of TSC patients. Mental retardation, cognitive dysfunction, autism, and other behavioral abnormalities are also common and may relate to the number and/or location of cortical tubers.

The cutaneous manifestations in TSC, which are typically the first clue to the diagnosis, include hypomelanotic macules (ash leaf spots), facial angiofibromas, forehead plaques, shagreen patches, and ungual fibromas. The renal manifestations of TSC, which are also found in a majority of patients, include angiomyolipomas (AMLs), simple cysts, polycystic kidney disease, and renal cell carcinoma.

Cardiac rhabdomyomas are highly associated with TSC and found in 30% to 50% of affected individuals. They are usually asymptomatic but can cause outflow tract obstruction, congestive heart failure, and a variety of dysrhythmias. They also have a unique ability to regress and completely resolve during the first years of life.

Lymphangiomyomatosis (LAM) is caused by proliferation of atypical smooth muscle cells in lung tissue. It occurs almost exclusively in young women, presenting between 30 and 35 years of age, and is highly associated with TSC. Clinically, LAM is a progressive disorder of the lung, causing dyspnea, spontaneous pneumothorax, hemoptysis, cough, chylothorax, cor pulmonale, and chest pain. Progressive respiratory failure and death eventually occur.

Retinal hamartomas are identified in approximately 40% to 50% of individuals; other pigmentary abnormalities also may be seen. Fortunately, ophthalmologic findings rarely cause visual symptoms in patients with TSC.

Summary   The patient is a 6-year-old girl with a history of complex partial seizures and cognitive delay who now presents with the subacute development of headaches and vomiting. Her general exam demonstrates hypopigmented macules and facial angiofibromas that are consistent with a diagnosis of tuberous sclerosis complex. Her neurologic examination is significant for bilateral papilledema, brisk reflexes, and bilateral plantar extensor responses.

Localization   The patient's headache localizes to the intracranial pain-sensitive structures (cerebral arteries, dural arteries, large veins, venous sinuses) that are innervated through the trigeminal nerve. The headache, vomiting, and bilateral papilledema are caused by increased intracranial pressure. Brisk reflexes and bilateral plantar extensor responses are caused by pyramidal tract involvement associated with hydrocephalus. Her prior right focal seizures localize to the left cerebral hemisphere. Her cognitive delay represents a generalized cerebral dysfunction and is caused by her underlying diagnosis of TSC.

Differential Diagnosis This child's symptoms are highly suggestive of elevated intracranial pressure. Her headache is constant, severe, and progressively worsening. It is associated with persistent vomiting and awakens her from sleep. In a patient with TSC, a SEGA obstructing the flow of CSF is the most likely etiology. Other intracranial neoplasms are rare in this population.

However, were signs of TSC not present, other etiologies of hydrocephalus would need to be considered. More specifically, her history is most consistent with noncommunicating hydrocephalus, which is frequently caused by a mass lesion obstructing the flow of CSF through the ventricular system. This may occur with a wide range of pediatric brain tumors, especially those located in the posterior fossa (brainstem glioma, medulloblastoma, cerebellar astrocytoma, ependymoma).

Aqueductal stenosis is caused by partial or complete obstruction of the aqueduct of Sylvius. It may be hereditary or acquired as a consequence of hemorrhage, infection, a vascular malformation, or a neoplasm. It represents another type of obstructive hydrocephalus that may occur. The patient in this case is Mexican and experienced seizures as a young child. An alternate diagnosis might include neurocysticercosis that resulted in seizures with a new lesion that is now causing obstructive hydrocephalus.

Communicating hydrocephalus causes impairment of CSF absorption through the arachnoid granulations and is seen in conditions such as meningitis, encephalitis, subarachnoid hemorrhage, and intraventricular hemorrhage. The patient has no history of fevers, photophobia, or nuchal rigidity that would suggest a central nervous system infection.

The headache described in this case is not consistent with a tension-type or migraine headache. Pseudotumor cerebri causes headaches and papilledema but typically does not cause other signs of hydrocephalus, such as vomiting and nocturnal pain.

Evaluation The presentation in this case represents a neurologic emergency. The patient should undergo an emergent head CT with and without contrast. Neurosurgery should also be contacted immediately. Further imaging with a brain MRI with and without gadolinium will be necessary preoperatively if the patient is stable. Basic laboratory studies, such as a basic chemistry panel, CBC, and PT/PTT, also should be done.

Because her TSC has not yet been diagnosed, she will require a complete workup for associated complications. Guidelines for the evaluation of a newly diagnosed patient with TSC and family members have been published. An ophthalmology evaluation should be performed to monitor for resolution of papilledema and for retinal abnormalities seen in TSC. She should undergo an ECHO and ECG to investigate possible cardiac rhabdomyomas and arrhythmias. A renal ultrasound must be performed to rule out renal angiomyolipomas and cysts.

Management This child should be placed on a cardiorespiratory monitor and pulse oximeter immediately. An intravenous line should be placed and she should be made NPO in preparation for surgery. Her hydrocephalus can likely be managed surgically with prompt resection of her SEGA.

Once discharged from the hospital, discussion of her diagnosis with the school system is also necessary. She likely has cognitive delays associated with TSC and will require formal psychological/educational testing. Because she is not currently having seizures, an EEG is unlikely to be helpful at this point. However, the risk of recurrent seizures in this child with TSC is high and general seizure precautions should be reviewed with the family.

The involvement of a geneticist also might be helpful in the long-term management of this patient. Both parents and all siblings should be evaluated for clinical manifestations of TSC. It is recommended that both parents also undergo a neuroimaging study and a renal ultrasound in the event that there is occult disease. Currently, clinical genetic testing is available for patients with TSC and 80% of affected individuals will demonstrate a mutation in *TSC1* or *TSC2*. As genotype-phenotype correlations are becoming possible, this may be clinically important. This also may help in genetic counseling for the family.

Additional Questions

1. Discuss the appropriate therapeutic interventions for a child presenting with acute hydrocephalus and signs of herniation.

2. Describe the motor response, pupillary findings and respiratory patterns associated with progressive herniation.

3. Describe how to perform cold caloric testing in a comatose patient. What is the normal response with an intact brainstem?

References

Ashwal S. Congenital structural defects. In: Swaiman KS, Ashwal S, eds. *Pediatric Neurology: Principles and Practice*. 3rd ed. St. Louis, Mo: Mosby; 1999:234–300.

Cheadle JP, Reeve MP, Sampson JR, et al. Molecular genetic advances in tuberous sclerosis. *Hum Genet*. 2000;107:97–114.

Dabora SL, Jozwiak S, Franz DN, et al. Mutational analysis in a cohort of 224 tuberous sclerosis patients indicates increased severity of TSC2, compared with TSC1, disease in multiple organs. *Am J Hum Genet*. 2001;68:64–80.

Fenichel GM. *Clinical Pediatric Neurology: A Signs and Symptoms Approach*. 4th ed. Philadelphia, Pa: WB Saunders; 2001:77–89.

Franz DN. Non-neurologic manifestations of tuberous sclerosis complex. *J Child Neurol*. 2004;19:690–698.

Goh S, Butler W, Thiele EA. Subependymal giant cell tumors in tuberous sclerosis complex. *Neurology*. 2004;63:1457–1461.

Roach ES, DiMario FJ, Kandt RS, et al. Tuberous sclerosis consensus conference: recommendations for diagnostic evaluation. *J Child Neurol*. 1999;14:401–407.

Roach ES, Gomez MR, Northrup H. Tuberous sclerosis complex consensus conference: revised clinical diagnostic criteria. *J Child Neurol*. 1998;13:624–628.

A 10-year-old girl presents to the neurology office for evaluation of abnormal movements. Approximately 3 years ago, she began to have intermittent difficulty holding utensils, such as a spoon, with her right hand. Over the following months, she developed persistent right upper extremity posturing that extended from her hand up to her elbow and shoulder. Within 1 year, the patient's right lower extremity became involved. Right-sided stiffness now causes her to swing her leg out while walking. A noticeable head tilt to the right also has developed and is becoming progressively worse. She has adapted by writing and feeding herself with her nondominant left hand, which has not been affected. The patient has no past medical history and has had normal development. There is no family history of movement disorders.

Physical Examination General Examination: Normal with the exception of severe dextroscoliosis. Neurologic Examination: Mental Status: Alert and cooperative. Language: Her speech is fluent without dysarthria. Cranial Nerves: Her pupils are equal, round, and reactive to light. Her extraocular muscles are intact. Her face is symmetric. The tongue is midline without fasciculations. Motor: Her neck is flexed to the right. She has normal bulk with increased tone in the right upper and lower extremities. The right arm alternates between a flexed and extended posture. The right leg is maintained with an extended posture with ankle inversion and plantar flexion. She has normal tone and strength on the left. Coordination: Finger-to-nose testing is normal on the left. Sensory: Light touch, temperature, and vibration are intact. Gait: She ambulates independently but her gait is unsteady because of intermittent, involuntary movements on the right side. Reflexes: 2+ throughout. She has bilateral plantar flexor responses.

Guide to Case Discussion

  ▨ Briefly summarize this case.

  ▨ Localize the examination findings.

  ▨ Give the most likely diagnosis and provide a differential diagnosis.

  ▨ Discuss an appropriate diagnostic work-up.

  ▨ Discuss the management of this patient.

Diagnosis Idiopathic torsion dystonia.

Discussion Dystonia describes a movement disorder characterized by sustained, involuntary muscle contractions. The simultaneous involvement of both agonist and antagonist muscle groups produces characteristically abnormal, often bizarre postures and movement patterns. Idiopathic torsion dystonia (ITD) is the most common form of primary dystonia. It is also known as dystonia musculorum deformans and DYT1 dystonia. It accounts for 40% to 60% of early onset limb dystonia in non-Jewish populations, and for almost 90% of cases in Ashkenazi Jews of Eastern European descent. There is a reduced penetrance of approximately 30% to 40%, which leads to significant clinical variability.

ITD is an autosomal dominant genetic disorder caused by a GAG deletion in the *TOR1A* gene on chromosome 9q34.1. The deletion results in the loss of a single glutamic acid residue in the torsin A protein. The functions of torsin A are incompletely understood but the protein is expressed in especially high levels in the pars compacta of the substantia nigra. Research suggests that abnormal torsin A interferes with the functions of the endoplasmic reticulum, membrane trafficking, and vesicular release in neurons. This has lead to the theory that torsin A could produce functional aberrations in dopaminergic pathways implicated in several movement disorders.

Patients with ITD typically present in early adolescence with involvement of one limb. Affected children have a normal birth and developmental history. They do not experience cognitive, cerebellar, sensory, or pyramidal symptoms. Inversion of one foot is a common initial complaint. However, craniocervical and axial onset have been described. At first, abnormal movements may be intermittent and only seen with specific activities. Further progression to a more persistent and generalized dystonia occurs in most children (80%), but the course is highly variable. Progression in an "N-shaped" pattern from a leg to the unilateral arm to the contralateral leg followed by the contralateral arm has been described in many cases. Truncal dystonia also occurs and causes abnormal postures that result in lordosis, scoliosis, and kyphosis. Approximately 20% of affected children may experience a focal dystonia that does not generalize. In general, patients with an early age of onset of dystonia and involvement of the legs tend to have more rapid progression of symptoms and more severe disease.

Pathology and neuroimaging are normal in ITD. This again supports the theory of a functional disturbance in the nigrostriatal dopaminergic pathways as the underlying etiology of this disorder.

Summary The patient is a previously healthy, developmentally normal 10-year-old girl who presents with a progressive right hemidystonia. Her exam is significant for scoliosis as well as dystonia of the right cervical, upper, and lower extremity musculature.

Localization The patient's neurologic exam is consistent with a right hemidystonia. These signs can be accounted for by a lesion involving the left basal ganglia.

Differential Diagnosis Dystonias are typically classified as primary and secondary disorders (Table 46.1). By definition, primary disorders have dystonia as their only

TABLE 46.1

Differential Diagnosis of Generalized Dystonia in Childhood

Primary Dystonia
 Primary dystonias (DYT 1–13)
 Dopa-responsive dystonia (DYT5)

Secondary Dystonia
 Basal ganglia structural abnormalities
  Tumor
  Trauma
  Hemorrhage
  Infarction
  Arteriovenous malformation
  Central nervous system infection
  Demyelinating disease
 Genetic and hereditary disorders
  Wilson disease
  Huntington disease
  Neuroacanthocytosis
  Juvenile Parkinson disease
  Benign familial chorea
  Rett syndrome
  Ataxia-telangiectasia
  Spinocerebellar ataxias
 Inborn errors of metabolism
  Glutaric aciduria type 1
  Pantothenate kinase-associated neurodegeneration
  Mitochondrial disorders
  Leukodystrophies
  Lysosomal storage diseases
  Neuronal ceroid lipofuscinosis
  Lesch-Nyhan syndrome
  Hartnup disease
 Other
  Toxins/drugs
  Psychiatric/conversion reaction
  Endocrine abnormalities

clinical feature, although some may also be accompanied by tremor. Secondary dystonias result from well-defined acquired or exogenous causes. In these cases, dystonia is typically accompanied by other neurologic abnormalities.

Recent advances in the field of medical genetics have changed the way that primary dystonias are characterized and classified. Autosomal dominant, autosomal recessive, and X-linked recessive inheritance patterns have been described (Table 46.2). The associated chromosomal location and related proteins have been identified in many of these disorders. A wide variety of presentations throughout childhood and adulthood are now recognized. Some have been described only in

TABLE 46.2		
Classification of Primary Dystonias		
Designation	**Name**	**Inheritance**
DYT1	Idiopathic torsion dystonia	AD
DYT2	Autosomal recessive dystonia	AR
DYT3	X-linked dystonia-parkinsonism (lubag)	XR
DYT4	Torsion dystonia 4	AD
DYT5	Dopa-responsive dystonia (Segawa disease)	AD
DYT6	Adult-onset idiopathic torsion dystonia of mixed type	AD
DYT7	Focal, adult-onset idiopathic torsion dystonia	AD
DYT8	Paroxysmal nonkinesigenic dyskinesia	AD
DYT9	Paroxysmal dyskinesia with spasticity	AD
DYT10	Paroxysmal kinesigenic dyskinesia	AD
DYT11	Myoclonic dystonia	AD
DYT12	Rapid-onset dystonia with parkinsonism	AD
DYT13	Cranial-cervical-brachial dystonia	AD

AD = Autosomal dominant
AR = Autosomal recessive
XR = X-linked recessive

isolated families or certain populations. Idiopathic torsion dystonia (DYT1) as described in this patient accounts for the majority of childhood-onset primary dystonia. DYT1, DYT2, and DYT4 are predominantly generalized dystonias. DYT7 is predominantly a focal or segmental dystonia. DYT6 and DYT13 are mixed dystonias. DYT3, DYT5, DYT11, and DYT12 are considered dystonia-plus syndromes because they are associated with other abnormal movements such as parkinsonism and myoclonus. The paroxysmal dyskinesias (DYT8, DYT9, DYT10) are also included in this group of disorders.

Among the primary dystonias, dopa-responsive dystonia (DRD) is the most important alternate diagnostic consideration in a child presenting with an idiopathic dystonia. DRD is also known as hereditary progressive dystonia with marked diurnal fluctuation, Segawa syndrome, and DYT5. It is an autosomal dominant disorder caused by a mutation in the guanosine triphosphate cyclohydrolase-1 (*GCH1*) gene on chromosome 14q22.1. GCH1 is the rate-limiting enzyme in the synthesis of tetrahydrobiopterin, a cofactor for the enzymes that synthesize monoamines (dopamine, adrenaline, serotonin). Other enzymes in the dopamine synthesis pathway (tyrosine hydroxylase, 6-pyruvoyltetrahydropterin synthase) can cause the same clinical picture. These defects follow an autosomal recessive inheritance pattern and are rare.

DRD usually presents in mid-childhood, between the ages of 1 and 12 years. It has a female predominance. The initial symptoms begin insidiously with clumsiness, gait abnormalities, and dystonic posturing. The legs tend to be more affected than the arms. Neck and truncal dystonia are not characteristic of this disorder. DRD is progressive and with time involves dystonic movements of all four extremities if not treated. Parkinsonian symptoms such as rigidity and postural tremor may also be seen. Hyperreflexia is another recognized feature of this disease.

However, diurnal variation is the hallmark of DRD. Symptoms may be relatively mild in the morning but worsen throughout the day. It is important to recognize that almost 25% of patients do not describe fluctuating symptoms and an absence of diurnal variation does not rule out the diagnosis. Many children are misdiagnosed as having more common disorders, such as spastic cerebral palsy, for this reason.

DRD is important to recognize because it is a treatable condition. Affected children respond dramatically to low-dose levodopa. The response is sustained. Treatment with anticholinergic medications may also be helpful.

A wide variety of disorders may be responsible for secondary dystonias. They commonly result from underlying structural abnormalities of the basal ganglia. Neoplasms, vascular malformations, hemorrhage, and hypoxic-ischemic insults to the basal ganglia may produce dystonia. Posttraumatic hemidystonia can arise with injury to the contralateral basal ganglia. Central nervous system infections, such as bacterial meningitis, encephalitis, and HIV, can affect the basal ganglia. Demyelinating diseases like multiple sclerosis and acute disseminated encephalomyelitis can result in movement disorders. Medications (anticonvulsants, neuroleptics, levodopa) and toxins (carbon monoxide, cyanide, methanol) can also affect the basal ganglia. Endocrine disorders such as hypoparathyroidism must be considered. Psychogenic disorders and conversion reactions can also present with abnormal movements mimicking dystonia.

Multiple hereditary and metabolic disorders are associated with dystonic movements. However, these are secondary dystonias that are associated with other neurologic abnormalities such as impaired cognition, cerebellar signs, and pyramidal tract involvement. Other organ systems are also frequently involved, such as the eyes or liver. Hereditary and/or genetic diseases that are associated with dystonia may include Wilson disease, Huntington disease, neuroacanthocytosis, juvenile Parkinson disease, benign familial chorea, Rett syndrome, ataxia-telangiectasia, and spinocerebellar ataxias, among others. Inborn errors of metabolism causing dystonia include glutaric aciduria type 1, pantothenate kinase-associated neurodegeneration, mitochondrial disorders (Leigh disease, MELAS [mitochondrial encephalomyopathy, lactic acidosis, and stroke-like episodes]), leukodystrophies (Krabbe disease), lysosomal storage diseases (Niemann-Pick type C, GM_1 and GM_2 gangliosidosis, metachromatic leukodystrophy), neuronal ceroid lipofuscinosis, Lesch-Nyhan syndrome, and Hartnup disease. This is not an exhaustive list.

Evaluation   The approach to the evaluation of a child presenting with a dystonia depends on the age of the child, course of the disease, family history, associated symptoms, presence of other neurologic abnormalities, and evidence of other organ involvement. A brain MRI with and without gadolinium can be a helpful initial screening tool to evaluate for underlying structural abnormalities. Magnetic resonance (MR) spectroscopy is an adjunctive procedure that can help exclude metabolic disorders. When the clinical picture is consistent with a primary dystonia, specific genetic testing should be done for a mutation in the *DYT1* gene. If this is negative, a trial of levodopa is indicated to evaluate for DRD. If there is a response to levodopa, other confirmatory tests for DRD may also need to be performed. If there is no response to levodopa, a more exhaustive work-up is required. Additional testing is also necessary in any patient with a suspected secondary dystonia.

Screening lab tests might include a CBC with smear (neuroacanthocytosis), basic chemistry panel, liver function tests, copper, ceruloplasmin (Wilson disease), plasma amino acids, urine organic acids, serum lactate/pyruvate (mitochondrial disorders), serum mitochondrial DNA, alpha-fetoprotein (ataxia-telangiectasia), and serum lysosomal enzymes. EMG and NCS can help document peripheral nerve involvement. A formal ophthalmologic exam evaluates for the presence of Kayser-Fleischer rings, as well as for retinal abnormalities or optic nerve atrophy, which may suggest certain inborn errors of metabolism. An electroretinogram can also assess retinal involvement. An EEG may rule out suspected seizure activity. A lumbar puncture may be useful in the evaluation of central nervous system infection and/or inflammation. Muscle, skin, and nerve biopsy can be useful in arriving at a diagnosis in certain cases. Finally, specific molecular genetic testing is also often available and can simplify the work-up in a wide variety of these disorders.

Management The goals of treatment in patients with ITD are to reduce spasms, decrease abnormal posturing, prevent contractures, and restore functional abilities as much as possible. Response to medical management is highly variable and there are no standard protocols. In general, dopaminergic (levodopa), anticholinergic (trihexyphenidyl, benztropine), and antidopaminergic medications are used, as are benzodiazepines (clonazepam, diazepam, lorazepam) and baclofen. Botulinum toxin has become the treatment of choice in focal and segmental dystonias, although its use remains limited by the physician's expertise with injections and by the development of neutralizing antibodies in up to 10% of patients.

There is general consensus that a trial of levodopa is warranted in all children with primary dystonias. However, patients with a variety of dystonias may respond to levodopa and the drug is relatively well tolerated. Also, DRD sometimes occurs without fluctuating symptoms, so a trial of levodopa might aid in making this diagnosis. Small doses are initiated, often in association with a peripheral carboxylase inhibitor (carbidopa), and slowly titrated up while monitoring for a response.

Surgical interventions hold promise for patients with medically refractory ITD as well as other forms of primary and secondary dystonia. Deep brain stimulation (DBS) is the preferred procedure. It can be reversed and can be safely performed bilaterally. Stimulation of the globus pallidus internus is most frequently done and the results have been encouraging. Ablative procedures of pallidotomy and thalamotomy have also been used but are now less common because of the availability and success of DBS.

Finally, patients with ITS should receive physical and occupational therapy to maintain mobility. Adaptive equipment and bracing might also be required. Many patients also learn to accommodate for their dystonia by developing sensory tricks to facilitate movement. If scoliosis and/or contractures develop, referral to an orthopaedist is necessary. Patients should also be referred to a geneticist when the diagnosis of ITD is made to discuss the implications for the family.

Additional Questions

1. Describe the clinical and radiographic features of pantothenate kinase-associated neurodegeneration.
2. Describe the clinical features of Lesch-Nyhan syndrome.
3. How does Wilson disease present? How is it treated?

References

Fernandez-Alvarez E, Aicardi J. *Movement Disorders in Children*. London, UK: Mac Keith Press; 2001:79–129.

Goldman JG, Comella CL. Treatment of dystonia. *Clin Neuropharmacol*. 2003;26(2):102–108.

Müller U, Steinberger D, Németh AH. Clinical and molecular genetics of primary dystonias. *Neurogenetics*. 1998;1:165–177.

Németh AH. The genetics of primary dystonias and related disorders. *Brain*. 2002;125:695–721.

Uc EY, Rodnitzky RL. Childhood dystonia. *Semin Pediatr Neurol*. 2003;10(1):52–61.

A **4-year-old African girl** is brought to your office for the evaluation of new-onset staring spells. Shortly after arriving in the United States 2 months ago, her parents report the onset of 1- to 2-minute long spells of unresponsiveness, staring, drooling, and body stiffness associated with perioral cyanosis and sleepiness afterwards. She has otherwise been well without fever, illness, or head trauma. On review of her development, she appeared to be a normal child until approximately 18 months of age at which point she stopped gaining new abilities. She crawled at 9 months and walked at 16 months. She had learned approximately 10 words but at 18 months, stopped using these words and became disinterested in her environment. Around this same time, she started frequently clapping her hands together and stopped feeding herself. There is no family history of seizures, autism, or developmental delay.

Physical Examination General examination: Head circumference = 46 cm. Small, thin, 4-year-old girl with no dysmorphic facial features. Neurologic Examination: Mental Status: She is alert but makes poor eye contact. Language: She does not say any words or follow commands. Cranial Nerves: Her pupils are equal, round, and reactive to light. She tracks objects in all directions without nystagmus. Her face is symmetric. Her tongue is midline without fasciculations. Motor: She has normal bulk with diffusely increased tone that is more prominent in the lower extremities. She moves all extremities against gravity and is not weak. Coordination: She does not show interest in grabbing toys. Her hands are held together. Gait: She has a slightly ataxic gait. Reflexes: 3+ throughout with bilateral plantar flexor responses.

Guide to Case Discussion

- Briefly summarize this case.
- Localize the examination findings.
- Give the most likely diagnosis and provide a differential diagnosis.
- Discuss an appropriate diagnostic work-up.
- Discuss the management of this patient.

Diagnosis Rett syndrome.

Discussion Rett syndrome is a genetic neurodevelopmental disorder that primarily affects females. It has a variable clinical expression but is characterized by progressive cognitive impairment, speech/language disabilities, loss of purposeful hand use with stereotypic hand movements, and deceleration of head growth.

In its classic presentation, affected individuals have a normal birth and early developmental history until approximately 6 months of age. This is followed by a period of developmental arrest and often frank regression (ages 1 to 4 years) associated with social withdrawal, autistic behaviors, loss of purposeful hand use, and stereotypic hand movements (hand wringing, clapping, rubbing, tapping), as well as communication and cognitive impairments. Deceleration of head growth occurs during this time. An apraxic or ataxic gait may also develop. A period of stabilization then occurs during the preschool years. In later childhood and adolescence, social and communication skills may improve, but progressive decline in motor function occurs. Affected individuals subsequently demonstrate decreased mobility and spasticity.

Epilepsy occurs in approximately 90% of patients with Rett syndrome. Seizure onset is usually between the ages of 3 and 5 years. A peak frequency of seizures occurs in late childhood to late adolescence, but decreases—or may even resolve—in later life. Partial seizures are the most common seizure type. Although most patients with Rett syndrome learn to walk, a gait apraxia is very common. Breathing irregularities, such as hyperventilation, breath holding, and air swallowing are also frequently seen. Kyphoscoliosis, screaming/laughing spells, sleep disturbance, and diminished response to pain are further variable characteristics of the disorder.

It has become clear that some patients experience variant clinical features of Rett syndrome. Consensus Rett and variant Rett diagnostic consensus criteria were established in 2001. Classic Rett diagnostic features are discussed above. Patients are excluded from the diagnosis of Rett syndrome if they have a history of head trauma, central nervous system infection, or perinatal/postnatal brain damage. Children with organomegaly, retinopathy, cataracts, optic atrophy, or an identifiable neurodegenerative disorder are also excluded from a diagnosis of Rett syndrome. To be considered a variant case of Rett syndrome, a patient must have 3 of 6 main criteria and 5 of 11 supportive criteria (Table 47.1). These clinical features are very similar to those of Rett syndrome. Other Rett phenotypes have also been recognized and include normal female carriers, females with learning disabilities, females with Angelman syndrome, males with fatal infantile encephalopathy, males with typical Rett syndrome and Klinefelter syndrome, males with Rett syndrome-like features with X chromosome mosaicism, and males with X-linked cognitive impairment.

The genetic abnormality responsible for Rett syndrome lies in the methyl-CpG binding protein 2 gene (*MECP2*) on the long arm of the X chromosome (Xq28). The majority of cases are sporadic, although several familial cases have been reported. More than 200 different mutations in the *MECP2* gene have been described. The *MECP2* gene codes for two isoforms of the MeCP2 protein. The MeCP2 protein suppresses DNA transcription. Although the specific functions of this protein are still under investigation, evidence suggests that MeCP2 is involved in the maturation and maintenance of neurons, including dendritic arborization and axonal projections.

Longevity data in Rett syndrome is not yet available but patients may live to middle age. In the later stages of life, patients need significant supportive care.

> **TABLE 47.1**
>
> ## Variant Rett Syndrome 2001 Consensus Criteria
>
> Three main criteria and five supportive criteria are required for diagnosis of
>   a variant of Rett syndrome.
>
> **Main Criteria**
>   Absence of or reduction in hand skills
>   Reduction in or loss of babble speech
>   Reduction in or loss of communication skills
>   Deceleration of head growth from early childhood
>   Monotonous pattern of hand stereotypies
>   Regression stage followed by recovery of interaction contrasting with slow
>   neuromotor regression
>
> **Supportive Criteria**
>   Breathing irregularities
>   Bloating or air swallowing
>   Intense eye contact or pointing
>   Abnormal locomotion
>   Scoliosis
>   Lower-limb amyotrophy
>   Diminished response to pain
>   Laughing or screaming spells
>   Cold, purplish feet
>   Sleep disturbances
>   Bruxism

Summary   The patient is a 4-year-old girl with a history of developmental regression and new-onset, unprovoked, complex partial seizures. Her examination is remarkable for microcephaly, autistic features, hand stereotypies, spasticity, hyperreflexia, and an ataxic gait.

Localization   The patient's underlying neurologic disorder affects multiple areas of the central nervous system. The patient is experiencing complex partial seizures that localize to the cortex in one of the cerebral hemispheres. The history of developmental regression, autistic features, lack of speech, microcephaly, and hand stereotypies suggests diffuse involvement of cerebral gray matter. Spasticity and hyperreflexia denote involvement of pyramidal white matter tracts. Ataxia suggests involvement of the cerebellum.

Differential Diagnosis   The presentation and natural history of the disease process in this case is pathognomonic for the diagnosis of Rett syndrome. However, misdiagnosis of Rett syndrome can occur as the disease progresses through the stages outlined above. For example, a 2-year-old girl with delayed communication skills might be labeled as simply having an autistic spectrum disorder. A school-age girl in the stagnant phase of the disease might be diagnosed with cerebral palsy, mental retardation, epilepsy, and/or an ataxia syndrome. Adolescent girls might have significant spasticity and be wheelchair bound. They might be diagnosed with spastic cerebral palsy. The pattern of neurologic deterioration that occurs over the first several years of life is the key to making this diagnosis and a high suspicion for the disorder must be maintained.

In more general terms, in the case of a child with a chronic, progressive encephalopathy, several other metabolic and genetic disorders must be considered in the differential diagnosis. It should first be determined whether there is primary involvement of gray matter or white matter. Gray matter diseases tend to present with seizures and cognitive decline, whereas white matter diseases cause progressive spasticity and vision loss. Second, it is important to note whether there is other organ involvement. Lysosomal storage diseases, mitochondrial disorders, and peroxisomal disorders can involve organs outside of the central nervous system (liver, spleen, eyes). Whether there is peripheral nervous system in addition to central nervous system involvement is also important. Lysosomal storage diseases and mitochondrial disorders may also cause peripheral neuropathy. The inheritance pattern is also relevant. The child in this case is female and there is no family history of seizures, autism, or developmental delay. Thus, this may represent an X-linked, sporadic disorder.

The overall presentation in this case is one of a female child with a neurodegenerative process that primarily affects the gray matter but also has white matter involvement. She does not have dysmorphic facial features and there is no other apparent organ involvement. Her reflexes are increased, which excludes a concomitant peripheral neuropathy. Thus, disorders that deserve the highest consideration include mitochondrial diseases and neuronal ceroid lipofuscinosis (NCL), in addition to genetic disorders such as Angelman syndrome. Mitochondrial disorders vary widely in their clinical presentations but may present with developmental regression, seizures, and autistic features. NCL is caused by the accumulation of lipopigment in neurons and other cells. It occurs in multiple forms and presents with cognitive decline, epilepsy, vision loss/blindness, and motor disabilities. Angelman syndrome results from a mutation on chromosome 15 and demonstrates considerable overlap with Rett syndrome. Microcephaly, seizures, ataxia, gait abnormalities, and autistic features may be seen. Finally, given that the patient in this case was not born in the United States, TORCH infections, especially HIV, are an important additional consideration.

Evaluation The diagnostic approach to the patient presented in this case involves investigation of both her progressive developmental disability as well as her new-onset epilepsy. A detailed birth, developmental, medical, and family history is an essential first step to forming a useful differential diagnosis in these cases. Physical examination findings such as an abnormal head circumference, dysmorphic facial features, neurocutaneous stigmata, and/or hepatosplenomegaly are relevant. Ophthalmologic, cardiac, or musculoskeletal abnormalities might also be detected on a routine physical examination, pointing toward a specific diagnosis.

The presentation in this case is highly suggestive of Rett syndrome and an exhaustive work-up is not necessary now that the causative gene has been identified. Clinical genetic testing for the *MECP2* mutation can be performed to confirm the diagnosis. This patient also presents with multiple unprovoked complex partial seizures and she requires an EEG as well as neuroimaging. Brain MRI is superior to head CT in identifying underlying structural abnormalities that might explain the etiology of focal seizures.

If the diagnosis is less clear, a screening metabolic and genetic work-up for a chronic, progressive encephalopathy may include a basic chemistry panel, CBC, liver function tests, thyroid function tests, HIV testing, plasma amino acids, urine organic acids, serum lactate/pyruvate, serum mitochondrial DNA, serum lysosomal enzymes, and high-resolution karyotype. Specific genetic testing can be performed to exclude Angelman syndrome. Clinical genetic testing is available for certain forms of NCL. However, skin or conjunctival biopsy may be necessary to make the diagnosis in some forms of the disease. A formal ophthalmologic examination can also be very helpful in a screening evaluation.

Management The patient in this case first requires management of her epilepsy. Appropriate epilepsy teaching should be provided to the family. Given that the patient is having frequent complex partial seizures, an anticonvulsant should be started after her EEG is performed. Either carbamazepine or oxcarbazepine would be an appropriate initial medication choice.

Referral to a geneticist is appropriate to review the genetic basis of the disease and to provide genetic counseling were the parents to consider having additional children. Referral to a developmental pediatrician might also be appropriate to help with anticipated behavioral issues, screaming spells, and sleep disturbances. Although this patient currently has no musculoskeletal problems, in general, early referral to an orthopaedist should be considered as scoliosis and contractures develop.

There are no specific therapies for Rett syndrome. Clinical trials using folate and betaine (trimethylglycine) showed no objective improvement in participating patients. As the pathophysiology of Rett syndrome is increasingly understood, other biologically targeted interventions or gene therapies may be on the horizon.

References

Fenichel GM. *Clinical Pediatric Neurology: A Signs and Symptoms Approach*. 4th ed. Philadelphia, Pa: WB Saunders; 2001:117–147.

Hagberg B. Rett syndrome: long-term clinical follow-up experiences over four decades. *J Child Neurol*. 2005;20:722–727.

Ham AL, Kumar A, Deeter R, et al. Does genotype predict phenotype in Rett syndrome? *J Child Neurol*. 2005;768–778.

Kishi N, Macklis JD. Dissecting *MECP2* function in the central nervous system. *J Child Neurol*. 2005;20:753–759.

Nomura Y, Segawa M. Natural history of Rett syndrome. *J Child Neurol*. 2005;20:764–768.

Percy AK, Lane JB. Rett syndrome: model of neurodevelopmental disorders. *J Child Neurol*. 2005;20:718–721.

An 8-year-old boy is seen in the emergency room for neurologic consultation. He originally presented 3 days prior with complaints of headache and fatigue. He was also experiencing intermittent nausea. He was diagnosed with a nonspecific viral illness and discharged home. The parents bring him back today for complaints of increasing sleepiness and confusion. He is still complaining of nausea with a worsening headache. Both parents also have been feeling unwell recently, but no one in the family has had fever, cold symptoms, vomiting, or diarrhea. The family lives in a one-bedroom house that was built 37 years ago. They have been using a wood-burning fireplace and gas-operated heater to keep warm through the night.

Physical Examination Vital Signs: Afebrile. General Examination: There is no papilledema or nuchal rigidity. Neurologic Examination: Mental Status: The patient is lethargic and confused. He is oriented only to his name. Language: He follows simple commands intermittently. He is able to speak fluently. Cranial Nerves: His pupils are equal, round, and reactive to light. His extraocular muscles are intact. There are no visual field defects. His face is symmetric. His palate elevates symmetrically and his tongue is midline. Motor: He has normal bulk and tone. He has trouble cooperating with formal motor testing but there is no weakness. Coordination: No dysmetria is noted. Sensation: He withdraws to painful stimuli in all extremities. Gait: He is able to ambulate independently without ataxia. Reflexes: 2+ throughout with bilateral plantar flexor responses.

Guide to Case Discussion

- Briefly summarize this case.

- Localize the examination findings.

- Give the most likely diagnosis and provide a differential diagnosis.

- Discuss an appropriate diagnostic work-up.

- Discuss the management of this patient.

Diagnosis Acute carbon monoxide poisoning.

Discussion Carbon monoxide (CO) results from the incomplete combustion of hydrocarbons. It is odorless, colorless, nonirritating, and toxic. Common sources of CO include car exhaust, paint removers containing methylene chloride, and smoke from fires, furnaces, wood-burning stoves, and gas-powered engines. Carbon monoxide is the leading cause of death from poisoning in the United States, and the leading cause of poisoning death in childhood. The true incidence is unknown as many cases are misdiagnosed or not reported. It is estimated that approximately 5,000 individuals in the United States die from CO poisoning each year. Those younger than 15 years of age and older than 75 years of age are especially at risk. The number of cases increases during the winter months because of the use of indoor heating and closed windows.

CO toxicity may be acute or chronic. Mildly affected individuals may have non-specific complaints such as malaise, headache, dizziness, nausea, and/or vomiting. Signs and symptoms of moderate toxicity include weakness, confusion, syncope, dyspnea, tachycardia, tachypnea, chest pain, rhabdomyolysis, and visual distur-bances. Severe poisoning can result in seizures, coma, palpitations, hypotension, cardiopulmonary arrest, and death. Other neurologic findings can include agitation, hallucinations, confabulation, incontinence, and memory problems, as well as gait disturbances. The "classic" triad of cherry-red lips, cyanosis, and retinal hemor-rhages is rarely seen.

A neuropsychiatric syndrome develops 3 days to 8 months after exposure in 10% to 30% of cases. Almost any neurologic or psychiatric symptom can result. Common symptoms include memory loss, parkinsonism, dementia, psychosis, and incontinence. There can also be subtle personality or cognitive changes. Chronic low-level CO exposure can present with any of the preceding symptomatology. Severe acute exposure or chronic exposure can also cause cerebral edema or focal lesions, especially in the basal ganglia.

Several theories have been proposed for the pathophysiology of CO poisoning. The most widely accepted is that CO causes hypoxia by competitively binding to hemoglobin in the place of oxygen. Hemoglobin's affinity for CO is 200 to 250 times greater than its affinity for oxygen. Consequently, hemoglobin's capacity to carry and release oxygen to tissues is greatly reduced, resulting in cellular hypoxia. The brain and circulatory system are particularly vulnerable because of their high oxygen needs. In severe toxicity, resultant myocardial depression, peripheral vasodilatation, and ventricular dysrhythmia causing hypotension can also cause tissue ischemia.

Summary The patient is an 8-year-old boy who presents with a 3-day history of worsening fatigue, headache, nausea, and declining mental status. His neurologic exam shows decreased responsiveness and cognitive impairment, but no focal neu-rologic findings. Other family members may also be experiencing similar but milder symptoms. The fact that the family uses indoor heating in an older house is likely relevant.

Localization Fatigue, headache, nausea, and progressive mental status changes are relatively nonspecific symptoms, but in combination usually indicate diffuse cerebral dysfunction. There are no focal features on his neurologic exam.

Differential Diagnosis   The differential diagnosis of this child's symptoms can include many different processes. The fact that other family members seem to be affected suggests a local environmental exposure. Given that they use a wood-burning stove as well as a gas heater at night, carbon monoxide poisoning should be the first consideration. Lead toxicity might be an additional diagnostic possibility. Lead causes damage to the central and peripheral nervous systems, as well as to other organs. Symptoms at low levels of lead toxicity include anorexia, abdominal pain, constipation, nausea, vomiting, and lethargy. Higher doses can produce seizures, apathy, cognitive decline, ataxia, papilledema, and even death. Lead exposure from old house paint contaminating house dust or soil usually occurs in young children who frequently ingest lead when placing dirty objects in their mouths. Lead-based house paint has been banned since 1977. Preparation or storage of food in lead-containing pottery also can cause exposure.

Acute viral syndromes can cause fatigue, headache, and nausea but would likely be associated with other signs of illness, such as fever, cough, vomiting, and/or diarrhea. Central nervous system infections (bacterial meningitis, encephalitis) can cause similar symptoms in addition to mental status changes, but would also be expected to cause fever, meningismus, and/or photophobia. Primary headache disorders, such as migraine, may produce headache and nausea, but are not usually associated with mental status changes as seen in this patient. Additional findings of photophobia and sonophobia would also support a diagnosis of migraine.

Causes of increased intracranial pressure, such as brain tumors and subarachnoid bleeding, should be excluded. In addition, psychiatric illness, such as depression, or psychosis, or drug use, can present with similar nonspecific symptoms. There is no history of head trauma but a postconcussive syndrome or subdural hematoma might also present with headache, nausea, fatigue, and mental status changes.

Evaluation   A careful history and physical examination is essential when making the diagnosis of CO poisoning. The use of gas stoves for heating, exposure to open fires, the presence of a furnace or fireplace, and other environmental exposures should be investigated. Exposure to certain machinery in the workplace may also be relevant. The clinician should also ask about other ill persons or pets in the house.

If CO poisoning is suspected, a serum carboxyhemoglobin (COHB) level should be obtained. A level higher than 3% in a nonsmoker is consistent with CO poisoning. Long-term smokers can have baseline COHB levels up to 12%. Although levels greater than 60% are usually fatal, intermediate levels do not correlate with prognosis. Pulse oximetry is not a reliable measure of hypoxia in CO poisoning and may be falsely elevated as it cannot distinguish between COHB and oxyhemoglobin.

Additional diagnostic work-up may be required but depends on the individual patient's presentation and the severity of symptoms. Laboratory work-up might include a CBC, arterial blood gas, basic chemistry panel, creatine kinase, and cardiac markers. Arterial blood gas measurement can assess true oxygen delivery and the presence of acidosis. Lactate can be elevated in acute severe exposure.

A chest radiograph may show evidence of pulmonary edema in cases of severe toxicity. An ECG can show nonspecific changes, dysrhythmias, or evidence of myocardial ischemia. Neuroimaging should be obtained in patients with severe intoxication or persistent neurologic deficits. Although a head CT with and without contrast may be most easily obtained in the acute setting, a follow-up brain MRI with and without contrast may be more helpful at delineating cerebral involvement. Diffuse, symmetric white matter lesions occur predominantly in the periventricular white matter but may also involve the centrum semiovale and subcortical white matter. Focal findings may be seen and likely result from hypoxic-ischemic injury. In addition, the finding of bilateral globus pallidus involvement is highly suggestive of CO intoxication, although it may also be seen in other types of poisoning. Finally, when mental status is affected, neuropsychometric testing should be performed to assess cognition and to establish a baseline.

Management   The level of treatment required depends on the degree of toxicity a given patient has experienced. It is important to realize that COHB levels do not correlate with clinical symptoms and may be misleading. Supportive care should be instituted immediately when CO poisoning is diagnosed and begins with the administration of 100% high-flow oxygen. Providing oxygen improves hypoxia and helps eliminate CO from the circulatory system. However, there is no standard protocol regarding the dose or length of time for oxygen treatment.

More severely affected patients and/or those with underlying medical problems require hospitalization for monitoring of respiratory and cardiac status. Patients who are unable to protect their airway or who are at risk for aspiration require intubation. Complications such as seizures, arrhythmias, and cerebral edema should be medically managed when present.

The use of hyperbaric oxygen therapy in the management of CO toxicity is controversial but can be considered in certain situations. Pure oxygen is provided in a pressurized chamber and increases the amount of dissolved oxygen in the blood. Indications for hyperbaric treatment include severe poisoning with a COHB greater than 25%, persistent or severe neurologic dysfunction (coma, seizures, focal deficit), loss of consciousness, and myocardial dysfunction. It is often considered when there is cardiovascular compromise or metabolic acidosis, or when symptoms persist despite other measures.

Prevention is an additional important intervention. Patients should be educated about risk factors for CO poisoning such as poor ventilation, indoor combustion, and running motor vehicles. Appropriate local officials (the gas company, firefighters) should investigate the cause of the elevated environmental CO level. CO detectors should be installed in areas where combustion appliances are used.

Additional Questions

1. What toxin frequently affects the putamen?
2. What are the neurologic symptoms of arsenic poisoning? Mercury poisoning?

References

Abelsohn A, Sanborn MD, Jessiman BJ, et al. Identifying and managing adverse environmental health effects: 6. Carbon monoxide poisoning. *CMAJ*. 2002;166(13):1685–1690.

Kao LW, Nanagas KA. Carbon monoxide poisoning. *Med Clin North Am*. 2005;89(6):1161–1194.

Laraque D, Trasande L. Lead poisoning: success and 21st century challenges. *Pediatr Rev*. 2005;26(12):435–443.

Raub JA, Benignus VA. Carbon monoxide and the nervous system. *Neurosci Biobehav Rev*. 2002;26(8):925–940.

Varon J, Marik PE, Fromm RE Jr, et al. Carbon monoxide poisoning: a review for clinicians. *J Emerg Med*. 1999;17(1):87–93.

An **8-year-old girl** is brought to the emergency room by ambulance during her second seizure of the day. Her first seizure occurred 30 minutes earlier and was described as rhythmic, whole-body jerking with her eyes rolling back in her head and lasting approximately 8 minutes. After the first seizure stopped, she was very sleepy and unarousable. She has now been seizing for 15 minutes. You give her lorazepam intravenously followed by an intravenous fosphenytoin load and her seizure stops. She is an otherwise healthy child but her mother reports brief episodes of behavioral arrest that have been increasing in frequency over the past 4 months. They are now occurring a few times per day. There is no family history of epilepsy.

Physical Examination Vital Signs: Tachycardia. General Examination: Unremarkable. There is no meningismus, papilledema, or evidence of trauma. Neurologic Examination: Mental Status: Her eyes are closed and she is unarousable. Cranial Nerves: Her pupils are equal, round, and reactive to light. Continuous, repetitive, low-amplitude, jerky eye movements are noted bilaterally. Oculocephalic, corneal, and gag reflexes are intact. Facial movements are symmetric. Her tongue is midline. Motor: She has normal bulk with mild diffuse hypotonia. There are no spontaneous movements of the extremities. Sensory: There is no purposeful withdrawal to painful stimuli. Reflexes: 2+ throughout with bilateral plantar extensor responses.

Guide to Case Discussion

- Briefly summarize this case.
- Localize the examination findings.
- Give the most likely diagnosis and provide a differential diagnosis.
- Discuss an appropriate diagnostic work-up.
- Discuss the management of this patient.

Diagnosis   Childhood absence epilepsy presenting with convulsive status epilepticus and subsequent nonconvulsive status epilepticus provoked by fosphenytoin.

Discussion   Status epilepticus (SE) is defined as a seizure lasting more than 30 minutes or recurrent seizures during a 30-minute time span without recovery of consciousness between episodes. However, SE is a neurologic emergency and this definition is not universally accepted because significant morbidity and mortality are associated with ongoing seizure activity. Aggressive treatment is usually initiated within 5 to 10 minutes of continuous seizing. SE exhibits a bimodal age distribution with the highest rates in toddlers (younger than 5 years of age) and the elderly (older than 55 years of age). There is a remarkably increased incidence in children younger than 1 year of age.

SE classification is determined by the location of onset (focal versus generalized) and by etiology. SE can be further subdivided into generalized convulsive status epilepticus (GCSE) and nonconvulsive status epilepticus (NCSE) subtypes. Untreated GCSE can evolve into subtle GCSE where there are more subtle movements (such as slight finger or face twitches or nystagmus-type eye movements) as the seizure continues. Treatment of GCSE can also result in NCSE, and this should be suspected in patients who do not recover appropriately after the overt movements have stopped.

NCSE can occur with both generalized (absence) and focal (complex partial) epilepsy and is clinically distinguished from GCSE by a lack of limb-jerking movements. NCSE may manifest with subtle eye movements or solely unexplained unresponsiveness. The most common form of NCSE is recurrent or prolonged complex partial SE. NCSE can also occur when patients with idiopathic generalized epilepsy are given phenytoin or carbamazepine.

Mortality from SE in children ranges from 3% to 11% and is most closely linked to etiology. In children, acute symptomatic GCSE is consistently associated with the highest mortality rates, whereas children with febrile SE have minimal mortality and no morbidity, even in cases where SE lasts more than an hour. Morbidities associated with SE include the development of epilepsy as well as motor and cognitive disabilities.

Summary   The patient is a healthy 8-year-old girl with a 4-month history of spells of behavioral arrest who presents with new-onset generalized convulsive status epilepticus. Anticonvulsants stopped her second generalized tonic-clonic seizure but she is now comatose with continuous, rhythmic eye movements.

Localization   The patient's generalized tonic-clonic seizures localize to the cerebral cortex bilaterally. Her nonfocal neurologic exam with intact brainstem function also localizes her coma to the cerebral cortex diffusely. Plantar extensor responses denote bilateral corticospinal tract involvement.

Differential Diagnosis   The child in this case presents with a 4-month history of brief spells of behavioral arrest. These spells have increased in frequency and are now occurring on a daily basis. This history is highly suggestive of an underlying diagnosis of primary generalized epilepsy with absence seizures. The diagnosis

TABLE 49.1

Etiologies of Status Epilepticus in Childhood

Acute
 Metabolic disturbance (hypoglycemia, hypocalcemia, hyponatremia)
 Infection (meningitis, encephalitis, sepsis)
 Fever (febrile seizures)
 Intracranial hemorrhage
 Hypoxic-ischemic encephalopathy
 Ischemic stroke (arterial, venous)
 Intracranial tumor
 Anticonvulsant noncompliance
 Anticonvulsant withdrawal or dosage change
 Medication overdose
 Toxins
 Head trauma
 Hydrocephalus

Chronic
 Epilepsy (idiopathic, remote symptomatic)
 Neurodegenerative disorders

---

of absence seizures can easily be delayed as the characteristic staring spells are mistaken for daydreaming or a silly behavior. It also appears that this child has experienced unprovoked GCSE in this clinical setting. She is now comatose with rhythmic eye movements, which is consistent with NCSE. The possibility that her NCSE was iatrogenically induced by fosphenytoin must be considered as the most likely cause of her current condition in the emergency room.

Other possible acute and chronic causes of SE and coma must also be considered but seem much less likely in this otherwise normal, healthy child (Table 49.1). Metabolic disturbances such as hypoglycemia, hypocalcemia, and hyponatremia can result in seizures and mental status changes. Central nervous system (meningitis, encephalitis) and systemic infections (sepsis) can cause seizures and/or coma. Febrile seizures may be a cause. A multitude of cerebral injuries (stroke, hemorrhage, hypoxic-ischemic encephalopathy) can also result in these neurologic abnormalities. Head trauma and acute hydrocephalus must also be considered. Medication overdoses, ingestions, and toxins may cause seizures and/or coma. Finally, for patients already taking anticonvulsants, medication noncompliance, withdrawal, or dosage change may contribute to the development of SE.

Patients with chronic neurologic disorders are also at risk of developing SE. Underlying diagnoses such as primary generalized epilepsy, remote symptomatic seizure disorders, and neurodegenerative disorders can also be associated with SE.

Evaluation   SE is a neurologic emergency. Treatment of SE (whether convulsive or nonconvulsive) involves rapid medical stabilization of the patient and the stopping of the seizure itself. Because stopping the seizure can be dependent on correcting the underlying etiology, initial history, exam, and studies should target the reversible causes of SE. Although the child in this case is suspected to have an underlying idiopathic generalized epilepsy, this diagnosis needs to be confirmed with an appropriate work-up.

In general, studies to be obtained immediately with SE include blood glucose, electrolytes, calcium, magnesium, arterial blood gas, liver function tests, renal function tests, and a CBC. If a patient has refractory SE, or if there is a suspicion of other underlying diagnoses based on history and/or examination, antiepileptic drug levels, cultures, toxicology screening, and possibly other laboratory tests may need to be done. Neuroimaging with a head CT is appropriate in patients with new-onset SE when there is no identifiable cause, as in this child, or if the SE is refractory. This patient has not had symptoms of meningitis or encephalitis, but when a central nervous system infection is suspected, a lumbar puncture should be performed after neuroimaging is complete.

In addition, an emergent EEG is indicated in this child, given that she is experiencing NCSE. An EEG can help to establish whether SE is a result of absence or complex partial seizure activity. An immediate EEG is also necessary in cases of refractory SE, neuromuscular paralysis for SE, when mental status is still impaired after controlling overt seizure activity with SE, and for unexplained mental status/coma (to exclude NCSE).

Management Management of SE begins with assessment and stabilization of the airway, breathing, and circulation (the ABCs). This involves placing the patient on a cardiorespiratory monitor and pulse oximeter. An intravenous line also needs to be placed immediately. In several regimens, providing 2 mL/kg of 50% glucose is recommended early in the course of SE. Aggressive respiratory support or elective intubation should be considered in many cases.

Many protocols for the successful treatment of SE exist. In general, patients are initially given a benzodiazepine. Lorazepam (0.1 mg/kg) can be given intravenously or diazepam (0.5 mg/kg) can be given rectally if intravenous access has not been established. These doses may be repeated within 5 to 10 minutes if the patient continues to seize. This is followed by an intravenous load of fosphenytoin (20 phenytoin equivalents/kg) if the seizure is ongoing after 10 to 15 minutes. Intravenous phenobarbital (20 mg/kg) is the third-line drug after 15 to 20 minutes of seizure activity. After 20 to 30 minutes of seizing, an additional bolus of fosphenytoin (10 phenytoin equivalents/kg) may be given.

If these agents fail to resolve the seizure, underlying causes of SE (infection, increased intracranial pressure, hypoglycemia, or pyridoxine dependency) that will only respond to specific therapies should be reconsidered. Additional treatment for refractory SE then involves variable degrees of brain suppression with agents that include pentobarbital, phenobarbital, propofol, high-dose benzodiazepines, or other anesthetic agents (isoflurane, halothane), usually in an intensive care unit setting. These therapies generally need to be delivered as continuous intravenous infusions to obtain sufficient brain concentrations for prolonged suppression of brain electrical activity. Ideally, continuous EEG monitoring is in place to constantly monitor whether the desired level of cerebral suppression is achieved.

Valproic acid should be considered a first-line medication for patients already on valproic acid and for children in whom a generalized epilepsy syndrome is suspected. In these children, nonconvulsive seizures and NCSE can be provoked by phenytoin/fosphenytoin. There is a 1:600 risk of fatal hepatotoxicity in children age

2 years and younger on anticonvulsant polytherapy, so valproic acid should be used with caution in these children. Children who have suspected mitochondrial or fatty acid oxidation disorders should not be given valproic acid because of the high risk of hepatotoxicity.

More specifically for the child in this case, once an EEG and initial work-up are performed, management of her ongoing nonconvulsive seizure activity might include the intravenous administration of phenobarbital, valproic acid, or additional benzodiazepines. After she has been stabilized, she will need to be started on an appropriate long-term anticonvulsant for her absence seizures. Epilepsy teaching should also be done with the family.

Additional Questions

1. Which medication used for the treatment of status epilepticus in adults is potentially harmful to children? Why is it potentially harmful to children?

2. Why is intravenous fosphenytoin preferable to phenytoin in the treatment of seizure disorders?

3. What are the clinical features of childhood absence epilepsy?

4. What anticonvulsants are used in the treatment of childhood absence epilepsy?

References

Leszczyszyn DJ, Pellock JM. Status epilepticus. In: Pellock JM, Dodson WE, Bourgeois BFD, eds. *Pediatric Epilepsy: Diagnosis and Therapy.* 2nd ed. New York: Demos Medical; 2001:275–289.

Manno EM. New management strategies in the treatment of status epilepticus. *Mayo Clin Proc.* 2003;78:508–518.

Ramsay RE. Treatment of status epilepticus. *Epilepsia.* 1993;34(suppl 1):S71–S81.

Riviello JJ Jr, Holmes GL. The treatment of status epilepticus. *Semin Pediatr Neurol.* 2004;11:129–138.

Shneker BF, Fountain NB. Assessment of acute morbidity and mortality in nonconvulsive status epilepticus. *Neurology.* 2003;61:1066–1073.

A previously healthy 14-year-old boy is brought to the emergency room for complaints of the acute onset of left-sided face, arm, and leg weakness. His symptoms began after awakening from a nap during the day and have been progressing. The patient also complains of a worsening headache with nausea and emesis. On further questioning, the review of systems is remarkable for a 5-month history of an enlarging left scrotal mass that he had not disclosed to anyone.

Physical Examination General Examination: Notable for a large, nontender, left scrotal mass. There is no papilledema. Neurologic Examination: Mental Status: Alert and cooperative. Language: He has normal fluency and comprehension. Cranial Nerves: His pupils are equal, round, and reactive to light. His extraocular muscles are intact. His visual fields are intact. His forehead movement is symmetric but there is flattening of the left nasolabial fold. The tongue is midline. Motor: He has normal bulk with flaccid tone and minimal movement in the left upper and lower extremities. His strength on the right is 5/5 throughout. Coordination: No dysmetria or tremor is noted on the right. Sensory: Light touch, temperature, vibration, and proprioception are normal throughout. Gait: Unable to assess. Reflexes: 2+ on the right and 3+ on the left. Right plantar flexor and left plantar extensor response.

Guide to Case Discussion

- Briefly summarize this case.
- Localize the examination findings.
- Give the most likely diagnosis and provide a differential diagnosis.
- Discuss an appropriate diagnostic work-up.
- Discuss the management of this patient.

Diagnosis   Testicular germ cell tumor with a hemorrhagic cerebral metastasis.

Discussion   Brain metastases develop in 20% to 30% of adult patients with systemic cancers such as lung, breast, melanoma, renal, and colon cancer. In fact, 100,000 adult patients develop symptomatic brain metastases each year, making them the most common intracranial malignancy. The spectrum of pediatric tumors differs markedly, so one cannot simply extrapolate from adult data. Currently, approximately 5% to 10% of pediatric patients with solid tumors develop brain metastases at some point in their course. The pediatric solid tumors associated with the highest rate of brain metastasis include sarcomas (Ewing sarcoma, rhabdomyosarcoma, osteosarcoma), peripheral neuroectodermal tumors, germ cell tumors, retinoblastomas, and neuroblastomas.

Most brain metastases arise from hematogenous spread from the arterial circulation through pulmonary circuits. Rarely, metastases can arise from the Batson venous plexus. For tumor cells to reach the brain, they must possess certain neurotropic properties. To successfully form brain metastases, tumor cells must attach to and penetrate microvessel endothelium and degrade the extracellular matrix. They then respond to autocrine and brain-derived growth factors within the CNS. Pathologically, lesions are characteristically found at the gray–white junction and at arterial border zones, consistent with embolic phenomena. Eighty percent of brain metastases are located in the cerebral hemispheres, 15% in the cerebellum, and 5% in the brainstem.

Two-thirds of patients with brain metastases have neurologic symptoms at some point in their course. This means that most children with brain metastases will experience neurologic problems. More than 80% of brain metastases are discovered after the diagnosis of a systemic cancer. The clinical presentation is dependent on the size, location, and number of metastatic lesions. Nonetheless, patients often complain of generalized symptoms such as headache, fatigue, and altered cognition. Focal symptoms include seizures, hemiparesis, and numbness. Five percent to 10% of adult and pediatric patients present with acute neurologic symptoms caused by hemorrhage into a metastasis. Such acute presentations classically have been described in adult cases involving metastatic choriocarcinoma, renal cell carcinoma, and melanoma, and may be the result of a tendency for neovascularization or tumor invasion into blood vessels.

Unfortunately, the prognosis for most children with brain metastases remains dismal. Overall treatment results have been disappointing. In many cases, pediatric patients presenting with brain metastases have additional metastases in other locations, which worsens their prognosis. Except in rare cases, most children die weeks to months after their initial presentation.

Summary   The patient is a previously healthy 14-year-old boy with a 5-month history of a left scrotal mass who presents with the acute onset of left-sided weakness (involving the face, leg, and arm), headaches, and vomiting. His neurologic exam is remarkable for a central left facial nerve palsy, dense left hemiparesis, left hyperreflexia, and left plantar extensor response.

Localization   The child's neurologic exam is notable for a dense left hemiparesis with ipsilateral facial involvement, left hyperreflexia, and a left plantar extensor response. These signs are consistent with an upper motor neuron lesion localizing to the motor strip (precentral gyrus) of the right frontal lobe. A lesion involving the right internal capsule could also produce these findings. There does not appear to be spinal involvement as the face is involved and there is no apparent dermatomal level on sensory testing. No brainstem signs exist given the normal cranial nerve exam.

Differential Diagnosis Several underlying diagnoses need to be considered in a child presenting with an acute hemiparesis. Although arterial and venous ischemic stroke are important and more common causes, the possibility of a metastasis with or without hemorrhage should be considered high on the differential diagnosis in this adolescent presenting with a scrotal mass.

Arterial stroke may be seen in cardiac disorders, vasculitis, vasculopathies (moyamoya disease), inborn errors of metabolism (mitochondrial disease, homocystinuria), vasospastic disorders (migraine), arterial dissection, hematologic conditions with a hypercoagulable state (protein C deficiency, factor V Leiden mutation), and with trauma. Venous infarction from cerebral sinus venous thrombosis commonly occurs with localized infections (sinusitis, mastoiditis) as well as with a hypercoagulable state (malignancy, coagulation disorders). Given that this patient appears to have a malignancy, cerebral sinus venous thrombosis with a venous infarction secondary to a hypercoagulability is another important possible diagnosis. It might also explain findings such as headache and emesis. Other hemorrhagic conditions, such as a ruptured arterial venous malformation or bleeding into a primary brain tumor, could also be considered.

A focal seizure with a resulting Todd paralysis may present with unilateral weakness but would be unlikely in this patient as he has not had a witnessed seizure. Demyelinating disorders, such as acute disseminated encephalomyelitis and multiple sclerosis, can cause the acute onset of neurologic deficits. Again, these seem unlikely as there was no preceding viral illness to predispose him to acute disseminated encephalomyelitis (ADEM) and multiple sclerosis is uncommon in adolescence.

Evaluation In the emergency room, the patient will require an emergent head CT with and without contrast to evaluate for ischemic stroke, primary brain tumor, abscess, hemorrhage, and metastases. Basic laboratory work including a CBC, PT/PTT, chemistry panel, and liver function tests should be done.

Further evaluation will include a brain MRI with and without gadolinium. MRI findings that favor metastases include a multiplicity of lesions, location at the gray–white junction, a lesion in the border zone between two major arterial distributions, and a small tumor nidus with a large amount of associated vasogenic edema. Nevertheless, brain biopsy is still sometimes required for confirmation of pathology. Brain magnetic resonance angiography (MRA) can also be useful with focal hemorrhage to help rule out an underlying arteriovenous malformation. Catheter angiography may be needed for a more detailed evaluation in some cases. Consultation from neurosurgery can also be helpful when there is evidence of hemorrhage or metastasis.

A diagnostic work-up is also required for his scrotal mass. Appropriate testing should be guided by an oncologist. An initial search for other metastases might include a chest radiograph and bone scan.

Management The acute onset of a hemiparesis and intracranial hemorrhage represents a neurologic emergency. The patient's airway, breathing, and circulation should immediately be assessed. He should be placed on a cardiorespiratory monitor and pulse oximeter. An intravenous line should be placed. He will likely require further monitoring in the intensive care unit until he is medically stable and his diagnosis is clarified.

Symptoms such as vomiting and headache are suggestive of some degree of increased intracranial pressure. He should be followed closely for signs of progression and herniation, such as declining mental status or a unilateral dilated pupil. For an acutely deteriorating patient, intubation with hyperventilation to an arterial carbon dioxide pressure ($PaCO_2$) of approximately 30 mm Hg should be performed. Intravenous mannitol, an osmotic diuretic, can also be given to reduce intracranial pressure. Input from neurosurgery is important in the management of a patient with intracranial hemorrhage. Measures such as external ventricular drainage and hematoma evacuation are sometimes required. Serial head CTs will also be necessary to monitor for progression or resolution of the bleed. Complications of intracranial hemorrhage such as seizures, hyperglycemia, and hyponatremia should be appropriately medically managed.

Management decisions in the context of brain metastases can be quite complicated and depend on the tumor type and the patient's clinical status. It is now accepted that adult patients with surgically accessible single brain metastases and well-controlled systemic cancer should undergo resection of the brain lesion. This might also be true in some pediatric cases. Certain cancers are quite sensitive to radiation therapy and there are ongoing debates regarding indications for whole-brain radiotherapy. Stereotaxic radiosurgery with multiple convergent beams offers the benefits of delivering a high single dose of radiation to often surgically inaccessible metastases. Metastases in eloquent cortex, basal ganglia, thalamus, and the brainstem have been treated this way with a much lower risk when compared to invasive methods.

The care of any patient with brain and/or systemic metastases must also address the needs for supportive care. The overall goal of treatment is to maintain the highest quality of life, not just to eradicate the primary cancer. Corticosteroids are beneficial in treating symptomatic tumorigenic edema. In addition to their ability to stabilize the blood–brain barrier and thus reduce edema, steroids have many more beneficial effects; for example, they can help to mitigate nausea and emesis, increase the patient's appetite, provide pain relief, and prevent some hypersensitivity to radiation and chemotherapy.

Additional Questions

1. Describe three brain herniation syndromes and their associated neurologic findings.

2. What is the syndrome of inappropriate antidiuretic hormone (SIADH) secretion? What is cerebral salt-wasting syndrome? How are these disorders diagnosed and managed?

References

Becker KJ, Tirschwell DL. Intracerebral hemorrhage. In: Johnson RT, Griffin JW, McArthur JC, eds. *Current Therapy in Neurologic Disease*. 6th ed. St. Louis, Mo: Mosby; 2002:209–214.

Bouffet E, Doumi N, Thiesse P, et al. Brain metastases in children with solid tumors. *Cancer.* 1997;79(2):403–410.

Dropcho EJ. Brain metastases. 2001. Available at: http://www.medlink.com. Last accessed December 12, 2005.

El Kamar FG, Posner JB. Brain metastases. *Semin Neurol.* 2004;24(4):347–362.

Roach ES. Etiology of stroke. *Semin Pediatr Neurol.* 2000;7(4):244–260.

Schiff D, Wen P. Nervous system metastases. In: Bradley WG, Daroff RB, Fenichel GM, et al., eds. *Neurology in Clinical Practice.* 4th ed. Philadelphia, Pa: Butterworth-Heinemann; 2004:1441–1459.

Voloschin AD, Batchelor TT, Allen JC. Management of primary nervous system tumors in infants and children. In: Bradley WG, Daroff RB, Fenichel GM, et al., eds. *Neurology in Clinical Practice.* 4th ed. Philadelphia, Pa: Butterworth-Heinemann; 2004:1423–1440.

A healthy 16-year-old boy presents to the emergency room for complaints of headache and diplopia. He developed a severe, left-sided, throbbing headache associated with nausea, vomiting, and photophobia approximately 1 week ago. Three days after his symptoms began, he started to complain of diplopia. Two days later, his mother noted that his left pupil was larger than the right. There is no history of recent trauma, fever, or illness.

Physical Examination Vital Signs: Afebrile. General Examination: There is no papilledema or nuchal rigidity. Neurologic Examination: Mental Status: Alert and cooperative. Language: He has fluent speech without dysarthria. Cranial Nerves: His left pupil is 6 mm and reacts sluggishly to light, constricting to 4 mm. His right pupil is 4 mm and reacts briskly to light. There is a mild left-sided ptosis. Movements of the right eye are normal. He is able to completely abduct the left eye but has difficulty with adduction as well as upgaze and downgaze. His face is symmetric with normal sensation. His palate elevates symmetrically and his tongue is midline. Motor: He has normal bulk and tone with 5/5 strength throughout. Coordination: Finger-to-nose testing is intact bilaterally. Sensory: Normal light-touch, temperature, and vibration. Gait: He has a normal heel, toe, flat, and tandem gait. Reflexes: 2+ throughout with bilateral plantar flexor responses.

Guide to Case Discussion

- Briefly summarize this case.
- Localize the examination findings.
- Give the most likely diagnosis and provide a differential diagnosis.
- Discuss an appropriate diagnostic work-up.
- Discuss the management of this patient.

Diagnosis Ophthalmoplegic migraine.

Discussion Ophthalmoplegic migraine had been considered to be a subtype of migraine but more recently has been classified as a cranial neuralgia. It is a rare condition. Affected individuals experience recurrent attacks of migrainous type headaches associated with paresis of one or more ocular cranial nerves. The headache is usually severe and ipsilateral to the eye findings. Paresis of the ocular cranial nerves occurs within 4 days of the onset of the headache. The oculomotor nerve is most commonly affected, but trochlear and abducens nerve palsies have also been reported. The pupil is usually, but not always, involved. MRI changes may be seen in the affected nerve but other structural abnormalities must be appropriately ruled out to make the diagnosis.

Ophthalmoplegic migraine is typically considered to be a pediatric phenomenon, occurring primarily in children younger than 10 years old, but it has been reported in adolescents and adults. There may be a male predominance. Very young children may not provide a history of headache and may present with symptoms such as recurrent ophthalmoplegia with nausea, vomiting, and/or irritability. Painless ptosis or ophthalmoplegia can also occur.

The pathophysiology of ophthalmoplegic migraine is still poorly understood. It is now suspected to represent an inflammatory cranial neuropathy. It also has been hypothesized that symptoms may be caused by recurrent oculomotor nerve demyelination or by vascular dilatation causing compression of the oculomotor nerve. In addition, ischemic and other vascular mechanisms have been proposed.

The overall prognosis of ophthalmoplegic migraine is generally good. Headaches typically remit within 1 week. However, ophthalmologic abnormalities can take days to weeks to resolve. Recovery is usually complete, but after several episodes neurologic deficits may persist.

Summary The patient is a healthy 16-year-old boy who presents with a 1-week history of a migrainous headache in addition to left-sided ptosis and ophthalmoplegia with a dilated, sluggish pupil, which is consistent with an isolated oculomotor nerve palsy.

Localization The patient's headache localizes to the supratentorial pain-sensitive structures (cerebral arteries, dural arteries, large veins, venous sinuses) that are mediated through the trigeminal nerve. The findings of ptosis with impairment of eye adduction in addition to upgaze and downgaze are consistent with an isolated oculomotor nerve palsy. Pupillary motor fibers are also involved causing mydriasis.

In general, the oculomotor nerve may be affected along its course in several locations, including the brainstem (nucleus or fascicle), subarachnoid space, cavernous sinus, superior orbital fissure, and orbit. In this case, there are none of the additional cranial neuropathies that are often seen with involvement of the brainstem, cavernous sinus, or superior orbital fissure. There has been no vision loss, proptosis, or chemosis that would suggest an orbital lesion. Thus, involvement of the portion of the nerve within the subarachnoid space seems most likely.

Differential Diagnosis This patient's history and physical exam are most consistent with a diagnosis of ophthalmoplegic migraine. The diagnosis of a migraine is supported by the fact that the headache is characterized by unilateral throbbing pain and is associated with symptoms of nausea, vomiting, and photophobia. The physical exam demonstrates an isolated oculomotor nerve palsy that fits this definition. However, ophthalmoplegic migraine is a diagnosis of exclusion.

The most concerning cause of an isolated oculomotor nerve palsy is an aneurysm of the posterior communicating artery, but this is rare in childhood. Tumors, infectious (meningitis, Lyme disease, fungal infection, tuberculosis) and inflammatory processes (sarcoidosis) in the parasellar region, superior orbital fissure, and posterior fossa also need to be considered. Tolosa-Hunt syndrome and other cavernous sinus lesions are also in the differential diagnosis. Tolosa-Hunt syndrome is suspected to have clinical overlap with ophthalmoplegic migraine. This condition is caused by an inflammatory granulomatous lesion of the cavernous sinus that produces episodes of periorbital pain and ophthalmoplegia. Symptoms typically respond to steroids.

In older patients, dysfunction of cranial nerves III, IV, and VI may be caused by ischemic diabetic neuropathy, but the pupil is usually spared in these cases. Nerve sheath tumors of these same nerves may produce similar symptoms. Trauma may cause an isolated oculomotor nerve palsy, but is not present in this case. Idiopathic intracranial hypertension (pseudotumor cerebri) can cause headache and diplopia because of an abducens nerve palsy. Myasthenia gravis can cause diplopia and ptosis but is not associated with headache or pupillary abnormalities.

Evaluation   In the emergency room, the patient's evaluation should begin with a head CT, with and without contrast, to rule out larger structural abnormalities. However, additional neuroimaging is warranted to provide a more detailed evaluation of the oculomotor nerve, brainstem, and posterior fossa. A brain MRI with and without gadolinium should be performed in addition to magnetic resonance angiography (MRA). In some cases of ophthalmoplegic migraine, transient enhancement of the oculomotor nerve can be seen on MRI in the acute period and supports the diagnosis. Although a CT angiogram may also be helpful in ruling out vascular abnormalities, a four-vessel catheter angiogram is the gold standard when a posterior communicating artery aneurysm is suspected.

This adolescent should also be evaluated by ophthalmology to formally document the eye findings. Laboratory tests, including a CBC, basic chemistry panel, erythrocyte sedimentation rate, and liver function tests, help to screen for infectious and inflammatory disorders. The erythrocyte sedimentation rate is often elevated in Tolosa-Hunt syndrome. A lumbar puncture should also be performed to exclude infectious and inflammatory disorders. An opening pressure should be measured. Cell count, glucose, protein, and bacterial culture should be sent.

Management   This adolescent should be admitted to the hospital for work-up and management of his headache and isolated third cranial nerve palsy. Because of the rarity of this condition, treatment of ophthalmoplegic migraine is not standardized. Because permanent ocular nerve palsies have been documented, headache prophylaxis may be important when episodes are frequent. As with other migraines, treatment with beta blockers and calcium channel blockers has been used in some patients. Treatment with a course of corticosteroids also has been beneficial in some cases. Patients also need follow-up with ophthalmology to monitor for resolution of their symptoms.

Additional Questions

1. Review the anatomic course of the oculomotor nerve.
2. Which cranial nerves run through the cavernous sinus? How do disorders affecting the cavernous sinus present?

References

Brazis PW, Masdeu JC, Biller J. *Localization in Clinical Neurology*. 3rd ed. Philadelphia, Pa: Lippincott Williams & Wilkins; 1996:155–250.

Classification Committee of the International Headache Society. International classification of headache disorders II. *Cephalgia*. 2004;24(suppl 1):1–160.

De Silva DA, Siow HC. A case report of ophthalmoplegic migraine: a differential diagnosis of third nerve palsy. *Cephalgia*. 2005;25:827–830.

Fenichel GM. *Clinical Pediatric Neurology. A Signs and Symptoms Approach*. 4th ed. Philadelphia, Pa: WB Saunders; 2001:77–89.

Levin M, Ward TN. Ophthalmoplegic migraine. *Curr Pain Headache Rep*. 2004;8(4):306–309.

Weiss AH, Phillips JO. Ophthalmoplegic migraine. *Pediatr Neurol*. 2004;30:64–66.

The attending physician on your pediatric neurology rotation asks you to see **a 7-year-old girl** admitted to the general pediatric ward for management of aspiration pneumonia. There are currently no active neurologic issues but the child is well known to the neurology service. You are told that her brain MRI helped make her diagnosis 3 years previously. The patient was born at full term to a 32-year-old G_3P_2 mother by an uneventful vaginal delivery. Her development was slow in all areas but she walked independently with a stiff and awkward gait at 2 years of age. She spoke her first words around the same time. At 3 years of age, she developed abnormal stiffness and posturing of the left arm and leg. Shortly thereafter, the abnormal movements generalized, limiting her ambulation. Her speech became slurred and she experienced cognitive decline. There is no family history of neurologic disease.

Physical Examination General Examination: Normal. Neurologic Examination: Mental Status: Alert. Language: She follows some simple commands. She says several words with dysarthria but does not form sentences. Cranial Nerves: Her pupils are equal, round, and reactive to light. Her extraocular muscles are intact. Her face is symmetric. The tongue is midline. Motor: She has decreased bulk with increased tone and significant spasticity throughout. Coordination: There is frequent dystonic posturing of all four extremities. Sensory: She responds to tactile stimulation throughout. Gait: She is nonambulatory. Reflexes: Hard to assess because of spasticity and dystonia, but they are very brisk at the patellas. She has bilateral plantar extensor responses.

Guide to Case Discussion

- Briefly summarize this case.

- Localize the examination findings.

- Give the most likely diagnosis and provide a differential diagnosis.

- Discuss an appropriate diagnostic work-up.

- Discuss the management of this patient.

Diagnosis Pantothenate kinase-associated neurodegeneration.

Discussion Pantothenate kinase-associated neurodegeneration (PKAN) is a hetero-geneous autosomal recessive disorder characterized by focal iron accumulation in the basal ganglia. PKAN is now considered to be one of several disorders of neurodegen-eration with brain iron accumulation (NBIA). This category of diseases also includes two other autosomal recessive disorders, aceruloplasminemia and neuroferritino-pathy. Aceruloplasminemia is caused by a defect in the ceruloplasmin gene whereas neuroferritinopathy is associated with mutations in the ferritin light chain gene. NBIA was previously known as Hallervorden-Spatz syndrome but Hallervorden's involve-ment with Nazi activities during World War II and the discovery of the underlying genetic defects in several of these diseases have prompted new nomenclature.

PKAN is caused by a mutation in the pantothenate kinase 2 (*PKAN2*) gene on chromosome 20p12.3-p13. Pantothenate kinase is an important enzyme in the biosynthesis of coenzyme A from pantothenate (vitamin B_5). The protein product is targeted to mitochondria but how this abnormality causes the underlying pathogenesis of this disorder is not yet understood. Early-onset cases tend to be associated with more severe mutations that cause truncation of the protein product whereas muta-tions in later-onset cases are due to smaller amino acid changes.

Clinically, PKAN is typically characterized by a progressive dystonia. The onset of PKAN varies widely from early childhood through adulthood. Several clinical forms have been described (early versus late-onset forms, typical versus atypical forms) but these designations are frequently changing as more is learned about this disease.

In general, the early-onset form presents in children younger than 10 years of age with gait disturbance caused by spasticity. Other corticospinal tract signs are usually also present. Very early development may be normal but developmental delay is usually apparent by early childhood. There may be a period of stagnation but dystonia and other movement disorders (choreoathetosis, tremor) subse-quently follow with rapid progression. Ambulation is lost by the adolescent years (age 10 to 15 years), if not sooner. Retinitis pigmentosa and other retinal abnor-malities frequently occur, clinically resulting in vision loss. Optic atrophy has also been reported. Cognitive decline is common. Acanthocytes have been reported in a subset of patients. Juvenile cases typically present with the onset of dystonia. The later-onset form of the disease presents primarily with parkinsonism (tremor, bradykinesia) but speech and psychiatric abnormalities are also common. Disease progression is slower than in early onset cases. Dystonia, dementia, and motor impairment may occur with time. Retinal abnormalities are rare.

The brain MRI in PKAN demonstrates classic findings of the "eye-of-the-tiger" sign. T_2-weighted imaging shows bilateral, symmetric hyperintensity in a region of hypointensity in the medial globus pallidus. The areas of low signal are a result of iron accumulation, whereas high signal areas likely represent edema or reactive change. To date, all patients with the characteristic MRI findings have been found to have a mutation in the *PKAN2* gene. Thus, the MRI is virtually diagnostic in both early- and late-onset disease. Pathologically, significant iron deposition is found in the globus pallidus and the substantia nigra.

Summary The patient is a 7-year-old girl with a history of global developmental delay who experienced developmental regression as well as progressive spasticity, dystonia, and dysarthria. Her neurologic exam is remarkable for impaired cognition, dysarthria, spasticity, generalized dystonia, hyperreflexia, and bilateral plantar extensor responses. She is now admitted for aspiration pneumonia. Her brain MRI was an important factor in determining her underlying diagnosis.

Localization This child's findings of spasticity, dysarthria, hyperreflexia, and bilateral plantar extensor responses localize to the corticospinal tracts. Progressive dystonia is caused by basal ganglia involvement. There also appears to have been cognitive regression, which suggests involvement of the cortical gray matter.

Differential Diagnosis The differential diagnosis of PKAN primarily includes numerous neurodegenerative disorders, as well as inborn errors of metabolism causing dystonia and other movement disorders. Although acquired conditions, such as basal ganglia infection (meningitis, encephalitis), ischemia, vasculitis, structural abnormalities (tumor, arteriovenous malformation), and toxins can cause a progressive dystonia, they would be unlikely to explain this child's constellation of symptoms.

First, PKAN should be distinguished from other disorders of NBIA. This group of diseases is characterized by progressive extrapyramidal symptoms and iron deposition in the basal ganglia. Aceruloplasminemia and neuroferritinopathy do not produce the classic "eye-of-the-tiger" MRI findings and have different genetic defects. They also tend to present in later life. HARP (hypobetalipoproteinemia, acanthocytosis, retinitis pigmentosa, pallidal degeneration) syndrome is now considered to be part of the PKAN spectrum of disorders. Mutations in the *PKAN2* gene have been identified in affected families.

Juvenile Huntington disease can manifest with a rigidity and choreoathetosis that sometimes resembles PKAN. The MRI may show caudate atrophy and retinal abnormalities; optic atrophy and acanthocytosis do not occur. Juvenile forms of GM_1 and GM_2 gangliosidoses may present with features similar to PKAN but can be distinguished by brain MRI and laboratory abnormalities. Neuronal ceroid lipofuscinosis (NCL) can also present with rapidly progressive dystonia, spasticity, rigidity, and retinal abnormalities, but seizures are also common in NCL. Mitochondrial disorders, primary dystonias (idiopathic torsion dystonia, dopa-responsive dystonia), and Wilson disease deserve consideration. As PKAN is associated with acanthocytosis, the neuroacanthocytosis syndromes are also in the differential diagnosis. Finally, MRI T_2 hyperintensity in the globus pallidus can be seen in other disorders such as Leigh disease, alpha-fucosidosis, organic acidurias, postinfectious dystonia, as well as postinfarction dystonia, and can occasionally be confused with PKAN.

Evaluation The patient in this case apparently has undergone an evaluation and the diagnosis has already been made. However, her work-up certainly began with basic lab work as well as neuroimaging. An initial evaluation for a child presenting with a progressive dystonia, developmental regression, and spasticity may include a CBC (neuroacanthocytosis, PKAN), basic chemistry panel, liver function tests, thyroid function tests, copper, and ceruloplasmin. A work-up for inborn errors of metabolism may include plasma amino acids, urine organic acids, serum lactate/pyruvate, and lysosomal enzymes. As results return, more detailed testing for specific diseases is usually warranted.

Evaluation by an ophthalmologist is also required to document any associated retinal pigmentary abnormalities or optic atrophy. Electroretinograms and VERs are sometimes performed to better assess the visual pathway.

Fortunately, in the case of PKAN, the MRI is virtually diagnostic. If an "eye-of-the-tiger" sign is seen, the diagnosis may be confirmed with molecular genetic testing. Sequence analysis of the *PKAN2* gene is now clinically available and has greatly simplified the diagnosis of this disorder.

Management There are no specific treatments for PKAN at this time. Attempts at iron chelation with desferrioxamine have not altered the clinical course of the disease. Thus, management is primarily symptomatic. Dystonia is often treated with levodopa/carbidopa, bromocriptine, or anticholinergic agents (trihexyphenidyl), but medications ultimately have limited benefit as the disease progresses. Transient improvement in symptoms has been reported with ablative pallidotomy and thalamotomy, as well as with deep brain stimulation, in some cases.

Physical and occupational therapists are needed to help maintain mobility and to maximize developmental potential. As symptoms progress, an orthopaedist may be needed to help manage contractures and spasticity. Rehabilitative specialists also may help to prescribe appropriate adaptive equipment, as well as therapies for spasticity such as baclofen or botulinum toxin injections. Given the associated retinal abnormalities, long-term monitoring by ophthalmology might be required. A nutritional specialist and gastroenterologist may become involved when dysphagia prevents adequate oral intake. Finally, any child diagnosed with a neurodegenerative disease should be referred to a geneticist for family genetic counseling.

Additional Questions

1. Describe the clinical features of dopa-responsive dystonia.
2. Describe the clinical features of juvenile Huntington disease.

References

Coryell J, Gregory A, Hayflick SJ. Pantothenate kinase-associated neurodegeneration. 2004. Available at: http://www.genetests.org. Last accessed January 16, 2005.

Hayflick SJ. Pantothenate kinase-associated neurodegeneration (formerly Hallervorden-Spatz syndrome). *J Neurol Sci.* 2003;207:106–107.

Mink JW. Basal ganglia motor function in relation to Hallervorden-Spatz syndrome. *Pediatr Neurol.* 2001;25:112–117.

Swaiman KF. Hallervorden-Spatz syndrome. *Pediatr Neurol.* 2001;25:102–108.

Thomas M, Hayflick SJ, Jankovic J. Clinical heterogeneity of neurodegeneration with brain iron accumulation (Hallervorden-Spatz syndrome) and pantothenate kinase-associated neurodegeneration. *Mov Disord.* 2004;19(1):36–42.

A 9-year-old boy without significant past medical history presents to the neurology clinic with complaints of jerking spells. The patient has experienced frequent brief twitching of his extremities for several months. He frequently drops things and has had many falls, some of which have resulted in bruises on his face. He has otherwise been a healthy child and had done well in school until recently. Since the onset of his symptoms, his grades have fallen and he has become very forgetful. The family moved to the United States from Guatemala when he was 3 years old. He received all of his immunizations shortly after arrival. There is no family history of neurologic disease.

Physical Examination General Examination: Normal. Neurologic Examination: Mental Status: Alert and cooperative. He has difficulty recalling his home phone number and address. Language: He speaks in full sentences without dysarthria but his speech is slow. Cranial Nerves: His pupils are equal, round, and reactive to light. His extraocular muscles are intact and his visual fields are full. His face is symmetric. The tongue is midline. Motor: He has normal bulk with slightly increased tone diffusely and mild rigidity of the upper extremities. His strength is 5/5 throughout. Coordination: There is no dysmetria. Sensory: Light-touch, temperature, and vibration are intact. Gait: He has a slightly wide-based, clumsy gait. Reflexes: 3+ throughout with bilateral plantar extensor responses.

Guide to Case Discussion

- Briefly summarize this case.
- Localize the examination findings.
- Give the most likely diagnosis and provide a differential diagnosis.
- Discuss an appropriate diagnostic work-up.
- Discuss the management of this patient.

Diagnosis   Subacute sclerosing panencephalitis.

Discussion   Subacute sclerosing panencephalitis (SSPE) is a progressive central nervous system disorder caused by a defective measles virus. SSPE is primarily a pediatric disorder, most commonly occurring in children who experienced a primary measles virus infection while younger than 2 years of age. Males are affected more than females. There is a latency period of 6 to 8 years prior to the onset of symptoms, with most children presenting between 10 and 14 years of age. In industrialized nations, widespread immunization programs have helped to eliminate this devastating disease, but in less-developed countries, measles continues to cause significant morbidity and mortality. When SSPE occurs in immunized individuals, it is thought to result from a subclinical infection prior to the immunization. There is no evidence that the attenuated measles vaccine causes sporadic cases of SSPE.

Measles is a type of ribonucleic acid (RNA) paramyxovirus. It likely enters the brain during an acute, primary measles infection. The precise mechanisms involved in the spread of measles virus through the brain and the virus' ability to lie dormant for many years are still poorly understood. Pathologically, there is a preference for the parietal and occipital lobes of the brain, but involvement of the anterior cerebral hemispheres, brainstem, subcortical structures, and spinal cord also occurs. Gray and white matter are affected.

Clinically, SSPE initially manifests with subtle behavior change and cognitive decline. School performance may deteriorate. Affected children may appear forgetful or confused. As these are very nonspecific symptoms, SSPE is often difficult to diagnose in the early stages of the disease. Myoclonus subsequently follows and is characterized by rapid jerks of the head, trunk, or limbs. Myoclonic jerks may also present as head drops, falls, or gait abnormalities, so there must be a high clinical suspicion for possible seizure activity. Generalized tonic-clonic and complex partial seizures can also occur. Motor abnormalities, such as pyramidal and extrapyramidal signs, can develop. Some children experience ataxia or dystonia. Ophthalmologic abnormalities are seen in 10% to 50% of affected patients. They include chorioretinitis, papillitis, papilledema, optic atrophy, and cortical blindness.

With time, patients develop progressive spastic quadriplegia, intellectual deterioration, and autonomic failure. Myoclonus may abate or stop completely. The disease is uniformly fatal, with life typically ending in a vegetative state. Most patients survive 1 to 3 years after the diagnosis is made. However, there is an acute fulminant form of the disease that progresses very rapidly and can result in death within 3 months of onset.

The diagnosis is usually confirmed when patients fulfill three of the following five standard diagnostic criteria: (a) an appropriate clinical presentation with progressive cognitive decline and myoclonus; (b) an EEG showing periodic, stereotyped, high-voltage discharges; (c) CSF demonstrating raised immunoglobulins or oligoclonal bands; (d) elevated serum and CSF measles titers; (e) a brain biopsy consistent with panencephalitis.

Summary   The patient is a previously healthy 9-year-old boy who presents with a subacute progressive encephalopathy and myoclonic seizures. Immunizations were delayed until 3 years of age. His neurologic exam is remarkable for encephalopathy, slow speech, increased tone with upper-extremity rigidity, wide-based gait, hyper-reflexia, and bilateral plantar extensor responses.

Localization   Symptoms of cognitive difficulties and slow speech suggest involvement of the cortical gray matter. Increased tone, hyperreflexia, and bilateral plantar extensor responses localize to the corticospinal tracts. Rigidity suggests involvement of the extrapyramidal tracts. A wide-based, clumsy gait is a nonspecific finding but it could be caused by spasticity or cerebellar involvement. Myoclonic seizures are a form of generalized epilepsy and localize to the cortex bilaterally.

Differential Diagnosis   Children often present with very nonspecific cognitive or behavioral abnormalities in the early phases of the disease, making the diagnosis challenging. In these cases, other acquired conditions may be higher on the differential diagnosis. A chronic meningitis (tuberculosis), encephalitis, HIV encephalopathy, brain tumors, central nervous system vasculitis, or toxic exposure may present with a chronic encephalopathy. However, when myoclonus becomes apparent, a broad range of neurodegenerative myoclonic conditions need to be considered. These disorders can be divided into progressive myoclonic epilepsies, progressive myoclonic encephalopathies, and progressive myoclonic ataxias.

The progressive myoclonic epilepsies include Lafora body disease, neuronal ceroid lipofuscinosis (NCL), myoclonic epilepsy with ragged red fibers (MERRF), Unverricht-Lundborg syndrome, sialidosis, and dentatorubral-pallidoluysian atrophy. Lafora body disease is caused by a mutation on chromosome 6q23-25. It presents in adolescence with generalized tonic-clonic and myoclonic seizures. Dementia, ataxia, and cognitive decline occur rapidly after onset. The diagnosis can be made through a biopsy of axillary skin. NCL describes a large, heterogeneous group of disorders associated with progressive vision loss, intellectual deterioration, and intractable seizures of varying types. NCL is caused by the accumulation of autofluorescent pigment in many different cell types. The diagnosis is made through molecular genetic testing or conjunctival biopsy.

MERRF is a form of mitochondrial cytopathy associated most frequently with myoclonic seizures and ataxia. However, affected individuals also may exhibit dementia, deafness, optic atrophy, peripheral neuropathy, or dystonia. A muscle biopsy is required to make a definitive diagnosis. Unverricht-Lundborg disease is the most common cause of progressive myoclonic epilepsy. It is an autosomal recessive disorder caused by an abnormality in the cystatin B gene on chromosome 21. It presents with myoclonus between 8 and 13 years of age. Affected individuals also may have ataxia and tremor, but intellectual decline is less common and progression is slower than with Lafora disease. The diagnosis can now be made with mutation analysis.

Myoclonus is often present, but a less significant feature of the progressive myoclonic encephalopathies, which include Creutzfeldt-Jakob disease, juvenile Huntington disease, GM_2 gangliosidosis, and Niemann-Pick disease. Several of the progressive ataxias also can cause myoclonus and can present with features similar to SSPE. The hereditary spinocerebellar ataxias, Wilson disease, Whipple disease, and celiac disease also deserve consideration.

Evaluation   The child in this case obviously has a progressive neurodegenerative disorder and requires an extensive work-up. Blood tests, CSF analysis, electrodiagnostic testing, and neuroimaging are warranted to exclude other possible diagnoses. Thus, hospitalization to initiate the process is appropriate given the presentation.

Initial screening blood work might include a CBC, basic chemistry panel, liver function tests, thyroid function tests, copper, ceruloplasmin, and an erythrocyte sedimentation rate. Preliminary screening for inborn errors of metabolism might include plasma amino acids, urine organic acids, serum lactate/pyruvate, very-long-chain fatty acids, and lysosomal enzymes. If the diagnosis of SSPE is considered early, serum measles titers can also be sent. Elevated titers of 1:256 or greater are consistent with the diagnosis. If other forms of encephalitis are entertained, serum titers of common pathogens such as *Mycoplasma pneumoniae*, Epstein-Barr virus, varicella virus, herpes simplex virus, and cytomegalovirus can also be done.

Many of the progressive myoclonic epilepsies and other neurodegenerative disorders in the differential diagnosis are associated with retinal pigmentary changes and/or optic atrophy, so a formal ophthalmology consult early in the work-up can also be very helpful. Additional testing with an electroretinogram and VERs might detect subtle abnormalities in the visual pathway, supporting a diagnosis with ophthalmologic involvement.

The child in this case appears to be having myoclonic seizures so an EEG or video EEG needs to be promptly performed. Early in the disease, the EEG might be normal or show nonspecific slowing. The clinician must keep a very high suspicion for SSPE during this time. Once myoclonus begins, the classic pattern is frequently seen, consisting of bilaterally symmetric, synchronous, high-voltage, periodic complexes of sharp and slow waves repeating every 4 to 10 seconds. The bursts correlate with myoclonus. This EEG finding is essentially diagnostic, and if found, may eliminate the need for an exhaustive work-up to rule out other neurodegenerative disorders and disease processes. As the disease progresses, the interval between complexes can shorten and eventually the EEG may become disorganized and slow.

Neuroimaging with a brain MRI is also warranted in this child, preferably with and without gadolinium. Early in the course of SSPE, T_2-weighted imaging may show nonspecific hyperintensity in the subcortical occipital white matter. With time, more diffuse white matter demyelination is usually seen, often resembling a leukodystrophy or acute disseminated encephalomyelitis. Severe cortical atrophy eventually occurs.

Finally, a lumbar puncture should also be performed. Cell count, glucose, protein, and bacterial culture should be sent. They are typically normal in SSPE, although a slight elevation in protein might be seen. If SSPE is suspected, CSF immunoglobulin IgG, oligoclonal bands, and measles titers should also be sent. Elevated levels of IgG are usually seen and indicate the presence of an infectious process. The presence of oligoclonal bands also supports the diagnosis. CSF measles titers of 1:4 or greater are consistent with the diagnosis. PCR analysis for the measles virus, which can confirm the diagnosis, can also be performed on CSF. As discussed above with serum testing, often other infections are excluded and antibody titers or PCR testing can also be done for these pathogens on CSF.

Management There are no definitive treatments for SSPE. Many antiviral and immunomodulatory therapies have been tried, including corticosteroids, amantadine, cimetidine, alpha-interferon, beta-interferon, isoprinosine, ribavirin, and intravenous immunoglobulin. At this time, a combination of oral isoprinosine and intraventricular alpha-interferon appears to be the most effective treatment for SSPE. Isoprinosine is an antiviral medication that works by activating the patient's immune system against the measles virus. It increases production of interleukins in addition to CD4+ lymphocytes, and boosts the function of natural killer cells. Alpha-interferon is a naturally occurring substance that is produced in response to infection. Interferon levels are reported to be low in patients with SSPE and delivery of the drug directly to the brain is more effective than other modes of administration. One clinical trial demonstrated that the use of both of these drugs can stabilize progression of the disease and induce remission in a subset of patients.

Myoclonic seizures are treated with traditional anticonvulsants such as valproic acid and clonazepam. Monitoring by an ophthalmologist may be necessary given the frequency of visual abnormalities. Physical and occupational therapists should be involved to help manage worsening spasticity and contractures. Nutritional status needs to be monitored closely as the disease progresses and referral to a nutritionist and to a gastroenterologist is eventually warranted.

Additional Questions

1. What other neurodegenerative disorder preferentially affects the parietal and occipital lobes?
2. What are the clinical features of measles virus infection?
3. How do the EEG findings in SSPE and Creutzfeldt-Jakob disease differ?

References

Campbell C, Levin S, Humphreys P, et al. Subacute sclerosing panencephalitis: results of the Canadian pediatric surveillance program and review of the literature. *BMC Pediatr.* 2005;5(1):47.

Garg RK. Subacute sclerosing panencephalitis. *Postgrad Med J.* 2002;78:63–70.

Honarmand S, Glaser CA, Chow E, et al. Subacute sclerosing panencephalitis in the differential diagnosis of encephalitis. *Neurology.* 2004;63:1489–1493.

Leppik IE. Classification of the myoclonic epilepsies. *Epilepsia.* 2003;44(suppl 11):2–6.

You are asked to evaluate **a 1-week-old girl** in the neonatal intensive care unit for microcephaly. The patient was born at full term to a 17-year-old G_1P_0 mother by an uneventful vaginal delivery. The mother rarely went to her prenatal visits but she reports an uncomplicated pregnancy. However, she did experience a flu-like illness around 5 months of gestation. The patient developed a petechial rash, hepatic dysfunction, jaundice, and thrombocytopenia shortly after birth. She has a small head size but is not otherwise dysmorphic. The neonatologist is also concerned because she has failed her newborn hearing screen twice.

Physical Examination Head circumference = 31 cm. General Examination: She is an ill-appearing, small-for-gestational-age infant. Her liver and spleen are not palpable. She has a petechial rash but there are no birthmarks. Neurologic Examination: Mental Status: She is alert. Cranial Nerves: Her pupils are equal, round, and reactive to light. She is able to fix briefly. Her face is symmetric. She does not react to loud sounds. She has a strong suck and a gag reflex. The tongue is midline without fasciculations. Motor: She has normal bulk with slightly increased tone. She moves all four extremities well and has a symmetric Moro reflex. Sensory: She responds to tactile stimulation throughout. Reflexes: 3+ throughout with equivocal plantar responses.

Guide to Case Discussion

- Briefly summarize this case.

- Localize the examination findings.

- Give the most likely diagnosis and provide a differential diagnosis.

- Discuss an appropriate diagnostic work-up.

- Discuss the management of this patient.

Diagnosis   Congenital cytomegalovirus infection.

Discussion   Cytomegalovirus (CMV) is a ubiquitous herpes virus that infects individuals of all ages. CMV is spread from one person to another through body fluids such as blood, urine, and saliva. It can be vertically transmitted from mother to fetus, as well as acquired through blood transfusion and organ donation. The infection may be primary or recurrent. Recurrent infection can be caused by reactivation of the original endogenous strain or by reinfection with another strain of CMV.

CMV is the most common congenital infection, seen in 0.4% to 2.5% of livebirths. Maternal infection during pregnancy can be primary or secondary. Intrauterine infection may be as high as 40% with primary infections. Approximately 5% to 10% of affected infants will be symptomatic at birth, with the remaining 90% of infected neonates showing no signs of illness. These asymptomatic children often go on to develop hearing loss (15%) and developmental delays, but usually do not experience the profound neurologic sequelae experienced by symptomatic infants. Epidemiologic studies suggest that a congenital CMV infection accounts for a large portion of sensorineural hearing loss in childhood.

Symptomatic neonates present with intrauterine growth retardation, jaundice, hepatosplenomegaly, hepatitis, direct hyperbilirubinemia, thrombocytopenia, petechiae, purpura, and hemolytic anemia. Neurologic involvement also may be seen at birth. Microcephaly, chorioretinitis, increased or decreased tone, intracranial calcifications, and sensorineural hearing loss are common manifestations. Later neurologic manifestations of the disease include mental retardation, cerebral palsy, epilepsy, visual impairment, and profound deafness.

Summary   The patient is a small-for-gestational-age 1-week-old full-term infant with an acute illness involving rash, hepatic dysfunction, thrombocytopenia, and hearing loss. Her mother experienced a flu-like illness at 5 months of gestation. The infant's exam demonstrates microcephaly, hearing loss, slightly increased tone, and hyperreflexia, but is otherwise unremarkable.

Localization   The infant in this case has a nonfocal neurologic exam. Hearing loss localizes to the vestibulocochlear nerves. Her mildly increased tone and hyperreflexia suggest corticospinal tract or central nervous system dysfunction.

Differential Diagnosis   This infant's presentation is highly suggestive of a congenital infection, particularly in light of a maternal illness during the pregnancy. TORCH infections include toxoplasmosis, other infections (HIV, syphilis, varicella virus), rubella, CMV, and HSV1 and HSV2. These infections can present with a similar clinical picture in the neonatal period and may all result in long-term neurologic sequelae such as vision loss, deafness, and developmental delay. Symptoms of these congenital infections may include jaundice, hepatosplenomegaly, hepatic dysfunction, fever, hemolytic anemia, chorioretinitis, microcephaly, small gestational size, and thrombocytopenia.

It may be difficult to differentiate TORCH infections at initial presentation, but there may be some distinguishing features. CMV tends to cause microcephaly and sensorineural hearing loss, whereas toxoplasmosis produces hydrocephalus, seizures, and chorioretinitis. The incidence of congenital measles infection has been dramatically reduced since the advent of widespread vaccination in the United States, so this is now a rare cause of congenital infection. HSV most commonly presents with encephalitis and focal seizure activity. In addition, HIV needs to be considered in every infant with a congenital infection as it may also predispose to superimposed infections from other pathogens such as syphilis and CMV. The mother in this case received poor prenatal care and may be at risk for sexually transmitted diseases. However, congenital CMV seems most likely in this case, given that it is the most common congenital infection and the child already has apparent hearing loss.

Microcephaly is also an important finding on this neonate's examination. Microcephaly may be primary or secondary in etiology. Primary disorders include genetic syndromes, hereditary microcephaly, disorders of neuronal migration (lissencephaly, schizencephaly) and disorders of prosencephalization (holoprosencephaly). Secondary disorders are acquired and may include intrauterine, perinatal, or postnatal injuries from causes such as infection, toxic exposures, or hypoxic-ischemic injuries. Given this child's presentation with an acute illness, her microcephaly is most likely a consequence of intrauterine infection.

Evaluation This infant's constellation of symptoms is highly suggestive of a congenital infection. At initial presentation, a complete septic work-up is warranted, including a CBC, blood culture, urinalysis, and urine culture. CSF analysis should include cell count, glucose, protein, HSV PCR, VDRL, and bacterial culture. Additional studies to be performed include liver function tests, electrolytes, renal function tests, calcium, magnesium, phosphorus, and glucose. Given that a congenital infection seems likely, serum TORCH titers, VDRL, and HIV testing should also be performed. Screening for maternal drug abuse with a urine toxicology screen can also be considered.

Intrauterine CMV infection is best diagnosed by detecting the virus in urine or saliva within the first 3 weeks of life. Because infected infants shed enormous amounts of CMV in their urine, urine culture using a shell vial assay is the gold standard for the diagnosis of a congenital infection. CMV immunoglobulin IgM and IgG antibody titers can also be measured in the serum, but are less specific than urine culture. PCR testing for CMV DNA can also be performed on serum, saliva, or urine, but is typically unnecessary given the accuracy of the shell vial assay. A positive test for CMV, however, cannot determine whether the infection was contracted pre- or postnatally.

Given the suspicion for a congenital infection and the patient's microcephaly, neuroimaging is warranted. Approximately half of infants with congenital CMV have periventricular calcifications, which are best evaluated by a head CT scan. A brain MRI with and without gadolinium is more useful to evaluate for the numerous cortical malformations that are associated with congenital CMV. Disorders of neuronal migration reported in these children include polymicrogyria, pachygyria, lissencephaly, and focal cortical dysplasias. Periventricular leukomalacia also may be seen. It is likely that infection at an earlier gestational age correlates with more severe cortical malformations. Toxoplasmosis also may cause periventricular calcifications, but in contrast to congenital CMV, cortical malformations are rare.

This child should also be evaluated by an ophthalmologist to evaluate for an associated chorioretinitis. BAERs need to be performed to better evaluate her hearing loss.

Management This infant will require medical management through the acute phase of her infection. Although controlled, prospective studies have not been performed, symptomatic congenital CMV is often treated with a 6-week course of intravenous ganciclovir. There is some evidence that it may help to reduce the severity of long-term sensorineural hearing loss. However, ganciclovir is associated with bone marrow suppression and testicular atrophy in male infants, so the risks and potential benefits should be weighed carefully prior to its use.

This child will also be at risk for significant neurologic sequelae. After hospital discharge, she will require a formal hearing and speech evaluation, as well as long-term audiology follow-up. A formal developmental evaluation should also be performed as she will likely qualify for early interventional physical and occupational therapy. Long-term ophthalmology follow-up also might be required if her vision is affected.

Additional Questions

1. What is schizencephaly?
2. What cortical malformation should be suspected in a child with a midline facial deformity?
3. What disorders cause basal ganglia calcifications?

References

Bale JF. Congenital infections. *Neurol Clin.* 2002;20:1039–1060.

Barkovich AJ. *Pediatric Neuroimaging.* 3rd ed. Philadelphia, Pa: Lippincott Williams & Wilkins; 2000:715–770.

Demmler GJ. Congenital cytomegalovirus infection. *Semin Pediatr Neurol.* 1994;1(2):36–42.

Fenichel GM. *Clinical Pediatric Neurology: A Signs and Symptoms Approach.* 4th ed. Philadelphia, Pa: WB Saunders; 2001:353–370.

Pass RF. Congenital cytomegalovirus infection and hearing loss. *Herpes.* 2005;12:50–55.

A healthy 7-year-old boy presents to your office for concerns of difficulty in school. He was born at full term by a repeat cesarean section after an uneventful pregnancy. He met all developmental milestones on time. He is now repeating the first grade. Teachers complain that he frequently does not turn in his homework assignments and when he does it is full of careless mistakes. He often gets out of his chair during class and disrupts his classmates. Even when he raises his hand to answer a question, he usually ends up speaking out of turn. His family has to help him with his homework at night and he requires constant redirecting. His parents are currently separated and his grandmother provides much of his care as his mother works full-time. His father never finished high school but no one in the family has been diagnosed with a learning disability.

Physical Examination   General Examination: The child is a nondysmorphic 7-year-old boy. He cooperates with the examination but is very fidgety and distractible. Neurologic Examination: Mental Status: He is alert and cooperative. Language: He has fluent speech without dysarthria. Cranial Nerves: His pupils are equal, round, and reactive to light. His extraocular muscles are intact and there are no visual field cuts. His face is symmetric. The tongue is midline. Motor: He has normal bulk and tone with 5/5 strength throughout. Coordination: Finger-to-nose is intact bilaterally. Sensory: Normal light-touch, temperature, and vibration. Gait: He has a normal heel, toe, flat, and tandem gait. Reflexes: 2+ throughout with bilateral plantar flexor responses.

Guide to Case Discussion

- Briefly summarize this case.
- Localize the examination findings.
- Give the most likely diagnosis and provide a differential diagnosis.
- Discuss an appropriate diagnostic work-up.
- Discuss the management of this patient.

Diagnosis   Attention deficit hyperactivity disorder.

Discussion   Attention deficit hyperactivity disorder (ADHD) is a common neuro-behavioral syndrome seen in approximately 3% to 7% of school-age children. ADHD also can occur in adolescents and adults. ADHD is characterized by the core symptoms of hyperactivity, inattention, and impulsivity. Boys are more frequently affected than girls. Although the pathophysiology of ADHD is still incompletely understood, dopaminergic and norepinephrine neurotransmitter pathways in frontostriatal circuitry are suspected to be involved. Genetics also plays an important role in the development of ADHD but a consistent associated chromosomal region has not yet been identified. Current research supports the involvement of dopamine D4 and D5 receptor genes, as well as a dopamine transporter gene.

The diagnosis of ADHD is made based on the constellation of symptoms, the context in which they occur, and the degree to which they impair an individual.

The *Diagnostic and Statistical Manual of Mental Disorders* (4th ed., revised) (DSM-IV-R) lays out the standard diagnostic criteria (Table 55.1). Three types of ADHD are described: (a) combined inattentive, hyperactive, and impulsive (80%);

TABLE 55.1

Symptoms of Attention Deficit Hyperactivity Disorder from DSM-IV-R Diagnostic Criteria

Inattention (6 or more symptoms required)[a]
  Often fails to give close attention to details or makes careless mistakes
  Often has difficulty sustaining attention in tasks or play activities
  Often does not seem to listen when spoken to directly
  Often does not follow through with instructions and fails to finish assignments
  Often has difficulty with organizing tasks and activities
  Often avoids tasks that require sustained attention
  Often loses things necessary for activities
  Often is easily distracted by external stimuli
  Often is forgetful

Hyperactivity and Impulsivity (6 or more symptoms required)[a]
  Often fidgets with hands or feet
  Often leaves seat
  Often runs and climbs excessively
  Often has difficulty with quiet leisure activities
  Often seems "on the go" or "driven by a motor"
  Often talks excessively
  Often blurts out answers
  Often has difficulty awaiting turn
  Often interrupts or intrudes

---

[a]Symptoms must begin before 7 years of age and must be present in more than one environment (home and school). They must persist for more than 6 months. Symptoms must also be to a degree that is maladaptive and inconsistent with the child's developmental level.

(b) predominantly inattentive (10% to 15%); and (c) predominantly hyperactive and impulsive (5%). The diagnosis is most apparent in children with hyperactivity and impulsivity but can be missed in the primarily inattentive subtype that often manifests with more subtle symptoms of academic underachievement.

Information about symptoms must be obtained from the child, the parents, and the teachers. The presence of symptoms without functional impairment is inconsistent with the diagnosis. Several standardized clinical rating scales (Conners Rating Scale, National Initiative for Children's Healthcare Quality Vanderbilt Assessment Scale) can be used to reliably evaluate symptoms.

Summary The patient is a healthy 7-year-old boy who presents with poor school performance associated with an increased activity level (fidgety, inability to stay in his chair), impulsivity (speaks out of turn), and poor attention (needs excessive help to stay focused on assignments). He is disruptive in the classroom, does not follow through with assignments, and makes careless mistakes. A parental separation and a father who has not finished high school might be relevant factors. He has a normal neurologic exam but is fidgety and distractible.

Localization The child in this case has a normal neurologic examination. Behavioral abnormalities localize diffusely to the cerebral cortex but are a nonspecific finding.

Differential Diagnosis The child in this case exhibits many symptoms of ADHD. However, ADHD can mimic or coexist with many other psychiatric conditions and determining the etiology of underachievement in school can be challenging. As many as one third of children with ADHD may be affected by another mental health condition. Other disorders that need to be considered include learning disabilities, oppositional defiant disorder, conduct disorder, anxiety disorder, posttraumatic stress disorder, depression, bipolar disorder, tic disorder, and adjustment disorder.

The symptoms of learning disabilities usually manifest when a child is required to engage in academic work and are less likely to be present at other times. However, clinicians should maintain a high level of suspicion for learning disabilities as they are reported to occur in as many as 12% to 60% of children with ADHD. Oppositional defiant disorder can be associated with a high activity level, but the primary symptoms involve acting defiantly when asked to follow directions or rules. Children with conduct disorder have extreme behavior problems with frequent fighting, lack of remorse, intent to do harm, and antisocial tendencies. These behaviors often lead to involvement in the legal system. Anxiety, inattention, excessive worries, and fidgetiness may be associated with anxiety disorder. Posttraumatic stress disorder may have similar symptoms, in addition to re-experiencing the trauma and nightmares. Depression in childhood may present with nonspecific findings such as irritability and feelings of sadness. Phases of bipolar disorder have significant overlap with the symptoms of ADHD, causing an increased activity level, impulsivity, irritability, and an elated mood. Tic disorders can be associated with symptoms of ADHD and obsessive compulsive disorder. In addition, adjustment disorder as a result of chronic stressors should be excluded.

Finally, medical disorders need to be considered in the differential diagnosis of a child presenting with possible ADHD. Under certain circumstances, conditions such as absence epilepsy, sleep disorders, hyperthyroidism, brain tumors, genetic diseases (fragile X syndrome), and neurodegenerative disorders may enter the differential diagnosis.

Evaluation There are no specific laboratory tests for the work-up of ADHD. The child in this case obviously has several comorbid factors. There has been a disruption in his family environment with his parents' separation. His mother works full-time, which might cause additional stress. His father never completed high school, which raises the concern that he, too, might have ADHD, a learning disability, and/or a psychiatric illness. Thus, this child's evaluation should begin with a thorough birth, developmental, behavioral, and psychosocial history. A family history is also essential as there is a strong genetic component to many of the disorders in the differential diagnosis. Initial screening questions should assess the risk of psychiatric conditions such as depression, anxiety disorder, bipolar disorder, and oppositional defiant disorder. The child should be asked about relationships with family and friends, worries, moods, and sleep habits.

This child requires a formal assessment of achievement, intellectual abilities, and educational level. Testing is most often performed through the school system or by an independent psychologist. This should confirm or exclude the diagnosis of ADHD and/or a learning disability, as well as screen him for other psychiatric disorders. If there is a concern for a concomitant psychiatric condition, the child should be referred to a psychiatrist for further management. Complex cases may require referral to developmental or behavioral specialists.

Management Once the diagnosis has been confirmed, management of ADHD includes pharmacologic and nonpharmacologic therapies, and should be guided by a physician familiar with this condition. Stimulant medications are the first-line therapy for the treatment of ADHD. Methylphenidate and dextroamphetamine are safe and effective treatments for the symptoms of hyperactivity, impulsivity, and inattention. Approximately 70% to 80% of affected children will demonstrate a response to one of these medications. Short-, intermediate-, and long-acting preparations are available and dosing needs to be tailored to each child's individual needs. Stimulants are generally well-tolerated but parents need to be counseled regarding the possible side effects, which include appetite suppression, disruption of sleep, tics, headache, abdominal pain, and mild elevations of heart rate and blood pressure. There is some evidence that stimulants may affect growth parameters, so weight, height, blood pressure, and pulse should be monitored regularly during the course of treatment.

Several nonstimulant medications are also used. Atomoxetine is a norepinephrine reuptake inhibitor that is effective for the treatment of ADHD. It functions by increasing dopamine and norepinephrine in the prefrontal cortex. Typical side effects include sedation, headaches, appetite suppression and weight loss. Recent reports of severe liver injury have prompted a bolded warning label stating that atomoxetine should be discontinued in any patient with jaundice or evidence of hepatic disease. Because atomoxetine is less likely than stimulants to exacerbate tics, it may be a more appropriate treatment for children with tic disorders and/or Tourette syndrome. Additional alternative medications, including bupropion, tricyclic antidepressants (imipramine, desipramine), and alpha-adrenergic agonists (clonidine), also are prescribed but are not specifically FDA approved for the treatment of ADHD.

Behavioral therapy can be an important component in the management of a child with ADHD. However, behavioral therapy alone has been shown to be inferior to pharmacologic treatment alone. Measures such as structuring daily routines, providing a reward incentive program, and modifying the classroom environment may have an impact on symptoms. Accommodations within the school setting, such as placement in a smaller class or sitting at the front of the room, might help. In most cases, however, concomitant administration of an ADHD medication also is necessary to maximize an affected child's academic and social potential.

Finally, it is important to relay to the family that ADHD is a chronic condition that can extend into adolescence and adulthood. Recognition and proper treatment in childhood can help avoid long-term morbidities such as impaired family and peer relationships, academic underachievement, poor employment opportunities, poor self-esteem, and substance abuse.

Additional Questions

1. What are the diagnostic criteria for Tourette syndrome?
2. What medications are used to treat tics?

References

American Academy of Pediatrics, Committee on Quality Improvement, Subcommittee on Attention-Deficit/Hyperactivity Disorder. Clinical practice guideline: diagnosis and evaluation of the child with attention-deficit/hyperactivity disorder. *Pediatrics*. 2000;105: 1158–1170.

American Psychiatric Association. *Diagnostic and Statistical Manual of Mental Disorders.* 4th ed. Rev. Washington, DC: American Psychiatric Association; 2000.

Brown RT, Amler RW, Freeman WS, et al. Treatment of attention-deficit/hyperactivity disorder: overview of the evidence. *Pediatrics*. 2005;115(6):e749–e757.

Rappley MD. Attention deficit-hyperactivity disorder. *N Engl J Med*. 2005;352:165–173.

Thapar A, O'Donovan M, Owen MJ. The genetics of attention deficit hyperactivity disorder. *Hum Mol Genet*. 2005;14(2):R275–R282.

A **1-week-old male infant** is transferred from a local community hospital for management of seizures. He was born at 37 weeks to a 25-year-old G_2P_1 mother. The pregnancy and delivery were uncomplicated. On day 3 of life, prior to hospital discharge, he developed spells of rhythmic left face, arm, and leg jerking lasting 1 to 2 minutes. A septic work-up was normal. The EEG showed abnormal sharp activity more on the right than the left. The child was started on phenobarbital but has continued to have seizures. A head CT was read as possibly showing lissencephaly. The family history is unremarkable.

Physical Examination Head circumference = 32 cm. General Examination: The infant has a high forehead, micrognathia, a short, upturned nose, and low-set, posteriorly rotated ears. Neurologic Examination: Mental Status: The infant is alert. Cranial Nerves: His pupils are equal, round, and reactive to light. He is able to fix briefly on a face. His face is symmetric. He responds to loud sounds. He has a strong suck and a gag is present. The tongue is midline. Motor: He has normal bulk with a mild hypotonia. He moves all four extremities equally against gravity and does not appear to be weak. The Moro reflex is symmetric. Sensory: He withdraws to mild pain throughout. Reflexes: 3+ throughout with bilateral plantar extensor responses.

Guide to Case Discussion

- Briefly summarize this case.
- Localize the examination findings.
- Give the most likely diagnosis and provide a differential diagnosis.
- Discuss an appropriate diagnostic work-up.
- Discuss the management of this patient.

Diagnosis Miller-Dieker syndrome.

Discussion Lissencephaly (smooth brain) is one of several neuronal migrational disorders. It is characterized by effacement of the normal gyral and sulcal structure of the brain. Pachygyria (broad gyri) probably lies within the same spectrum of malformations. Formation of the normal six-layered cortex is an extremely complex process involving an interaction between the radial glia and migrating neurons. Any disruption of this process can result in significant brain malformation.

Two basic forms of lissencephaly have been described. Classic lissencephaly (type 1) is associated with Miller-Dieker syndrome and the isolated lissencephaly sequence, in addition to other X-linked forms and autosomal recessive lissencephaly. The cerebral cortex is extremely thick and formed of four (rather than six) abnormal layers. Underlying white matter is abnormally thin. The cortex to white matter ratio is approximately 4:1. To date, five genes have been associated with classic lissencephaly, including *LIS1*, *DCX*, *RELN*, *ARX*, and *14-3-3e*.

Cobblestone lissencephaly (type II) is associated with a different brain surface pattern that appears more like cobblestone paving. In these cases, the cortex shows no lamination and the cortex to white matter ratio is 1:1. Cobblestone lissencephaly is associated with the congenital muscular dystrophies, which include Walker-Warburg syndrome, muscle-eye-brain disease, and Fukuyama muscular dystrophy. The genes responsible for these conditions are *POMT1*, *POMGnT1*, and *fukutin*, respectively. Areas of cobblestone lissencephaly often alternate with regions of pachygyria. It is also occurs with other cerebral malformations including agenesis of the corpus callosum, cerebellar dysplasia, and Dandy-Walker malformation.

With regards to the classic lissencephalies, Miller-Dieker syndrome is caused by a mutation in the *LIS1* gene on chromosome 17p13.3. *LIS1* encodes for the platelet-activating factor acetyl-hydrolase-1 beta$_1$ subunit that inactivates platelet-activating factor (PAF). Research has shown that PAF is a required for normal neuronal migration. The MRI in Miller-Dieker syndrome shows a posterior-to-anterior gradient of abnormalities with more severe abnormalities in the posterior portion of the brain. Agyria is often seen in the occipital lobes with pachygyria found frontally. Affected patients have dysmorphic features including a thin upper lip, micrognathia, a short nose with upturned nares, temporal hollowing, and low-set, posteriorly rotated ears. Infants may demonstrate hypotonia at birth but later develop spasticity. Seizures may begin in the neonatal period but often present with infantile spasms in early infancy. Cardiac anomalies, such as ventricular septal defect and tetralogy of Fallot, occur in approximately 25% of patients. Cataracts, cryptorchidism, and kidney abnormalities are also occasionally seen. Affected children are profoundly developmentally delayed and experience a life with intractable epilepsy.

The clinical features of Miller-Dieker syndrome are much more severe than those seen in the isolated lissencephaly sequence. This is likely explained by the underlying genetic defects of these disorders. Miller-Dieker syndrome results from contiguous gene deletions on chromosome 17p13.3 in which *LIS1* as well as other neighboring genes are deleted. Infants with isolated lissencephaly sequence do not have facial dysmorphisms or other organ involvement. They also typically have milder cerebral dysgenesis. Mutations in these cases are limited to the *LIS1* gene or may be caused by other small deletions on chromosome 17p13.3.

The X-linked form of lissencephaly (XLIS) also causes a pattern of classic lissencephaly. The *XLIS* gene (also known as the *doublecortin* or *DCX* gene) codes for the protein product doublecortin, which stabilizes microtubules and likely interacts with the LIS1 protein. Males with X-linked lissencephaly are severely affected. In contrast to Miller-Dieker syndrome, the brain MRI demonstrates more severe structural abnormalities in the frontal lobes (anterior-to-posterior gradient). Females possessing the doublecortin mutation demonstrate a very unique brain MRI pattern with two apparent bands of cortex. Normal-appearing cortex lies on top of a layer of white matter that sits on top of another layer of gray and white matter. Most affected females experience mental retardation and epilepsy, but patients with normal intelligence have been reported.

Autosomal recessive lissencephaly with cerebellar hypoplasia is associated with mutations in the reelin (RELN) gene. Affected infants experience profound developmental delay, hypotonia, and intractable epilepsy. Mutations in the ARX gene are responsible for X-linked lissencephaly with corpus callosum agenesis and ambiguous genitalia (micropenis, cryptorchidism). Only male infants are affected. They demonstrate microcephaly, hypothalamic dysfunction, global developmental delay, and refractory seizures. Female carriers of the abnormal ARX gene are usually cognitively normal. The brain MRI may be normal or show absence of the corpus callosum (partial or complete).

Summary   The patient is a 1-week-old full-term male infant who presents with left focal seizures on day 3 of life and possible lissencephaly. The exam is remarkable for small head size, dysmorphic features, mild hypotonia, hyperreflexia, and plantar extensor responses.

Localization   The infant's left focal seizures localize to the right cerebral cortex. Hypotonia can be a result of central or peripheral causes. Given the presence of dysmorphic features, seizures, and lissencephaly, a central etiology is most likely. In addition, hyperreflexia is not consistent with a primary lower motor neuron disorder. Hyperreflexia and extensor plantar responses suggest corticospinal tract involvement.

Differential Diagnosis   When classic lissencephaly is seen on brain MRI, the diagnostic considerations typically include Miller-Dieker syndrome (LIS1 gene), isolated lissencephaly sequence (LIS1 gene), X-linked lissencephaly (DCX gene), autosomal lissencephaly with cerebellar hypoplasia (RELN gene), and X-linked lissencephaly with corpus callosum agenesis and ambiguous genitalia (ARX gene). Dysmorphic physical characteristics, other organ involvement, and the gradient of abnormalities seen on brain MRI help narrow the differential diagnosis. The LIS1 gene is responsible for all cases of Miller-Dieker syndrome and for 65% of patients with an isolated lissencephaly sequence, in addition to most cases with a posterior-to-anterior gradient of abnormalities on brain MRI.

The cobblestone lissencephalies (Walker-Warburg syndrome, muscle-eye-brain disease, Fukuyama muscular dystrophy) can usually be distinguished from the classic lissencephalies by the brain MRI as well as by the associated dysmorphic features, muscle weakness, and an elevated creatine kinase. Other genetic syndromes, as well as metabolic disorders, can be associated with lissencephaly and other neuronal migrational abnormalities. Zellweger syndrome is a peroxisomal disorder that is often associated with the lissencephaly/pachygyria. Glutaric aciduria type II, pyruvate dehydrogenase deficiency, sulfite oxidase deficiency, and molybdenum cofactor deficiency can be associated with cortical dysplasia. Thus, depending on the clinical presentation, metabolic diseases also may need to be considered in the differential diagnosis.

Evaluation The infant in this case needs further evaluation of both his seizure disorder and his suspected structural brain abnormality. Given his dysmorphic features, the possibility of an underlying genetic syndrome should strongly be considered.

With rare exception, a septic work-up should be performed in any neonate presenting with seizures. Even when another etiology may likely explain seizures (such as a cortical malformation), the sequelae of untreated sepsis and/or neonatal meningitis can be great. A CBC, blood culture, urinalysis, urine culture, and lumbar puncture should be done. Excluding HSV encephalitis also should always be considered in an infant with focal seizures. However, whether a CSF HSV PCR needs to be performed and intravenous acyclovir started is a matter of clinical judgment. A basic chemistry panel, glucose, calcium, magnesium, and phosphorus levels also need to be done at the onset of seizures as metabolic disturbances may be contributory.

For the infant in this vignette, at the time of transfer, it would be reasonable to perform a phenobarbital level and liver function tests as he is still having seizures. A repeat EEG or a video EEG should also be performed to reassess his seizure disorder. A video EEG may have the advantage of better characterizing seizure semiology. Given his presentation and head CT findings, a brain MRI is warranted to better evaluate his cerebral dysgenesis. The presence of classic or cobblestone lissencephaly as well as the identification of any additional malformations may help guide the remainder of his work-up.

In addition, this infant should be evaluated by a geneticist to confirm that his dysmorphisms are consistent with Miller-Dieker syndrome. A work-up for other organ involvement (cardiac, genitourinary) might be indicated. This infant should also be evaluated by an ophthalmologist as Miller-Dieker, as well as other lissencephaly syndromes, are associated with ocular abnormalities. As discussed above, the genetic defects have been identified in several lissencephaly syndromes and specific genetic testing is now clinically available for most of these disorders. In general, review of the case with a radiologist and a geneticist will help tailor the work-up for a given patient.

When Miller-Dieker syndrome is suspected, a standard karyotype analysis and fluorescent in situ hybridization (FISH) for a submicroscopic deletion in the *LIS1* gene on chromosome 17 should be performed. If these two tests are normal, Miller-Dieker syndrome is unlikely. However, if the brain MRI demonstrates a posterior-to-anterior gradient, additional testing with direct sequencing of the *LIS1* gene and Southern blot analysis can be worthwhile. In males with more severe cortical malformations anteriorly, sequencing of the *DCX* gene is indicated.

Management Because this infant is having frequent seizures, he should be placed on a cardiorespiratory monitor and a pulse oximeter. Monitoring in the NICU should be considered. Attempts should be made to control his seizures. This likely first involves maximizing his phenobarbital level. The need for additional anticonvulsants can then be assessed.

Most patients with a severe neuronal migrational disorder have abnormalities of tone and profound developmental delay that impairs the ability to feed orally.

Nutritional and feeding status need to be assessed. Often, feeding difficulties necessitate placement of a nasogastric tube and, ultimately, a gastrostomy tube. Finally, genetic counseling should be performed with the parents to review the recurrence risk with future pregnancies.

Additional Questions

1. What is the syndrome of bilateral periventricular nodular heterotopia? Describe its inheritance pattern and the associated genetic defect.

2. What is bilateral perisylvian syndrome and how does it clinically present?

3. Why is valproic acid rarely used in the management of neonatal seizures?

References

Golden JA. Cell migration and cerebral cortical development. *Neuropathol Appl Neurobiol.* 2001;27:22–28.

Guerrini R, Filippi T. Neuronal migration disorders, genetics, and epileptogenesis. *J Child Neurol.* 2005;20:287–299.

Jones KL. *Smith's Recognizable Patterns of Human Malformation.* 5th ed. Philadelphia, Pa: WB Saunders; 1997:194–195.

Kanatani S, Tabata H, Nakajima K. Neuronal migration in cortical development. *J Child Neurol.* 2005;20:274–279.

Leventer RJ. Genotype-phenotype correlation in lissencephaly and subcortical band heterotopia: the key questions answered. *J Child Neurol.* 2005;20:307–312.

You are asked to evaluate **a 6-month-old male infant** with suspected nonaccidental head trauma on the general pediatrics ward. He was transferred from an outside hospital after a routine head CT performed for macrocephaly and developmental delay showed bilateral subdural effusions with a variety of densities suggestive of chronic and acute hemorrhage in addition to enlarged tortuous vessels crossing the subdural space. A bone survey did not show any fractures, but metaphyseal widening was documented. The parents deny any history of trauma. His mother did not experience any pregnancy complications, and he was born at full term. He does not roll over or sit independently. He has no interest in grabbing toys. He occasionally smiles but does not babble.

Physical Examination His head circumference is greater than the 98th percentile. General Examination: The infant is cute with chubby cheeks. His anterior fontanelle is widely open and bulging. There is alopecia in the posterior regions of the head with patches of short, broken hair more anteriorly. No retinal hemorrhages are noted on funduscopic exam. Neurologic Examination: Mental Status: Alert. Cranial Nerves: His pupils are equal, round, and reactive to light. He occasionally fixes but has poor visual attention. His face is symmetric. His tongue is midline. Motor: He has significant axial hypotonia with poor head control. Appendicular tone is increased. He moves all four extremities well against gravity. Reflexes: 3+ throughout with bilateral plantar extensor responses.

Guide to Case Discussion

- Briefly summarize this case.
- Localize the examination findings.
- Give the most likely diagnosis and provide a differential diagnosis.
- Discuss an appropriate diagnostic work-up.
- Discuss the management of this patient.

Diagnosis Menkes disease.

Discussion Menkes disease is a rare X-linked recessive disorder of copper transport. It is caused by a mutation in the copper-transporting P-type adenosine triphosphatase (ATPase) gene (*ATP7A*). The mutation results in decreased intestinal copper absorption and abnormal distribution of copper in body tissues. Paradoxical copper accumulation occurs in the kidney, spleen, and pancreas, whereas the liver and brain demonstrate relative copper deficiency.

Male children with classic Menkes disease typically appear healthy until 2 to 3 months of age, at which point they start to demonstrate developmental delay, hypotonia, intractable seizures, and failure to thrive. Frank developmental regression may occur. Children often have a cherubic appearance with chubby or sagging cheeks. The skin is often pale. Sparse, course, short, twisted, and lightly pigmented hair is often a clue to the diagnosis. The hair is said to have the texture of steel wool cleaning pads. Light microscopy reveals the classic finding of pili torti (hair shaft twisting) as well as transverse fracture and longitudinal splitting of the hair shaft.

Other findings may include umbilical or inguinal hernia, joint laxity, skin laxity around the nape of the neck, metaphyseal flaring in long bones, Wormian bone in the cranial sutures, rib fractures, bladder diverticula, and gastric polyps. Autonomic instability and hypoglycemia can be seen in the neonatal period. Blood vessel tortuosity is also common and contributes to complications such as subdural hematomas and cerebral infarction. Optic atrophy, poor visual acuity, myopia, strabismus, and peripheral retinal hypopigmentation have been reported in Menkes patients. Most children experience progressive neurodegeneration and die prior to 3 years of age. However, milder variants of Menkes disease with a longer life expectancy have been reported.

Occipital horn syndrome (OHS) or Ehlers-Danlos type IX is another copper transport disorder representing the milder end of the clinical spectrum. Menkes disease and OHS are the only known phenotypes associated with mutations in the *ATP7A* gene. OHS is characterized by wedge-shaped calcifications (known as occipital horns) located where the trapezius and sternocleidomastoid muscles insert on the occipital bone. This disorder usually presents in mid-childhood with connective tissue abnormalities. Like Menkes disease, associated anomalies can include bladder diverticula, inguinal hernias, lax skin, tortuous vessels, and autonomic instability. Cognitive deficits are usually mild.

Summary The patient is a 6-month-old boy with a history of global developmental delay who was admitted with chronic and acute subdural hematomas in addition to metaphyseal widening. His examination is remarkable for cherubic appearance; macrocephaly with a bulging fontanelle; patchy, abnormal hair; poor visual attention; axial hypotonia; appendicular hypertonicity; hyperreflexia; and bilateral plantar extensor responses.

Localization Macrocephaly and the bulging fontanelle are explained by the presence of chronic and acute subdural hematomas. Global developmental delay suggests diffuse cortical involvement. Poor visual attention may be a result of involvement of the retina, optic nerve, or occipital cortex. Appendicular hypertonicity, hyperreflexia, and plantar extensor responses localize to the corticospinal tracts. Hypotonia can be central or peripheral in etiology. Given the presence of subdural hematomas, developmental delay, and upper motor neuron signs, a central process involving white and gray matter is most likely.

Differential Diagnosis There are many reports in the literature of children with Menkes disease presenting as cases of suspected child abuse. Any infant found to have subdural hematomas should be carefully examined for other evidence of nonaccidental trauma (retinal hemorrhages, broken bones, bruising). Bone abnormalities seen in Menkes disease, such as metaphyseal spurring or rib fractures, also may raise concerns for trauma. Certainly shaken baby syndrome is much more common than a rare genetic disease. However, by 3 to 6 months of age, classic findings of Menkes disease, including subdural hematomas, tortuous vessels, characteristic facies, hair abnormalities, seizures, and developmental regression, are rarely confused with other disorders.

With early symptoms, other neurodegenerative diseases occurring in this age group may need to be considered. The history and physical examination in Menkes disease typically suggest gray, as well as white, matter involvement. Disorders that enter the differential diagnosis include organic acidurias, aminoacidurias, mitochondrial cytopathies, and biotinidase deficiency. Menkes patients have been reported to have deficient cytochrome c oxidase (COX) activity and neuropathologic features similar to Leigh disease. Glutaric aciduria type 1 also may produce nontraumatic subdural hematomas. Hair abnormalities are specific for certain inborn errors of metabolism, such as biotinidase deficiency (alopecia), giant axonal neuropathy (kinky hair), and fine hair (homocystinuria).

The differential diagnosis for inborn errors of metabolism that cause facial dysmorphisms can also be considered for children with Menkes disease. These disorders include lysosomal storage diseases (mucopolysaccharidoses, GM_1 gangliosidoses, Gaucher disease), peroxisomal diseases (Zellweger syndrome and variants), mitochondrial disorders (glutaric aciduria type II, electron transport defects, pyruvate dehydrogenase deficiency), and biosynthetic defects (mevalonic aciduria, Smith-Lemli-Opitz syndrome, congenital disorders of glycosylation, homocystinuria). The specific clinical features, organ involvement, and results of initial screening tests may be required to differentiate these diagnostic possibilities.

Evaluation When the classic features of Menkes disease are present, a focused work-up can be performed to confirm the diagnosis. Consultation with a geneticist early in the hospital course will help guide necessary testing. Serum copper and ceruloplasmin levels are low in Menkes disease and should be obtained. Copper transport studies can be performed on cultured fibroblasts. Plasma and CSF catecholamine (homovanillic acid, vanillylmandelic acid) concentrations also are increased in most patients because of partial deficiency of copper-dependent enzymes (dopamine-beta-hydroxylase, lysyl oxidase). These tests are clinically available and can be used to screen for the disorder. Finally, molecular genetic testing for mutations in the *ATP7A* gene is clinically available and reveals an abnormality in approximately 95% of cases. A staged protocol with targeted mutational analysis, mutation scanning, and sequence analysis is performed.

The follow-up brain MRI and brain magnetic resonance angiography (MRA) is indicated in this child to further evaluate the abnormalities seen on his head CT scan. The brain MRI in Menkes disease demonstrates abnormal myelination, cerebral atrophy with compensatory ventriculomegaly, and tortuous vessels. MRA also shows the typical corkscrew vasculature.

Given his poor visual attention, a formal ophthalmologic exam is indicated to document ocular abnormalities seen with Menkes disease and to help exclude other diagnoses. VERs or an electroretinogram can also be helpful in assessing the visual pathway.

Children with Menkes disease are at increased risk of having intractable seizures. The parents should be specifically questioned about behaviors suggestive of seizure activity. An EEG should be performed when indicated.

Management Treatment with subcutaneous injections of copper histidine or copper chloride before 10 days of age has been reported to significantly improve or normalize developmental outcome in some, but not all, children with Menkes disease. Early diagnosis is often difficult, though, as infants may appear normal until 2 to 3 months of age. The use of aggressive copper replacement therapy in children who already manifest severe complications of the disease is controversial but often attempted.

Complications of Menkes disease also require monitoring or intervention. The presence of subdural hematomas and intracranial vascular abnormalities should be followed with serial head CTs or brain MRIs. Consultation with neurosurgery is also warranted as subdurals sometimes require drainage. Bladder and urethral diverticula are very common and predispose to frequent urinary tract infections. Referral to a urologist for appropriate diagnostic testing and/or surgical correction is appropriate. Antibiotic prophylaxis is often used to prevent bladder infections. An orthopaedist may need to evaluate a child with significant bone abnormalities.

Hypotonia and developmental delays may result in feeding difficulties. Thus, evaluation by a nutritionist and gastroenterologist is generally indicated. Most children require gastrostomy tube placement. This child should receive a comprehensive developmental evaluation with ongoing early interventional services to maximize his developmental potential. Additional genetic counseling is also needed to assess the mother's carrier status and to help guide decisions about future pregnancies. Prenatal diagnosis is available.

Additional Questions

1. What are the clinical features of the congenital disorders of glycosylation?

2. What are the clinical features of the glutaric aciduria type 1?

References

Clark JTR. *A Clinical Guide to Inherited Metabolic Diseases*. 2nd ed. Cambridge, UK: Cambridge University Press; 2002:134–168.

Gasch AT, Caruso RC, Kaler SG, et al. Menkes' syndrome: ophthalmic findings. *Ophthalmology*. 2002;109(8):1477–1483.

Hsich GE, Robertson RL, Irons M, et al. Cerebral infarction in Menkes' disease. *Pediatr Neurol*. 2000;23:425–428.

Kaler SG. *ATP7A*-related copper transport disorders. 2005. Available at: http://www.genetests. org. Last accessed January 20, 2005.

Kaler SG. Metabolic and molecular bases of Menkes disease and occipital horn syndrome. *Pediatr Dev Pathol.* 1998;1:85–98.

Nassogne MC, Sharrard M, Hertz-Pannier L, et al. Massive subdural hematomas in Menkes disease mimicking shaken baby syndrome. *Childs Nerv Syst.* 2002;18:729–731.

A previously healthy 6-year-old boy is brought to your office for neurologic evaluation. He did very well in kindergarten and had started to read three-letter words. He was also very social and enjoyed playing with his friends. His first grade teacher is now concerned because he is not keeping up with the rest of his class. Over the last 6 months, he has stopped reading and is now having difficulty identifying letters. He has become very clumsy when running. He avoids participation in physical activities and appears withdrawn. His mother is also worried that he may be having trouble seeing because he often bumps into things. He is frequently irritable and throws temper tantrums for no apparent reason. The child's maternal grandmother had a brother who died in late childhood, but the details of his illness are unknown.

Physical Examination General Examination: He is a well-appearing 6-year-old boy. There is mild optic disc pallor bilaterally. His skin tone is darker than his mother's with notable hyperpigmentation in the antecubital fossa and palmar creases. Neurologic Examination: Mental Status: He is alert but uncooperative and distractible. He has difficulty spelling his name and states that $2 + 3 = 7$. Language: His speech is fluent. Cranial Nerves: His visual acuity is 20/80 bilaterally. His pupils are equal, round, and reactive to light. There is no afferent pupillary defect. His extraocular muscles are intact. His face is symmetric. His tongue is midline. Motor: He has normal bulk. His tone is increased in the lower extremities but he has 5/5 strength throughout. Coordination: Finger-to-nose testing is intact bilaterally. Sensory: Light touch, temperature, and vibration are intact throughout. Gait: He can ambulate on his heels and toes, but has a clumsy and stiff, flat gait. Reflexes: 3+ throughout with bilateral sustained clonus at the ankles and plantar extensor responses.

Guide to Case Discussion

- Briefly summarize this case.
- Localize the examination findings.
- Give the most likely diagnosis and provide a differential diagnosis.
- Discuss an appropriate diagnostic work-up.
- Discuss the management of this patient.

Diagnosis Adrenoleukodystrophy.

Discussion Adrenoleukodystrophy (ALD) is an X-linked peroxisomal disorder occurring in approximately 1 in 17,000 boys. It is thought to be the most common leukodystrophy. The causative defect in the *ABCD1* gene localizes to Xq28 and results in abnormalities of ALDP, a peroxisomal membrane protein. ALD results in the accumulation of saturated very-long-chain fatty acids (VLCFAs) in the brain, adrenal glands, and plasma. The mechanisms by which elevated VLCFAs cause neurologic deficits are still poorly understood.

ALD has several clinical phenotypes in both males and carrier females. The two primary forms of the disease include cerebral ALD and adrenomyeloneuropathy (AMN). The childhood cerebral form of ALD is most common, seen in 40% of hemizygous males. It usually presents in boys between 3 and 11 years of age. It manifests with rapidly progressive inflammatory, demyelinating changes in the central nervous system white matter. The parietal and occipital white matter is affected first. Initial symptoms often involve subtle behavioral problems, social withdrawal, and cognitive decline. Affected boys are occasionally erroneously diagnosed as having attention deficit hyperactivity disorder when behavior and learning problems manifest at school. Neurologic deterioration inevitably ensues, resulting in spastic paraparesis, gait abnormalities, dysphagia, vision loss, and hearing loss. Seizures occur as a late manifestation in 30% of patients. Most children progress to a vegetative state within 3 years of the onset of symptoms. Approximately 70% of affected boys will also have adrenocortical insufficiency.

ALD in its cerebral form can also present in adolescent and young adult males, accounting for 4% to 7% of cases. Progression may occur more slowly than in the childhood form, but symptoms are essentially the same. Approximately 2% to 5% of adult males experience adult-onset of the cerebral form of ALD. Dementia, psychiatric disturbances, gait abnormalities, and other neurologic deficits occur in addition to typical brain MRI inflammatory demyelinating changes. A rare olivopontocerebellar (OPC) form occurs in adolescent and adult males. It manifests with cerebellar and brainstem signs. The Addison-only phenotype is seen in school-age boys without neurologic deficits. However, most go on to develop AMN later in life.

AMN is a chronic distal axonopathy that primarily affects the corticospinal tracts of the spinal cord. Peripheral nerves also may be involved, but to a lesser extent. An axonal neuropathy with distal sensory loss in the lower extremities is seen in approximately 40% of affected patients. Clinically, AMN presents in early adulthood with a slowly progressive paraparesis, often mimicking the symptoms of multiple sclerosis. Decline in function may occur over decades. AMN is found in males as well as carrier females. It may be seen in its "pure" form, or it can occur with cerebral involvement. Pure AMN affects only the spinal cord but approximately 20% of adult males also will develop rapidly progressive inflammatory changes in the brain (AMN-cerebral form). Approximately 50% of female carriers develop a pure AMN-like condition in middle age. The myelopathy can range in severity. In these individuals, adrenal and cerebral involvement is otherwise rare.

Summary The patient is a previously healthy 6-year-old boy who presents with a 6-month history of subacute cognitive decline, behavioral disturbance, clumsiness, and vision loss. The death of a male relative on the maternal side of the family is likely relevant. His exam is remarkable for darker skin color than that of his mother; uncooperative behavior; cognitive impairment; optic disc pallor; decreased visual acuity; increased tone in the lower extremities; a clumsy, stiff gait; hyper-reflexia; and bilateral plantar extensor responses.

Localization   The child's cognitive and behavioral abnormalities localize to the cerebral cortex diffusely. Although the finding of optic disc pallor points to optic nerve involvement as the cause for his decreased visual acuity, other parts of the visual pathway could be affected (occipital lobes). Increased lower-extremity tone, stiff gait, hyperreflexia, and plantar extensor responses are caused by corticospinal tract involvement and suggest spastic paraparesis.

Differential Diagnosis   The child in this case presents with a neurodegenerative disorder that primarily affects the white matter (pyramidal tract signs, optic atrophy), but which also demonstrates gray matter involvement (cognitive and behavioral abnormalities). Skin hyperpigmentation is fairly specific for adrenal insufficiency. The death of a male child on the maternal side of the family is consistent with an X-linked inheritance pattern. Thus, ALD is the most likely diagnosis.

Acquired disorders can also be considered but seem much less likely. For example, slow-growing brain tumors, hydrocephalus, chronic meningitis, encephalitis, central nervous system vasculitis, acute disseminated encephalomyelitis (ADEM), subacute sclerosing panencephalitis (SSPE), and toxic exposures can cause mental status changes, behavior problems, long tract signs, and vision loss. Other neurodegenerative diseases also enter the differential diagnosis. Disorders primarily affecting the white matter (the leukodystrophies) should be considered first (Table 58.1). The age at presentation, distinct clinical features, and brain MRI findings help to distinguish among these conditions.

Metachromatic leukodystrophy (MLD) is a lysosomal storage disease with three clinical variants characterized by onset in infancy, childhood, and adulthood. There

TABLE 58.1

The Classic Leukodystrophies

Disorder	Inheritance	Chromosome	Gene/Defect
Adrenoleukodystrophy	XR	Xq28	*ABCD1*
Metachromatic leukodystrophy	AR	22q13	*ARSA*/Arylsulfatase A
Krabbe disease	AR	14q31	*GLAC*/ Galactocerebrosidase
Alexander disease	SP AD	17q21	*GFAP*/Glial fibrillary acidic protein
Canavan disease	AR	17p13	*ASPA*/Aspartoacylase
Pelizaeus-Merzbacher disease	XR	Xq22	*PLP*/Proteolipid protein

AD = Autosomal dominant
AR = Autosomal recessive
SP = Sporadic
XR = X-linked recessive

is both central and peripheral nerve involvement. The juvenile form occurs in children between 5 and 10 years of age. Early development is normal until symptoms of progressive ataxia, spastic gait, dysarthria, cognitive decline, and seizures occur.

Alexander disease usually presents in infancy with megalencephaly, spasticity, seizures, and developmental regression. However, juvenile onset with ataxia, spasticity, and bulbar dysfunction can occur. The brain MRI usually features frontotemporal white matter signal abnormalities. Canavan disease is also typically considered to be a leukodystrophy of infancy. It is characterized by the onset of megalencephaly and hypotonia at several months of age. Irritability, spasticity, seizures, and optic atrophy develop with time. Rare juvenile cases have been described with slowly progressive dysarthria, developmental delay, and seizures beginning around 5 years of age. The brain MRI reveals diffuse white matter involvement, sparing the brainstem and cerebellum. Magnetic resonance (MR) spectroscopy can be diagnostic in Canavan disease, demonstrating an elevated N-acetylaspartate (NAA)-to-choline ratio.

Krabbe disease is a lysosomal storage disease that typically presents with developmental regression, irritability, spasticity, optic atrophy, and seizures before 6 months of age. Peripheral neuropathy also develops in early infancy and can result in hyporeflexia or areflexia in advanced disease. As with Alexander and Canavan disease, later-onset forms occur, but are much less common. In contrast to other leukodystrophies, Pelizaeus-Merzbacher disease is characterized by dysmyelination (rather than demyelination) and typically presents with pendular nystagmoid eye movements in male infants before 3 months of age. Spasticity, ataxia, and choreoathetosis develop with time.

More recently described leukodystrophies include childhood ataxia with central nervous system hypomyelination (CACH) or vanishing white matter disease, as well as megalencephalic leukoencephalopathy with subcortical cysts (MLC). CACH typically presents with new-onset ataxia in children 1 to 5 years of age. Symptoms can begin spontaneously, but often start after minor trauma or a febrile illness. Spasticity, tremor, hyperreflexia, and seizures occur with declining neurologic status. A distinctive pattern of diffuse white matter T_1-weighted hypointensity, and T_2-weighted hyperintensity is seen on brain MRI. Finally, MLC is an autosomal recessive disorder caused by a mutation on chromosome 22. Affected children experience macrocephaly, ataxia, spasticity, and cognitive deterioration. The brain MRI demonstrates diffuse white matter signal change and subcortical cysts.

Finally, numerous other metabolic diseases can affect central nervous system white matter and might deserve consideration with certain clinical presentations. These conditions include a variety of mitochondrial disorders, congenital muscular dystrophies, Aicardi-Goutières syndrome, cerebrotendinous xanthomatosis, Sjögren-Larsson syndrome, and GM_2 gangliosidosis, as well as many others.

Evaluation The child in this case presents with a neurodegenerative course and deserves a thorough diagnostic evaluation. ALD should be considered high in the differential diagnosis of any school-age boy presenting with behavioral and cognitive decline, long tract signs, and vision loss. Serum VLCFAs should be done early in his work-up. The presence of elevated VLCFAs is consistent with the diagnosis. Confirmatory mutational analysis can now be performed and is most useful for genetic counseling.

As other more common, acquired, infectious, inflammatory, and neoplastic diseases are also in the initial differential diagnosis, it is reasonable to do basic blood work, including a CBC, basic chemistry panel, liver function tests, thyroid function tests, erythrocyte sedimentation rate, and an ANA. Screening for other metabolic diseases (urine organic acids, plasma amino acids, serum lactate/pyruvate, lysosomal enzymes) also can be considered in some cases.

A brain MRI with and without contrast is indicated. The classic pattern demonstrates parieto-occipital white matter demyelinating lesions with a leading edge of contrast enhancement. With time, the changes spread anteriorly. Once an MRI is performed, the diagnosis is usually clear and an exhaustive work-up to exclude other conditions is unnecessary. MRI changes are typically seen prior to the onset of symptoms, which has prognostic value. The presence of contrast enhancement of white matter lesions is associated with rapid progression of disease. Thus, brain MRI is a useful tool for selecting appropriate children for treatments such as bone marrow transplant. The NAA-to-choline ratio on MR spectroscopy has also been used as a diagnostic and predictive tool in ALD.

Once the diagnosis of ALD is recognized, evaluation by an endocrinologist is necessary to assess adrenal insufficiency. An impaired cortisol response to adrenocorticotropic hormone (ACTH) stimulation is seen. Consultation by an ophthalmologist also is required to evaluate this child's vision loss and to document a baseline eye exam. VERs also may be helpful in assessing the visual pathway.

Management The management of children with ALD involves treating the underlying metabolic abnormality and controlling the anticipated complications. All boys with adrenal insufficiency should receive replacement adrenal hormone therapy, although this does not alter the neurologic course of the disease.

Bone marrow transplant (BMT) is now being used in boys in the early inflammatory stages of the disease. BMT stabilizes symptoms of the disease. Candidates must be chosen carefully, however, as BMT carries significant risks. Dietary restriction of VLCFAs is sometimes prescribed. Lorenzo's oil consists of a 4:1 mixture of glyceryl trioleate and glyceryl trierucate. It bypasses the metabolic defect and normalizes VLCFA levels in the blood within 4 weeks. Like BMT, Lorenzo's oil has shown little benefit in boys with advanced disease. However, a recent study has suggested that Lorenzo's oil might have a preventative effect if started in asymptomatic boys younger than 6 years of age who have normal brain MRI scans. Finally, clinical trials have investigated the use of lovastatin to lower serum VLCFA levels. The effect of lovastatin on the clinical course of the disease is still unclear.

Caring for a child with ALD involves multidisciplinary care as the disease progresses. Feeding difficulties ultimately occur and evaluation by a nutritionist and a gastroenterologist becomes necessary. Rehabilitation specialists may become involved in an affected child's care to help manage spasticity and to prescribe necessary adaptive equipment. Ongoing physical and occupational therapy may be beneficial. A geneticist should be involved early in an affected child's care to determine maternal carrier status, screen other family members, and help make decisions about future pregnancies.

Additional Questions

1. Which leukodystrophies are associated with peripheral nerve involvement?
2. How do disorders that primarily affect gray matter present? Describe the clinical features of three of these diseases.

References

Berger J, Moser HW, Forss-Petter S. Leukodystrophies: recent developments in genetics, molecular biology, pathogenesis and treatment. *Curr Opin Neurol.* 2001;14:305–312.

Kaye EM. Disorders primarily affecting white matter. In: Swaiman KS, Ashwal S, eds. *Pediatric Neurology: Principles and Practice.* 3rd ed. St. Louis, Mo: Mosby; 1999: 849–859.

Moser H, Dubey P, Fatemi A. Progress in X-linked adrenoleukodystrophy. *Curr Opin Neurol.* 2004;17:263–269.

Moser HW, Fatemi A, Zackowski K, et al. Evaluation of therapy of X-linked adrenoleukodystrophy. *Neurochem Res.* 2004;29(5):1003–1016.

Naidu S, Theda C, Moser HW. Peroxisomal disorders. In: Swaiman KS, Ashwal S, eds. *Pediatric Neurology: Principles and Practice.* 3rd ed. St. Louis, Mo: Mosby; 1999:510–529.

Schiffmann R, Boespflug-Tanguy O. An update on the leukodystrophies. *Curr Opin Neurol.* 2001;14:789–794.

Swaiman KF. Lysosomal diseases. In: Swaiman KS, Ashwal S, eds. *Pediatric Neurology: Principles and Practice.* 3rd ed. St. Louis, Mo: Mosby; 1999:438–482.

An 18-month-old boy presents to the emergency room for evaluation of generalized weakness and loss of developmental milestones. Ten days earlier he had developed an acute gastroenteritis with vomiting, diarrhea, and high fevers. These symptoms have since resolved. Prior to the viral illness, his development was relatively on track. He could say three words and understand basic commands. He rolled over at 4 months and sat well at 7 months. He cruised at 9 months, but has never been able to pull to a stand or walk independently. He had a poorly developed pincer grasp. Since his illness, however, he flops over when placed in a sitting position and cannot support himself on his legs. His parents have also noted abnormal left eye movement for the last 3 days. His birth history was unremarkable. There are no neurologic diseases in the family. A head CT in the emergency room demonstrates focal areas of hypodensity in the putamen and pons.

Physical Examination   General Examination: There are no dysmorphic features. There is no hepatosplenomegaly. Neurologic Examination: Mental Status: He is alert but not playful. Language: He does not say any words. Cranial Nerves: His pupils are equal, round, and reactive to light. He has difficulty laterally deviating his left eye. His face is symmetric with normal strength. He has an appropriate gag and his tongue is midline. Motor: He has normal bulk and significant axial hypotonia with fair head control. He does not sit independently. He is able to lift all extremities against gravity but mild weakness is suspected. Coordination: There is no dysmetria grabbing for toys. Sensory: He withdraws to mild pain throughout. Gait: He is unable to support himself on his legs or take steps. Reflexes: 3+ throughout with bilateral plantar extensor responses.

Guide to Case Discussion

- Briefly summarize this case.

- Localize the examination findings.

- Give the most likely diagnosis and provide a differential diagnosis.

- Discuss an appropriate diagnostic work-up.

- Discuss the management of this patient.

Diagnosis Leigh disease.

Discussion Leigh disease (subacute necrotizing encephalomyelopathy) is a heterogeneous neurologic disease that results from defects in mitochondrial respiratory chain abnormalities and from abnormalities in pyruvate metabolism. The respiratory chain consists of five multi-subunit enzymes whose components are encoded for by nuclear and mitochondrial genes. Many different enzyme deficiencies produce a similar constellation of symptoms. The inheritance pattern of Leigh disease is complex; autosomal recessive, maternal (mitochondrial DNA), X-linked, and sporadic cases have been reported. Autosomal recessive Leigh disease is caused by mutations in nuclear respiratory chain genes involving complex I, complex II, and complex IV (cytochrome c oxidase [COX]). Multiple causative mutations in maternally inherited mitochondrial DNA have also been reported. X-linked Leigh disease is caused by alterations in the gene encoding for a subunit of pyruvate dehydrogenase, representing a primary disorder of pyruvate metabolism.

The clinical presentation of Leigh disease is highly variable, which likely reflects the fact that multiple metabolic defects can be responsible for the syndrome. Both infantile and juvenile forms have been described. The infantile form typically has its onset in the first 2 years of life. There is often a history of developmental delay (of varying severity), hypotonia, and feeding problems. Neurologic deterioration is often associated with physiologic stress such as illness. Pyramidal tract signs, ataxia, and movement disorders (dystonia, choreoathetosis) subsequently occur. Brainstem involvement with eye-movement abnormalities (nystagmus, optic atrophy, progressive external ophthalmoplegia) and respiratory difficulties are also common. The juvenile form is much less common and presents in later childhood or adolescence. Dystonia and other extrapyramidal abnormalities are most prominent. Neurologic deterioration may occur much more slowly than in the early onset form.

Neuroimaging plays an important role in suggesting the diagnosis of Leigh disease. Bilaterally symmetric abnormalities of the basal ganglia, periaqueductal gray, and cerebral peduncles are characteristic. Within the basal ganglia, there is a predilection for the putamina, but the caudate nuclei and globi pallidi also may be affected. Brain magnetic resonance (MR) spectroscopy can also support the diagnosis when affected areas demonstrate a lactate peak and reduced N-acetylaspartate (NAA). White matter involvement is occasionally seen. The spinal cord also may be involved.

Summary The patient is an 18-month-old boy with a history of mild global developmental delay who presents with weakness and developmental regression with an acute viral illness. His exam is remarkable for encephalopathy, a left abducens nerve palsy, axial hypotonia, mild generalized weakness, hyperreflexia, and plantar extensor responses.

Localization His global developmental delay and encephalopathy suggest diffuse involvement of the cerebral gray matter. Difficulty abducting his left eye can be explained by an abducens nerve palsy and is likely the result of the lesion found in the pons. His hypotonia and generalized weakness localize to the muscle. Difficulty pulling to a stand indicates proximal weakness and is consistent with an underlying myopathy. Brisk reflexes and bilateral plantar extensor responses are a result of corticospinal tract involvement. Thus, this disease process appears to affect multiple levels of the peripheral and central nervous system. Non-nervous system organs are not involved by initial history and physical examination.

Differential Diagnosis   Many metabolic diseases can present with acute or subacute developmental regression with illness in this age group. Bilaterally symmetric findings on an MRI scan, as well as multisystem involvement, always raise concern for an inborn error of metabolism. Acquired disease processes (chronic meningitis, encephalitis, HIV, hydrocephalus, slow-growing neoplasm, central nervous system vasculitis, acute disseminated encephalomyelitis, head trauma, chronic subdural hematomas, endocrine abnormalities) can cause similar central nervous system symptoms but are less likely to result in a concomitant myopathy and/or acute/subacute deterioration with physiologic stress. These diagnoses are easily excluded by neuroimaging and/or basic laboratory work.

In general, progressive encephalopathy in children younger than 2 years of age can be caused by aminoacidopathies (maple syrup urine disease, phenylketonuria), lysosomal storage diseases (GM_1/GM_2 gangliosidoses, Krabbe disease, Gaucher disease, mucopolysaccharidoses, Niemann-Pick disease, metachromatic leukodystrophy), mitochondrial disorders, leukodystrophies (Canavan disease, Alexander disease), peroxisomal disorders (Zellweger syndrome and variants), and glycogen storage diseases (Pompe disease), as well as several others (ceroid lipofuscinosis, Menkes disease, biotinidase deficiency, Rett syndrome). Fatty acid oxidation defects, such as medium-chain acylcoenzyme A dehydrogenase (MCAD) deficiency, typically present in children younger than 2 years of age with signs of a metabolic crisis. Vomiting, lethargy, and coma occur with fasting or intercurrent illness. Developmental delay, epilepsy, and proximal weakness are frequent long-term sequelae of this group of disorders. These diseases can be differentiated based on the clinical presentation, presence or absence of dysmorphic features, other organ involvement (ophthalmologic abnormalities, organomegaly), and the results of initial screening tests.

Lactic acidosis can represent a primary defect of anaerobic metabolism or a secondary defect caused by other medical conditions such as multiorgan system failure or sepsis. Persistent lactic acidosis in a medically stable child suggests a primary disorder. Several other inborn errors of metabolism can be associated with lactic acidosis (fatty acid oxidation disorders, maple syrup urine disease, organic acidurias, biotinidase deficiency) but abnormalities are also seen on serum amino acid and urine organic acid studies in these conditions.

In addition, the patient in this case has a characteristic head CT finding of symmetric hypodensities in the putamina and the pons. Thus, the differential diagnosis of conditions that demonstrate basal ganglia abnormalities on neuroimaging studies can also be considered. Acute acquired abnormalities such as hypoxia, hypoglycemia, carbon monoxide poisoning, and encephalitis can preferentially affect the basal ganglia. Chronic neurodegenerative diseases, such as Huntington and Wilson diseases, may show basal ganglia involvement on brain imaging. In addition, inborn errors of metabolism causing basal ganglia abnormalities include mitochondrial disorders, glutaric aciduria (types I and II), maple syrup urine disease, Canavan disease, biotinidase deficiency, molybdenum cofactor deficiency, methylmalonic academia, and propionic acidemia, as well as many others. The putamen is most frequently involved in mitochondrial disease, Wilson disease, Huntington disease, molybdenum cofactor deficiency, and, to a lesser extent, the glutaric acidurias.

Thus, given this child's clinical picture in addition to his head CT findings, a mitochondrial disorder such as Leigh disease seems to be the most likely diagnosis. Few other diseases affect both the central nervous system and muscle tissue. He does not have organomegaly or dysmorphic facial features that might suggest a lysosomal storage disease or peroxisomal disorder. There is no macrocephaly that might point to Alexander or Canavan disease. There is no history of seizures that would suggest a disorder primarily affecting the gray matter. Other diseases that affect the basal ganglia on neuroimaging do not fit well with his presentation.

Evaluation   The evaluation of a child with a suspected neurodegenerative disorder begins with a thorough pregnancy, birth, developmental, and family history. Further details might be obtained from the family for the child in this case. A history of miscarriages in the mother or consanguinity may be relevant. It is important to inquire whether there is a family history of epilepsy, mental retardation, unexplained death in infants, developmental delay, autism, myopathy, peripheral neuropathy, migraine, diabetes, deafness, vision loss, or any other neurologic disease.

In the emergency room, in light of his recent illness, initial lab work should include a CBC, basic chemistry panel, glucose, liver function tests, and creatine kinase (given his apparent weakness). The presence of hypoglycemia, elevated liver function tests, elevated creatine kinase, or metabolic acidosis is important. A lumbar puncture should be considered to rule out central nervous system infection, although the child does not appear to have overt signs of meningitis or encephalitis (headache, photophobia, meningismus). If a lumbar puncture is done, CSF lactate should be measured.

Screening for metabolic diseases should begin with serum lactate/pyruvate, urine organic acids, plasma amino acids, ammonia, and urine ketones. Serum and CSF lactate are elevated in Leigh disease, as well as in other mitochondrial disorders. Persistent metabolic acidosis is also common. Lactate and pyruvate are in equilibrium with each other. Children with primary lactic acidosis either have normal or elevated pyruvate. The lactate-to-pyruvate ratio is calculated, with a normal value considered to be less than 20. Patients with proportionally elevated serum pyruvate and lactate values will also have an elevated ratio. These findings suggest a disorder of pyruvate metabolism like pyruvate dehydrogenase deficiency. If serum lactate is elevated and pyruvate is normal or decreased, the lactate-to-pyruvate ratio will be greater than 20. These lab results suggest a disorder of the mitochondrial respiratory chain. Blood can also be sent for commercially available analysis when a mitochondrial DNA mutation is suspected.

Given the head CT findings, a follow-up brain MRI with contrast should be promptly performed. As discussed above, Leigh disease demonstrates bilaterally symmetric signal abnormalities of the basal ganglia as well as brainstem involvement.

Brain magnetic resonance spectroscopy (MRS) can also be performed. The presence of a lactate peak and reduced N-acetylaspartate (NAA) in affected areas supports the diagnosis. MRS can help differentiate mitochondrial disorders from other diseases that affect the basal ganglia (maple syrup urine disease, Wilson disease) as these other disorders do not produce a lactate peak.

After the initial work-up is complete, histochemical and biochemical studies on a muscle biopsy specimen or skin fibroblasts are often required to evaluate for specific abnormalities of mitochondrial metabolism. Ragged red fibers are occasionally seen on the Gomori trichrome stain. However, a normal serum/CSF lactate and normal muscle biopsy do not rule out a diagnosis of a mitochondrial cytopathy because of the variable tissue distribution of abnormal mitochondria in these conditions.

The child in this case also requires a formal ophthalmologic examination, as many neurodegenerative disorders are associated with retinal pigmentary abnormalities, optic atrophy, and abnormal eye movements. Consultation with a geneticist early in the hospital course is also essential to help guide the work-up.

Management   The child in this case requires hospitalization for diagnosis and stabilization of his neurologic disorder. An intravenous line should be placed and fluids provided, given that he may be dehydrated from his recent illness. He should be placed on a cardiorespiratory monitor.

There are no standard treatments for children with Leigh disease. Vitamin replacement therapy with thiamine, riboflavin, coenzyme Q, and/or carnitine often is provided in an attempt to maximize oxidative abilities of the mitochondria. Children with pyruvate dehydrogenase deficiency often benefit from treatment with the carbohydrate-deficient ketogenic diet.

Genetic counseling in Leigh disease is complex and depends on the inheritance pattern. Thus, after a diagnosis is confirmed, the geneticist plays an important role in screening other family members and providing counseling. As an outpatient, the patient will need a comprehensive developmental evaluation, including hearing testing, given his speech/language delay. Ongoing physical, occupational, and speech therapy should be provided. The clinical course of Leigh disease is highly variable. Some patients quickly deteriorate whereas others may have a more stagnant course. If the disease progresses, multiple subspecialties (pulmonary, nutrition, gastroenterology, ophthalmology, rehabilitation medicine, orthopaedics) may need to become involved in an affected child's long-term care.

References

Banwell BL. Clinicopathologic conference: loss of milestones and failure to thrive in a 28-month-old boy. *J Pediatr.* 2002;140(6):759–765.

Barkovich AJ. *Pediatric Neuroimaging.* 3rd ed. Philadelphia, Pa: Lippincott Williams & Wilkins; 2000:71–156.

DeVivo DC, DiMauro S. Mitochondrial diseases. In: Swaiman KS, Ashwal S, eds. *Pediatric Neurology: Principles and Practice.* 3rd ed. St. Louis, Mo: Mosby; 1999:494–509.

Fenichel GM. *Clinical Pediatric Neurology: A Signs and Symptoms Approach.* 4th ed. Philadelphia, Pa: WB Saunders; 2001:117–147.

Huntsman RJ, Sinclair DB, Bhargava R, et al. Atypical presentations of Leigh syndrome: a case series and review. *Pediatr Neurol.* 2005;32(5):334–340.

Lerman-Sagie T, Leshinsky-Silver E, Watemberg N, et al. White matter involvement in mitochondrial diseases. *Mol Genet Metab.* 2005;84:127–136.

You are called to see **a 2-day-old girl** in the newborn nursery because of concerns of poor feeding. She is the product of a full-term, normal, spontaneous vaginal delivery. The prenatal course was uncomplicated. The mother had no infections and she did not take any medications other than prenatal vitamins. The delivery did not require any instrumentation and the infant had normal Apgar scores. The birth weight was 6 pounds, 3 ounces. Shortly after being taken to the nursery, the patient was noted to have bilateral adduction of her eyes. She has had difficulty latching on to the breast as well as sucking on a bottle. There is little facial movement when she cries. When asleep, her eyes do not fully close. She has not had any respiratory distress. There is no family history of neurologic disease.

Physical Examination Head circumference = 35 cm. General Examination: She is a healthy-appearing full-term infant without dysmorphic features. Neurologic Examination: Mental Status: She is awake and alert. Cranial Nerves: Her pupils are equal, round, and reactive to light. She responds to visual threat. She is unable to abduct her eyes. A corneal reflex is present bilaterally and she responds to noxious stimuli along the distribution of the trigeminal nerve. She has a paucity of facial expressions and poor movement of the face bilaterally with weak eye closure. Her gag reflex is intact and the tongue protrudes symmetrically without fasciculations. Motor: She has normal tone and moves all four extremities well against gravity. The Moro reflex is symmetric. Reflexes: 2+ throughout with equivocal plantar responses.

Guide to Case Discussion

- Briefly summarize this case.
- Localize the examination findings.
- Give the most likely diagnosis and provide a differential diagnosis.
- Discuss an appropriate diagnostic work-up.
- Discuss the management of this patient.

Diagnosis   Möbius syndrome.

Discussion   Möbius syndrome is typically characterized by congenital, nonprogressive, bilateral facial diplegia and abducens nerve palsies. Although cranial nerves VI and VII dysfunction is the hallmark of the syndrome, no clear diagnostic criteria have been defined. The facial paralysis is usually bilateral and incomplete, but can be unilateral. The abducens nerve palsy is bilateral in 90% of cases. However, other cranial nerves may be involved. The hypoglossal nerve is the third most commonly affected cranial nerve and tongue weakness can contribute to dysphagia. Hearing loss and congenital deafness have been reported in a minority of patients.

Associated limb deformities of the hands and feet, such as clubfoot, brachydactyly, syndactyly, and clinodactyly, are relatively common. Poland syndrome (unilateral aplasia or absence of the pectoralis muscle) has been reported in several patients. Cardiovascular malformations infrequently occur. Many patients have normal or near-normal intelligence. However, other neurologic complications have included poor coordination, motor delay, hypotonia at birth, long tract signs, mental retardation (10% to 75%), and autistic features. The morbidity and mortality of Möbius syndrome are primarily related to feeding problems, aspiration risk, and respiratory difficulties. A wide spectrum of severity exists.

The vast majority of reported cases of Möbius syndrome are sporadic. However, several familial forms have been described with autosomal recessive, autosomal dominant, and X-linked recessive inheritance patterns. Both sexes appear to be equally affected.

The pathogenesis of Möbius syndrome is still poorly understood. There is still debate as to whether the primary defect lies in the cranial nerve nuclei, nerve, or muscle. Two main hypotheses exist. Möbius syndrome may result from abnormal development of the rhombencephalon as the result of a genetic abnormality. However, it also has been postulated that Möbius syndrome arises from an interruption of the vascular supply to the brainstem during a critical period of development. This may be the result of an environmental, mechanical, or genetic cause. Toxins, including misoprostol, ergotamine, and cocaine, are associated with Möbius syndrome.

Summary   The child is a 2-day-old full-term infant with an unremarkable prenatal and birth history who presents with eye movement abnormalities, facial weakness, and difficulty feeding. On examination, she demonstrates facial diplegia (little facial expression, poor suck, difficulty closing her eyes) and bilateral abducens nerve palsies.

Localization   Facial weakness can be either supranuclear (pseudobulbar palsy) or nuclear in origin. Depending on the disease process, it can also be localized to the motor unit (cranial nerve, neuromuscular junction, muscles). In this case, the presence of congenital bilateral facial and abducens nerve palsies best localizes to the brainstem because of the proximity of these two cranial nerve nuclei in the caudal pons.

Differential Diagnosis   Congenital facial weakness can be unilateral or bilateral. Unilateral facial weakness is often caused by damage to the facial nerve during the birth process. The nerve is compressed against the sacrum in large infants while moving through the birth canal. Injury to the facial nerve can also be seen with forceps deliveries, but facial bruising is often present in such cases. Asymmetric crying facies is the most common cause of facial asymmetry in neonates. It is a sporadic condition caused by aplasia or hypoplasia of the depressor anguli oris muscle. The corner of the affected side of the mouth fails to turn down when the child cries, but other facial movements are normal. Genetic syndromes (Goldenhar syndrome, DiGeorge syndrome, trisomy 13, trisomy 18, osteopetrosis) also are associated with unilateral facial weakness, but other anomalies also are seen in these conditions.

Unilateral congenital ophthalmoplegia also can occur. For example, congenital oculomotor and trochlear nerve palsies are typically unilateral. Duane retraction syndrome is the result of aplasia of the abducens nuclei and may be unilateral or bilateral. The atrophic lateral rectus muscle is reinnervated by fibers from the oculomotor nerve, which results in ophthalmoplegia. On examination, a lateral rectus palsy and retraction of the globe with attempted adduction are seen. Finally, Brown syndrome results from congenital shortening of the superior oblique muscle or its tendon. There is relatively normal eye abduction but elevation is limited in adduction. Other cranial nerves are unaffected in these conditions but they are sometimes considered in the differential diagnosis of a child with Möbius syndrome.

Bilateral congenital facial weakness can be caused by a variety of other disorders, most of which are neuromuscular diseases. Congenital myasthenia gravis presents in infancy with ptosis, ophthalmoplegia, generalized weakness, hypotonia, as well as feeding and respiratory abnormalities. Fatigability is an important distinguishing feature. Transient neonatal myasthenia can cause similar symptoms in infants of mothers with myasthenia gravis, but these quickly resolve during the first few weeks of life. Congenital myotonic dystrophy is an autosomal dominant, triplet-repeat disorder caused by a mutation in chromosome 19. In the newborn, facial diplegia may be prominent. Other associated features include generalized weakness, areflexia, respiratory distress, feeding difficulties, and joint abnormalities (club foot, arthrogryposis). Myotonia is seen in the mother but not the affected infant.

Several of the congenital myopathies also can be associated with facial weakness. Most notably, nemaline myopathy and centronuclear myopathy have facial musculature involvement. Ocular weakness is often seen in centronuclear myopathy, but is rarely seen in nemaline myopathy. Other symptoms include expected features of muscle disease such as hypotonia, generalized weakness, and hyporeflexia. In contrast to the other congenital myopathies, central core disease is not associated with facial weakness or ophthalmoplegia. Mitochondrial myopathies and facioscapulohumeral dystrophy should be considered in the differential. Several mitochondrial diseases can produce ophthalmoplegia.

Facioscapulohumeral dystrophy is an autosomal dominant muscular dystrophy that can occasionally present with progressive facial diplegia in infancy. Ptosis, hyponasal speech, and proximal weakness develop with time.

Finally, bilateral perisylvian syndrome is a sporadic or X-linked disorder of neuronal migration that results in pachygyria of the sylvian fissures and rolandic cortices. Affected children present with pseudobulbar palsy, dysphagia, seizures, and mental deficiency. The diagnosis is easily confirmed with neuroimaging.

Acquired cranial nerve dysfunction has many etiologies but most of these would arise postnatally. These include trauma to the skull base/cranial nerves, basilar meningitis, demyelinating disease, brainstem glioma, and skull-based tumors.

The child in this case is nondysmorphic and has isolated sixth and seventh cranial nerve involvement. There is no evidence of neuromuscular, genetic, or other disease. Thus, Möbius syndrome is the most likely diagnosis.

Evaluation Möbius syndrome is usually a clinical diagnosis based on history and physical exam. There are no specific diagnostic lab tests. Neuroimaging with a brain MRI should be performed to look for associated cerebral malformations. Calcifications of the cranial nerve nuclei may be seen on head CT or brain MRI. Other associated structural abnormalities can include a hypoplastic brainstem or hypoplasia of affected cranial nerves.

The patient should also be evaluated by an ophthalmologist given her abducens nerve palsies. Consultation with a geneticist can also be helpful to assess any associated dysmorphic features and to rule out genetic syndromes. If limb deformities are present, an orthopaedist should be consulted. Hearing screening should also be performed as other cranial nerves can be affected.

Although challenging to perform in a neonate, EMG and NCS can be helpful in excluding other diagnoses. In Möbius syndrome, the damage occurs early in gestation and denervation potentials would not be present. However, they could be present with a perinatal nerve injury. Electrophysiologic testing can also help distinguish between nerve, neuromuscular junction, and muscle diseases in select cases.

Management The severity of cranial nerve impairment and other associated features guide the medical management of children with Möbius syndrome.

Feeding difficulties, especially in infancy, are often the biggest challenge. Supportive measures with a nasogastric or gastrostomy tube are often required. A nutritionist and gastroenterologist must be involved early in a patient's course. In some cases, plastic surgery using reanimation procedures, including using muscle and tendon transplants or the accessory nerve, have been successful in repairing the facial paralysis. Some children also may need to be followed by a pulmonologist if recurrent aspiration is a significant problem.

Incomplete eye closure can lead to corneal abrasions. Strabismus does not always require surgery as it can improve with age. However, long-term monitoring by an ophthalmologist is required. An orthopaedist should follow any child with limb deformities.

Finally, children with Möbius syndrome are at risk for developmental delays. A complete developmental evaluation is warranted once the child is medically stable. Ongoing physical, occupational, speech, and vision therapy helps to maximize the abilities of affected children.

Additional Questions

1. What does an asymmetric Moro reflex indicate?
2. Identify three causes of congenital deafness.

References

Fenichel GM. *Clinical Pediatric Neurology: A Signs and Symptoms Approach*. 4th ed. Philadelphia, Pa: WB Saunders; 2001:149–169, 299–316, 331–351.

Peleg D, Nelson GM, Williamson RA, et al. Expanded Möbius syndrome. *Pediatr Neurol*. 2001;24(4):306–309.

Riggs JE, Bodensteiner JB, Schochet SS. Congenital myopathies/dystrophies. *Neurol Clin.* 2003;21:779–794.

Sano M, Kaga K, Takeuchi N, et al. A case of Möbius syndrome—radiological and electro-physiological findings. *Int J Pediatr Otorhinolaryngol.* 2005;69(11):1583–1586.

Verzijl HTFM, Padberg GW, Zwarts MJ. The spectrum of Möbius syndrome: an electrophysi-ological study. *Brain.* 2005;128:1728–1736.

Verzijl HTFM, van der Zwaag B, Cruysberg JRM, et al. Möbius syndrome redefined: a syndrome of rhombencephalic maldevelopment. *Neurology.* 2003;61(3):327–333.

INDEX BY CATEGORY OF DISEASE

INDEX